WHEELS OF LIFE

LIBERATE YOUR SPIRIT, MANIFEST YOUR DREAMS

Journey through the progressively transcendent levels of spectrum consciousness with Anodea Judith's classic introduction to the chakras. Written in a practical, down-to-earth style, this fully illustrated book has sold over 100,000 copies, and has been completely updated and expanded.

Wheels of Life reveals how to use your chakras for better health, greater personal power, and expanded spiritual awareness. The physical exercises, poetic meditations, and visualizations will help you to:

- Ground and center your energy.

- Open, close, and balance your sexuality.

- Increase personal power and energy.

- Open your heart to love and compassion.

- Use sounds to open consciousness.

- Develop your intuition.

- Expand your awareness.

Together, the seven chakras form a profound formula for wholeness that integrates mind, body, and spirit. From liberating our spirits to manifesting our dreams, the chakras are the very wheels that carry us through life.

ABOUT THE AUTHOR

Anodea Judith, Ph.D. is a leading authority on the integration of chakras and therapeutic issues. Somatic therapist, counselor, yoga teacher, and workshop leader, she is the author of *Eastern Body, Western Mind: Psychology and the Chakra System as a Path to the Self*, and co-author with Selene Vega on *The Sevenfold Journey: Reclaiming Mind, Body, and Spirit through the Chakras*. She holds an M.A. in Clinical Psychology and a Ph.D. in Health and Human Services.

TO WRITE TO THE AUTHOR

If you wish to contact the author or would like more information about this book, please write to the author in care of Llewellyn Worldwide, and we will forward your request. Both the author and publisher appreciate hearing from you and learning of your enjoyment of this book and how it has helped you. Llewellyn Worldwide cannot guarantee that every letter written to the author can be answered, but all will be forwarded. Please write to:

Anodea Judith
℅ Llewellyn Worldwide
2143 Wooddale Drive
Woodbury, MN 55125-2989

Please enclose a self-addressed, stamped envelope for reply, or $1.00 to cover costs. If outside U.S.A., enclose international postal reply coupon.

For information on Anodea Judith's workshops, mail a request to:
PMB #109
708 Gravenstein Highway North
Sebastopol, CA 95472

Or check out Anodea Judith's Internet website at:
www.SacredCenters.com

WHEELS OF LIFE

A USER'S GUIDE TO THE CHAKRA SYSTEM

ANODEA JUDITH

Llewellyn Publications
Woodbury, Minnesota

SECOND EDITION
Seventeenth Printing, 2012

First edition, seventeen printings, 1987

Cover design: Adrienne W. Zimiga
Cover art: Women Meditating © photolibrary.com/Alfonse Pagano; Tranquil Lotus © photolibrary.com/stereohype
Figure illustrations: Mary Ann Zapalac
Second edition book design: Christine Nell Snow
Second edition editing: Christine Nell Snow and Kimberly Nightingale

Permissions:
"The Wheel of Life" by Paul Edwin Zimmer, 1981.
The Chakras by C.W. Leadbeater. Quest Books, Wheaton, IL, 1972.
The Black Pagoda by Robert Eversole. University Presses of Florida, Gainsville, FL, 1957.
Kundalini Yoga for the West by Swami Sivananda Radha. Timeless Books, Porthill, ID, 1981. Color plates of "Chakra Set" are available from Timeless Books.
Sexual Secrets by Nik Douglas and Penny Slinger. Destiny Books, Rochester, VT, 1979.
Energy Matter and Form by Christopher Hills. University of the Trees Press, Boulder Creek, CA, 1977.

Library of Congress Cataloging-in-Publication Data
Judith, Anodea
        Wheels of Life.
    (Llewellyn's new age series)
    Bibliography: p.
    Includes index.
        1. Chakras.   I. Title.   II. Series.
    BF1442.C53J83   1988   131   87-45110
    ISBN 13: 978-0-87542-320-3
    ISBN 10: 0-87542-320-5

Llewellyn Publications
A Division of Llewellyn Worldwide Ltd.
2143 Wooddale Drive
Woodbury, MN 55125-2989
www.llewellyn.com
Llewellyn is a registered trademark of Llewellyn Worldwide Ltd.

Printed in the United States of America.

FOR MY SON ALEX

OTHER WORKS BY THE AUTHOR

*Eastern Body, Western Mind: Psychology and
the Chakra System as a Path to the Self* (Celestial Arts)

*The Sevenfold Journey: Reclaiming Mind, Body, and Spirit
through the Chakras* with Selene Vega (Crossing Press)

The Truth About Chakras (Llewellyn Publications)

*Waking the Global Heart: Humanity's Rite of Passage from the Love of
Power to the Power of Love* (Elite Books)

Contact: The Yoga of Relationship (Insight Editions)

*Chakra Balancing: A Guide to Healing and
Awakening Your Energy Body* (Sounds True)

Wheels of Life (Llewellyn Publications)

The Illuminated Chakras: A Visionary Voyage into Your Inner World
(Sacred Centers)

The Chakra System: A Complete Course in Self-Diagnosis and Healing
(Sounds True)

ACKNOWLEDGMENTS

In the many years in which I have worked with the chakras, there have been numerous memorable people who have crossed my path and shared their wisdom. At the top of that list are the students and clients who have undertaken the daring work of healing and personal growth. Your struggles and triumphs, your questions and comments, have all been a guiding force in my work. May the words in this book help guide you in return.

Then there are those steadfast members of my personal life who have believed in me, worked with me, and supported me in a myriad of ways. Topping that list is my husband, Richard Ely, for loving me and cheering me on, for editing, and for making sure my science is accurate. I would like to thank my son, Alex Wayne, who contributes computer graphics and makes me laugh. And I would like to thank my long-time friend and teaching cohort, Selene Vega, who first inspired me to write a book about the chakras. She has helped develop the material shared in our workshops and was co-author of my second book, *The Sevenfold Journey.*

I would like to thank Carl Weschcke for publishing this book the first time around before chakras were popular, and the many fine folks at Llewellyn who have been part of this re-Vision: Jim Garrison, Christine Snow, Kimberly Nightingale, and Lynne Menturweck. I would also like to thank Mary Ann Zapalac for artwork, and Carlisle Holland, D. O., Robert Lamb, D. C., and Michael Gandy, L. Ac., for sharing their professional expertise.

Most of all I am grateful to the indelible spirit that keeps us alive and to the Chakra System itself, for being such a profound gateway to the mysteries of life.

It is a great honor to be of service to you all.

CONTENTS

PREFACE TO THE SECOND EDITION

IT HAS NOW BEEN TWENTY-FIVE years since I first discovered the word *chakra*. At that time I rarely found the word in an index or card catalog, yet there are now countless references and scores of New Age books on the subject, not to mention tuning forks, colored candles, incenses, t-shirts, and the usual paraphernalia that embellish any archetypal theme awakening in the collective consciousness. While I am duly flattered by those who credit the first edition of this book as seminal in that trend, I believe it is instead part of a larger cultural thirst for models of integration and wholeness. In short, the Chakra System is an idea whose time has come.

As we begin the third millennium of the current era, we are facing a time unparalleled in human development. Our history books have shown us that the systems we use to organize our lives have an enormous effect on our collective reality. This knowledge makes it imperative to innovate systems that serve us intelligently. As we pass through this particular cusp in history, we must build bridges between past and future, not only creating models that fit new realities, but continually updating old models to keep them viable in a rapidly changing culture. If the Chakra System is going to be meaningful in the twenty-first century, it must reflect the underlying fabric that has always existed, while still having the flexibility to be relevant to the demands of modern life. The ancients created a profound system. We can now marry its wisdom with modern information about the natural world, the body, and the psyche to create an even more effective system.

When I first injected chakra theory with such ideas as *grounding*, or proposed the idea of a downward current of consciousness, some were skeptical. Most interpretations of the chakras focused on transcending our physical reality, portraying it as inferior or degenerate. Life is suffering, we are told, and the transcendent planes are its antidote. If life is suffering and transcendence the antidote, the logic of this equation implies that transcendence is counter to life itself—a view that I seriously question in this book.

I do not believe that we need to sacrifice our zest for life and its enjoyment in order to advance spiritually. Nor do I see spirituality as antithetical to worldly existence, or that spiritual growth requires intense domination and control of our innate biological natures, hence of life itself. I believe this is part of a control paradigm, appropriate to a former age but inappropriate to the current challenges of our time. These challenges require models of integration rather than domination.

Since the early eighties, when I first wrote this book, the collective paradigm has shifted considerably. Emphasis on reclaiming the body and acknowledging the sacredness of Earth has increased exponentially, along with a recognition that matter has an innate spiritual value. We have learned that repression of natural forces creates unpleasant side effects and shadow energies. Ignoring the body creates illness. Devaluing the Earth creates ecological crisis. Repressed sexuality can explode in rape and incest.

It is now time to reclaim what we have lost and integrate it with new frontiers. It becomes both a personal and a cultural imperative to reweave the disparate concepts of East and West, spirit and matter, mind and body. As Marion Woodman said, "Matter without spirit is a corpse. Spirit without matter is a ghost."[*] *Both describe something that is dead.*

The Tantric philosophies, from which the chakras emerge, are a philosophy of weaving. Their many threads weave a tapestry of reality that is both complex and elegant. Tantra is a philosophy that is both pro-life and pro-spiritual. It weaves spirit and matter back into its original whole, yet continues to move that whole along its spiral of evolution.

It is at this time that we finally have the privilege to weave the knowledge of ancient and modern civilization into an elegant map for the evolutionary journey of consciousness. This book represents a map to that journey. Consider it the user's guide to the chakras. I suspect there will be many more editions, by many more authors in the future, but this is the current update from my perspective.

So what's different in this edition? It contains more references to the Tantric teachings, as I have had more time to study them, though I have still tried to keep my words as Western and non-esoteric as possible. I have also revised and shortened it a bit, as so many have told me they felt intimidated by the size of the previous version. Eliminated

---

[*]Lecture given at the "Fabric of the Future" conference, November 7, 1998, Palo Alto, CA.

was the ongoing political rhetoric so important to me in my twenties. Now, in my mid-forties, though my spiritual politics still hold, I prefer to let a system speak for itself. Some of the science has also been updated, as even our models for matter are rapidly changing.

I have tried to retain the original metaphysical flavor of this book, and keep it distinct from my subsequent books. *The Sevenfold Journey: Reclaiming Mind, Body, and Spirit through the Chakras* (written with Selene Vega, 1993) is the workbook that contains the "practice" to this book's "theory." It features the daily exercises, both mental and physical, that support personal progress through the Chakra System. My third book, *Eastern Body, Western Mind: Psychology and the Chakra System as a Path to the Self*, is a look at the psychology of the chakras, their developmental progression, the traumas and abuses that happen to us at each chakra level, and how to heal them. It weaves Western psychology and somatic therapies into the Eastern system of the chakras.

The book you now hold describes the underlying metaphysical theory behind the Chakra System. More than just an assemblage of energy centers located in the body, the chakras reveal a profound mapping of universal principles, intricately nested within each other as progressively transcendent planes of reality. The levels of consciousness that the chakras represent are doorways into these various planes. As these planes are embedded within each other, none can be eliminated from the system and still have it hold together theoretically or experientially. I do not believe that we would be given a system of seven chakras to merely discard the lower three.

This book looks at both outer and inner realities. It looks at the Chakra System as a profound system for spiritual growth, as well as a diagram of the sacred architecture in which we are embedded—the larger structure that holds us. If we are indeed "fashioned in the image of God," I believe the sacred architecture found in nature is the blueprint for our internal structures as well, both in the body and the psyche. When the bridge is made between our inner and outer worlds, they become seamlessly one, and inner growth is no longer antithetical to outer work in the world. Therefore this book uses many models that are scientific in nature, as a way of illustrating ancient wisdom with modern metaphors.

Tantric scholars and Kundalini gurus often draw a distinction between the chakras as witnessed through Kundalini experiences and the Westernized model of the chakras as a "personal growth system." Some claim that this distinction is so great that there is no meaningful relationship between the two, using either one to deny the validity of the other. There is without a doubt a marked difference, for example, between having an insight or vision (sixth chakra association) and experiencing the overwhelming inner luminescence associated with a Kundalini awakening. Yet I do not see these experiences as unrelated but existing on a continuum.

I firmly believe that clearing the chakras through understanding their nature, practicing related exercises, and using visualization and meditation, prepares the way for a spiritual opening that is apt to be less tumultuous than is so often the case for Kundalini awakenings. I believe this Westernization is an important step for speaking to the Western mind in a way that is harmonious with the circumstances in which we live, rather than antithetical to it. It gives us a context in which these experiences can occur.

Likewise, there are many who say that the chakras, as vortices in the subtle body, have nothing whatsoever to do with the physical body or the central nerve ganglia emanating from the spinal column, and that a spiritual awakening is not a somatic experience. Because an experience is not *entirely* somatic does not mean that its somatic aspect is negated. Anyone who has witnessed or experienced the physical sensations and spontaneous movements (*kriyas*) that are typical of a Kundalini awakening cannot deny that there is a somatic component. I believe this view is just more evidence of the divorce between spirit and body that I find to be the primary illusion from which we must awaken.

A man from India came to one of my workshops and told me that he had to come all the way to America to learn about chakras, because it was so esoteric in India that it was "secret knowledge," barred from anyone with a family and a job. I see "grounding" the chakras as allowing the material to be more accessible to more people. While Eastern gurus might warn that this is dangerous, I have found through my twenty-five years of working with the system that this common sense approach enables many to transform their lives without the dangerous and ungrounded symptoms so often associated with Kundalini. Far from diluting the spiritual base from which the chakras are rooted, this approach enlarges it.

Take your time reading this book. There is much to ponder. Let the chakras become a lens through which you can look at your life and world. The journey is rich and colorful. Let the Rainbow Bridge of the soul unfold before you as you walk your path.

—December, 1998

PREFACE TO THE FIRST EDITION

ONCE UPON A TIME, WHILE SITTING on my sheepskin rug in deep meditation, I had a strange experience. I was quietly and consciously counting my breaths when suddenly I found myself outside of my body—looking at another me sitting there in full lotus. No sooner did I realize who I was looking at (though she looked somewhat older) than I saw a book fall into her lap. As it landed, it jarred me back into my body and

I looked down and read the title: *The Chakra System* by A. Judith Mull (my name at the time).

That was 1975. I had only recently read the word "chakra" for the first time but it had obviously registered with some significance. I crawled out of my meditation and went to find the passage—a mere paragraph in a book by Ram Dass,[*] yet I turned almost directly to it. I read the passage several times and felt an immediate swirling of energy in my body—a deep inner churning—like the feeling a detective might have when finding an important clue. It was a feeling of conception, of something new starting to grow. I knew then I was to eventually write this book.

It took many years before the word chakra started appearing in book indexes and card catalogs. Information was scarce, so I was forced (fortunately) to develop my own theories through self-experimentation and the scrutiny of others to whom I taught yoga and administered bodywork. Before long, everything I saw seemed to fall into this neat little pattern of "sevenness": colors, events, behaviors, days—yet I could find little actual information to correlate my theories.

I gave it up, moved to the country, and began an earnest study of ritual magic—most notably working with the elements: earth, water, fire, and air. My meditations continued, my theories grew, and so did I. I still didn't have the words I wanted, so instead of writing about chakras, I found myself painting them. The process of visualization helped develop my thinking in a nonlinear way.

Two years later, forced to return to civilization, I found that the use of the word *chakra* had grown. I became part of a consciousness research group and went back to school. I returned to my bodywork practice. I underwent clairvoyant training and discovered others had independently come to see some of the same patterns. I was validated, and with my new-found clairvoyant sight, returned to this work.

Over the past ten years, I have developed these theories from the hundreds of clients I have seen for bodywork, psychic readings, counseling, and teaching. I have delved into Sanskrit literature, quantum

---

[*]Ram Dass, *The Only Dance There Is.*

physics, theosophy, magic, physiology, psychology, and personal experience to patch together a coherent system that bridges the old and the new. Both my work and I have undergone many changes.

Today, eleven years later, I finally give up being pregnant. Fully formed or not, this baby has decided to be born. I feel like I'm having septuplets—lots of pushing, long labor, yet impossible to stop once begun.

Each of these seven babies, called chakras, deserves to be a book of its own. I've given them English names—survival, sex, power, love, communication, clairvoyance, and wisdom—yet they go by many names, and most often, by numbers. In this work, however, they are represented as a family, an integral unit, working and growing together. The chapters couldn't possibly approach all there is to say about sex, power, or any of them—only what's relevant to follow branches of this particular family tree, with its roots in the Earth and its leaves in the heavens.

This book is a practical guide to a subject that is normally considered very spiritual. As "spiritual subjects" are so often considered impractical or inaccessible, this book attempts to re-examine the spiritual realms, showing how deeply they are embedded in each and every aspect of our daily lives. It is my belief that people will understand and value their spiritual natures only when it becomes practical to do so. Far more is accomplished when we want to do something than when we think we should.

When times are such that billions of people face the possibility of nuclear disaster, when men and women fear walking the streets at night, when alienation and disorientation are at an all-time high, then spirituality becomes very practical. The search for unifying factors in our daily existence, the search for understanding and direction, and the inevitable pull toward consciousness brings us to a critical evaluation of our spiritual natures. Too pragmatic and scientific to accept things on faith, Western peoples have lost touch with the world of spirit and the sense of unity it can bring. Ancient systems, couched in language and culture so different from ours, are often too alienating for the Western mind.

This book attempts to validate the needs facing us today physically, mentally, and spiritually. It contains theories for the intellectual, art for the visionary, meditations for the ethereal, and exercises for the body. Hopefully, it has something for everyone providing practicality without stifling the more important underlying essence.

To satisfy the Western mind (and my own), I've included some scientific theories, but my own background is not scientific, and I find that when you come right down to it, few people really think that way in their personal lives. For me, discovery of the chakras first came from an intuitive sense, later to grow and join with the rational. I would like to impart this order to the reader as well.

Literature tends to be linear and rational, while the states induced by the chakras require a different mode of consciousness. As a result, the information is presented in a variety of ways. To satisfy the rational mind, I have presented these theories with concrete scientific metaphors, popular paradigms from the fields of consciousness research and modern therapy techniques. This is the intellectual part. Its purpose is to transmit information and stimulate the thinking process.

To call to the other side of the brain, I have included guided meditations, exercises, artwork and personal anecdotes in hopes of making the chakras come more alive. This is the fun part. Its purpose is to bring the experience of being intuitively connected to the information at hand.

The meditations are written to be read slowly and poetically. I have not included a deep relaxation phase before each meditation for the simple reason that they are boring to read and would take away from the literary impact. However, if you plan to use the meditations yourself, or for a group experience, I strongly suggest taking time to relax the body and prepare yourself for entering slowly into a meditative state. The deep relaxation exercise or grounding meditation outlined in Chapter Two can be used as preparation, or you may wish to use your own technique. The meditations, professionally recorded with a musical background keyed to the chakras, can be obtained through Llewellyn Publications.

The physical exercises are of varying degrees of difficulty. Most of them can be done by the average person. A few, such as the headstand or the chakrasana[*], are for more flexible or developed bodies. It is strongly stressed that any physical exercises given in this book be done slowly and carefully, and that you take care not to push or strain muscles, or coerce the body into positions that are painful or uncomfortable in any way. If you experience discomfort, STOP.

If you are previously unfamiliar with chakras, or with metaphysics in general, give yourself time to assimilate each level. The associations are both broad and subtle. It cannot be attacked, like information in other disciplines. The most important thing is to enjoy the exploration. I know I did in writing this book.

—1987

Author's Note: These exercises are not featured in the Second Edition.

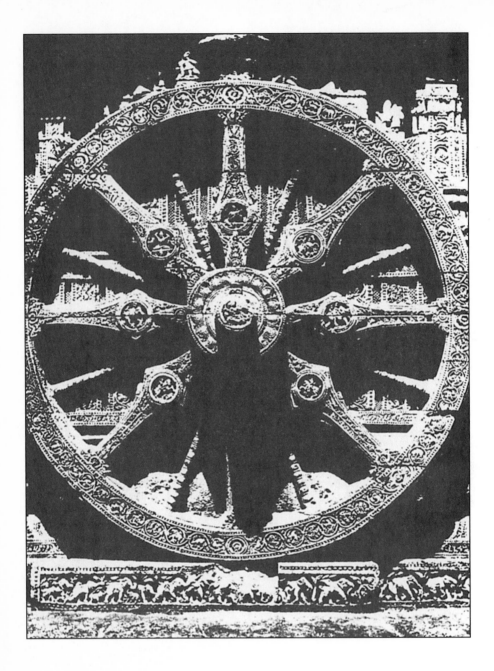

The Wheel of Salvation from the Temple of Konorak, India.

PART ONE

EXPLORING THE SYSTEM

THE WHEEL OF LIFE

Time is—
Love is—
Death is—
And the Wheel turns,
And the Wheel turns,
And we are all bound to the Wheel.

And the Sage said:
Lo, that which binds you to the Wheel
Is of your own making,
And the very Wheel
Is of your own making.
And the Wheel turns,
And the Wheel turns,
And we are all bound to the Wheel.

And the Sage said:
Know that we all are the One.
Know that the Wheel is of your own making
Know that the Wheel is of your own making,
And we are all bound to the Wheel.

And the Sage said:
Free yourself from the Wheel.
Know you are the One,
Accept your own work,
Free yourself from the Wheel.
Know that the Wheel is of your own making,
And we are all bound to the Wheel.

And the Sage freed himself from the Wheel,
And became the One,
The immortal God,
Freed from the Wheel,
Freed from illusion,
And knew then why the One had created the Wheel.
And the One became many,
And the One became we,
And we are all bound to the Wheel.

Time is—
Love is—
Death is—
And the Wheel turns,
And the Wheel turns,
And we are all bound to the Wheel.

Chapter 1

AND THE WHEEL TURNS

We are a circle within a circle ... With no beginning and never ending.[1]

FROM THE GREAT SPIRAL GALAXIES, thousands of light years across, to the trillions of atoms swirling in a grain of sand, the universe is composed of spinning wheels of energy. Flowers, tree trunks, planets, and people—each is made of tiny wheels turning inside, riding upon the great wheel of the Earth, spinning in its

3

orbit through space. A fundamental building block of nature, the wheel is the circle of life flowing through all aspects of existence. (See Figure 1.1, page 5 and Figure 1.2, page 6.)

At the inner core of each one of us spin seven wheel-like energy centers called chakras. Swirling intersections of vital life forces, each chakra reflects an aspect of consciousness essential to our lives. Together the seven chakras form a profound *formula for wholeness* that integrates mind, body, and spirit. As a complete system, the chakras provide a powerful tool for both personal and planetary growth.

Chakras are organizing centers for the reception, assimilation, and transmission of life energies. Our chakras, as core centers, form the coordinating network of our complicated mind/body system. From instinctual behavior to consciously planned strategies, from emotions to artistic creations, the chakras are the master programs that govern our life, loves, learning, and illumination. As seven vibratory modalities, the chakras form a mythical *Rainbow Bridge*, a connecting channel linking Heaven and Earth, mind and body, spirit and matter, past and future. As we spin through the tumultuous times of our present era, the chakras act as gears turning the spiral of evolution, drawing us ever onward toward the still untapped frontiers of consciousness and its infinite potential.

The body is a vehicle of consciousness. Chakras are the wheels of life that carry this vehicle about—through its trials, tribulations, and transformations. To run our vehicle smoothly, we need an owner's manual as well as a map that tells us how to navigate the territory our vehicle can explore.

This book is a map for the journey to consciousness. You can think of it as a "user's guide" to the Chakra System. This map, like any other, will not tell you where to go, but will help you navigate the journey you wish to take. Its focus is on integrating the seven archetypal levels that impact our lives.

With map in hand, we can embark on an exciting journey. Like all journeys, there is a certain amount of preparation needed in the form of background information: the psychological systems, the historical

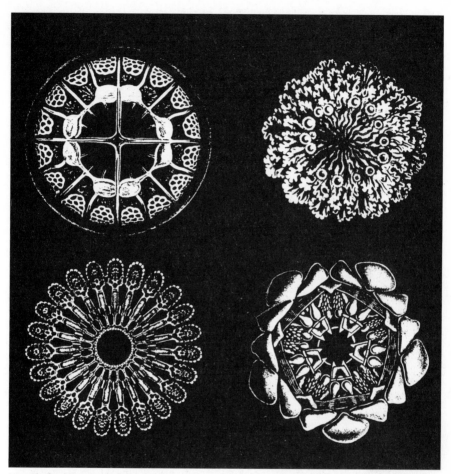

Top left: Species of rhizostomeae   Top right: Lichen
Bottom left: Gorgon-headed starfish   Bottom right: Sea urchin

FIGURE 1.1
Examples of the chakra forms found repeatedly in nature.

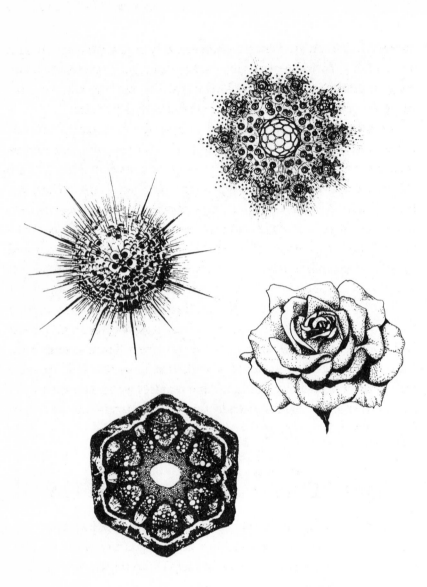

FIGURE 1.2
More examples of the chakra forms found repeatedly in nature.

context of the Chakra System, a deeper study of just what the chakras are, and the related energy currents they describe. This gives us a language to speak on our journey. We will then be ready to take the journey itself, climbing up the spinal column, chakra by chakra.

Each chakra we encounter is a step on the continuum between matter and consciousness. Therefore, this journey will encompass areas of our lives ranging from the somatic level of physical and instinctual awareness through the interpersonal level of social interaction, and finally to the more abstract realms of transpersonal consciousness. When all of the chakras are understood, opened, and connected together, we have then bridged the gulf between matter and spirit, understanding that we, ourselves, are the Rainbow Bridge that connects Earth and Heaven once again.

In a fragmented world where mind is severed from body, culture from planet, and the material from the spiritual, we have a deep need for systems that allow us to reclaim our wholeness. These systems must allow us to integrate mind and body and take us to new and expanded realms without denying the mundane realities we all face on a daily basis. I believe the chakras provide just such a system—one we cannot do without and one whose time has come.

APPROACHING THE SYSTEM

System—1) a complete exhibition of essential principles or
facts, arranged in a rational or organized whole, or
a complex of ideas or principles forming a coherent
whole.

—Webster's New Collegiate Dictionary

Imagine if you went to the library and found nothing but piles of books stacked helter-skelter across the floor. To find anything you would have to go through long and tedious hunting, with only a remote possibility of success. Ridiculously inefficient, you say.

Accessing consciousness without a system can be just as tedious. The circuitry in the brain allows for infinite possibilities of thought, and the manifestations of consciousness are far greater in number than the books in any library. Given the rhythm and speed of today's life, we certainly cannot access this information without efficient systems to streamline the process.

Many systems exist already, yet are insufficient for the changing culture of today. Sigmund Freud's division of the psyche into id, ego, and superego is a prime example of a simple system for studying human behavior, which formed the groundwork for psychotherapy in the early part of the twentieth century. Yet this model is now sorely inadequate, as it says little about the body, and even less about transcendent states of awareness.

Within the human potential movement, the need for new systems is quite evident. Clinics are opening to counsel people in psychic experiences as larger numbers are experiencing spontaneous awakenings of unusual spiritual energies. We are discovering ourselves confronted each day by new sets of problems. Biofeedback, Kirlian photography, acupuncture, homeopathy, Ayurvedic medicine, herbology, and myriads of New Age spiritual, verbal, and physical therapies are becoming more widely practiced each year. We now have so many options in healing, consciousness raising, religion, and lifestyles that the information and choices are overwhelming. The field has indeed opened up, and will certainly remain so if only we can derive some sense and order from the chaos. This is the purpose of a system. It gives us a systematic way to approach a complex task.

The logical way to build a system is to base it on the observation of persistent patterns. Many of these patterns have been described by our ancestors and passed down through the ages, shrouded in myth and metaphor, like dormant seeds waiting for the right conditions to sprout. Now, when we look for new directions for a changing age, perhaps it is time to archive the ancient systems of the past, dust them off, and upgrade them so that they are useful in the modern world in which we live. Before we do that, we must first examine the origin and evolution of that system, paying due respect to its ancient roots.

HISTORY OF THE CHAKRA SYSTEM

It is wonderful that the chakras, as archetypal components of consciousness, are finally gaining prominence in the collective mindset, with more books and references than ever before. While this popularity is making the chakras a household word, it is also spreading a lot of confusing and conflicting information. It is important to realize the chakras come from an ancient tradition, which many New Age teachers have barely explored. Here is a brief summary of the Chakra System's historical development for those who have an interest in its origin. (If you don't have an interest, feel free to skip to the next section.)

The chakras are inextricably linked with the science and practice of *yoga*. The word yoga means "yoke," and it is a system of philosophy and practice designed to yoke the mortal self to its divine nature of pure consciousness. The origin of yoga and earliest mention of the chakras[2] goes back to the *Vedas*, meaning "knowledges", a series of hymns that are the oldest written tradition in India. These writings were created from an even older oral tradition of the Aryan culture, believed to be an invading Indo-European tribe that swept into India during the second millenium B.C.E.[3]

The Aryans were said to have entered India on chariots, and the original meaning of the word chakra as "wheel" refers to the chariot wheels of the invading Aryans. (The correct spelling from Sanskrit is actually *çakra*, though pronounced with a "ch" as in church, hence the English spelling chakra.) The word was also a metaphor for the sun, that great wheel that rolls across the sky like a blazing chariot of a *cakravartin*, the name for the Aryan chariot-rulers. The wheel also denotes the eternal cycle of time called the *kalacakra*. In this way, the wheel represents celestial order and balance. One further meaning is that a chakra is a Tantric circle of worshipers.

It is said that the cakravartins were preceded by a glowing golden disk of light, much like the halo of Christ, only this spinning disk was seen in front of them. (Perhaps their powerful third chakras?)

The birth of a cakravartin was said to herald a new age, and it could be this time period that marked the dawning of the third chakra era of human history (see chapter 13, "Evolution"). It is also said that the god Vishnu descended to Earth, having in his four arms a chakra, a lotus flower, a club, and a conch shell.[4] This may also have referred to a chakra as a discus-like weapon.

Following the *Vedas* were the *Upanishads,* or wisdom teachings passed from teacher to disciple. There is some mention of the chakras as psychic centers of consciousness in the *Yoga Upanishads* (circa 600 B.C.E.) and later in the *Yoga Sutras of Patanjali* (circa B.C.E. 200). It is from Patanjali's sutras that we get the classic eightfold path of yoga tradition.[5] This tradition was largely dualistic, stating that nature and spirit were separate, and advised ascetic practices and renunciation of one's instinctual nature as a way to enlightenment.

It was in the non-dual Tantric tradition that the chakras and Kundalini came to be an integral part of yoga philosophy. The Tantric teachings are a syncretic weaving of many spiritual traditions of India, which came to popularity during the sixth and seventh century A.D., in reaction to the dualistic philosophy which preceded it. This tradition advised being in the world rather than separate from it. Tantra is commonly viewed in the West as primarily a sexual tradition, as Tantrism does put sexuality in a sacred context and regards the body as a sacred temple for the consciousness within. Yet this is actually only a small part of a broad philosophy which combines many practices of hatha and kundalini yoga, worship of deities, especially of the Hindu goddesses, and focuses on integrating universal forces.

The word tantra literally means "loom" and denotes a weaving of disparate threads into a tapestry of wholeness. Thus, the Chakra System, coming out of Tantric tradition, weaves the polarities of spirit and matter, mind and body, masculine and feminine, Heaven and Earth, into a single philosophy of many philosophical strands, reaching even back to the oral tradition that preceded the *Vedas.*

The main text about chakras that has come to us in the West is a translation of Tantric texts by the Englishman Arthur Avalon in his book *The Serpent Power* published in 1919.[6] These texts—the *Sat-Cakra-Nirupana*, written by an Indian pundit in 1577, and the *Padaka-Pancaka*, written in the tenth century—contain descriptions of the chakra centers and related practices. There is also another tenth-century text called the *Gorakshashatakam*, which gives instructions for meditating on the chakras. These texts form the basis of our understanding of chakra theory today.

In these traditions, there are seven basic chakras,[7] which exist within the subtle body, interpenetrating the physical body. The subtle body is the nonphysical psychic body that is superimposed on our physical bodies. It can be measured as electromagnetic force fields within and around all living creatures. Kirlian photography, for example, has actually photographed the emanations of the subtle body in both plants and animals. In the aura, which is the external manifestation of the subtle body, the energy field appears as a soft glow around the physical body, often made of spindle-like fibers. In yoga psychology, the subtle body is divided into five sheaths of varying refinement in the subtle body, called *koshas*.[8] At the core of the body, the subtle field appears as spinning disks—chakras. The chakras are the psychic generators of the auric field. The aura itself is the meeting point between the core patterns generated by the chakras and the influence of the external world.

Through modern physiology we can see that these seven chakras are located near the seven major nerve ganglia that emanate from the spinal column. (See Figure 1.3, page 12.) There are two minor chakras mentioned in the ancient texts, the *soma* chakra, located just above the third eye, and the *Anandakanda lotus*, which contains the Celestial Wishing Tree (*Kalpataru*) of the Heart Chakra (see further description, page 220). Some esoteric systems propose nine or twelve chakras,[9] while other traditions, such as Vajrayana Buddhism, describe only five centers.[10] Since a chakra is literally a vortex of energy, there is no limit to their number. However, the original seven "master" chakras form a profound and elegant system, one that maps logically onto the body through the nerve ganglia, yet connects our physical existence to higher and deeper non-physical realms. Mastering

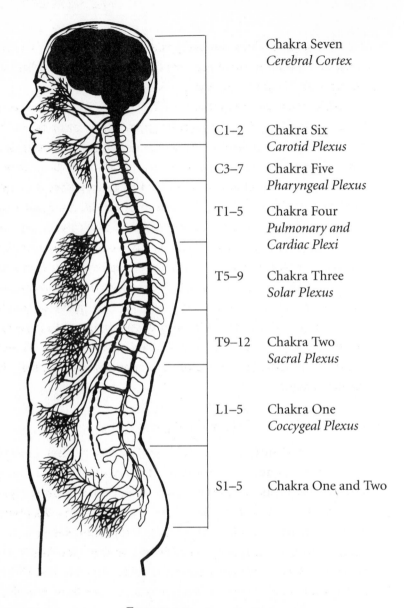

Chakra Seven
Cerebral Cortex

C1–2   Chakra Six
Carotid Plexus

C3–7   Chakra Five
Pharyngeal Plexus

T1–5   Chakra Four
*Pulmonary and
Cardiac Plexi*

T5–9   Chakra Three
Solar Plexus

T9–12   Chakra Two
Sacral Plexus

L1–5   Chakra One
Coccygeal Plexus

S1–5   Chakra One and Two

FIGURE 1.3
This diagram shows the vertebrae related to the different chakras
based on the spinal nerves which innervate the ganglia and various
organs. If these vertebrae are damaged in a way that affects the spinal nerves, the related chakras may be subsequently affected.

the first seven chakras can easily take a lifetime, and I advise people to work fully with these seven centers that relate to the body before undertaking more complex and obscure out-of-body systems.

While many interpretations on the chakras advise transcending the lower chakras in favor of the more expansive upper chakras, I do not agree with this philosophy, nor do I believe this is the intention of the Tantric texts. This view arose during a period in history where all the major patriarchal religions advocated the greater importance of mind over matter, thus denying the existence of the spiritual *within* the mundane realms. Careful reading of the Tantric texts does not imply the denial of the lower chakras in favor of the upper chakras, but merely an enfoldment, where each higher level is a transcendence, which *includes and is built on* the level below it. In this way, the lower chakras provide a *foundation* for our spiritual growth, much as the roots of a tree, which push downward, allow the tree to grow taller. We do not help the tree grow taller by pulling up its roots. This will be explored more fully as we explore the significance of the first chakra in the next chapter.

Systems From Other Cultures

Aside from Hindu literature, there are many other metaphysical systems featuring seven levels of man, nature, or physical planes. The Theosophists, for example, talk about seven cosmic rays of creation, with seven evolutionary races. The Christians talk about seven days of creation, as well as seven sacraments, seven seals, seven angels, seven virtues, seven deadly sins, and in Revelation 1:16 perhaps even seven chakras where it is said, "And He had in His right hand seven stars." Carolyn Myss has also correlated the chakras to the seven Christian Sacraments.[11]

The Kabbalistic Tree of Life, also a system of studying behavior and consciousness, has seven horizontal levels distributed among its three vertical pillars and ten Sephiroth. Similarly, the Tree of Life describes a path from Earth to Heaven as does the Chakra System. While the

Kabbalah is not an exact match to the Chakra System, it does have significant parallels in that it, too, describes an evolutionary journey from matter to supreme consciousness.[12] Using the Chakra System in conjunction with the Kabbalah helps map the Sephiroth onto the body and brings together two ancient traditions, which obviously have common roots. (See Figure 1.4, page 15.)

Seven-ness is also found outside of myth and religion. There are seven colors to the rainbow, seven notes in the Western major scale, seven days in the week, and it is believed that major life cycles run in periods of seven years each—childhood to age seven, adolescence at fourteen, adulthood at twenty-one, first Saturn return at twenty-eight. Arthur Young in *The Reflexive Universe* has described evolution in seven levels,[13] and the periodic table of elements can even be viewed as falling into a pattern of seven, by atomic weight.

Many cultures talk about energy centers or levels of consciousness similar to chakras, although there may not always be seven centers in their system. The Chinese have a system of six levels in the hexagrams of the I Ching, based on the two cosmic forces, yin and yang. There are also six pairs of organ meridians that correspond to five elements (fire, earth, metal, water, and wood). The Hopi Indians speak of energy centers in the body, as do the Tibetans.

There is little doubt that there is a basic key to understanding within the correlation of all this myth and data. Somewhere there lies a cosmic map for adventurers in consciousness. Hints have been dropped through the ages around the globe. Is it not time we pieced together these clues and began to navigate ourselves out of our present difficulties?

Fortunately, more and more research is being done now that supports the existence of chakras,[14] and their counterpart, the Kundalini energy. I hope that I can present enough of it within these pages to make this plain. I would prefer, however, to make this system believable to you primarily through your own personal experience and only secondarily through scientific evidence. The scientific aspects provide

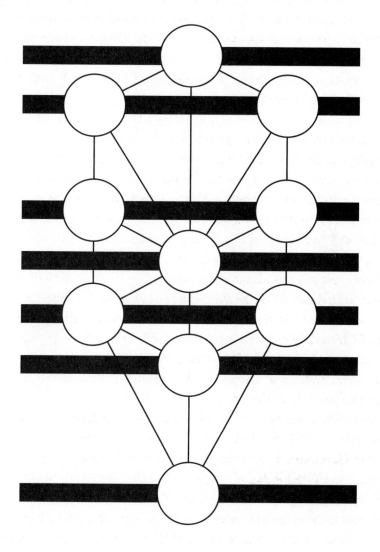

FIGURE 1.4
Kabbalistic Tree of Life, with its ten Sephiroth (circles),
twenty-two paths (lines connecting circles), three vertical pillars,
and seven levels (horizontal bars).

little practical value in actually using the system other than intellectual reassurance, since the chakras are ultimately an interior subjective experience. Knowing about the chakras is only part of the journey. The real challenge is to experience them.[15]

So, in order to understand the merits of this most ancient and now modernized system, I urge the reader to suspend disbelief within whatever parameters they find comfortable, jump aboard the mystic bandwagon of personal experience, and judge their truths from within. After all, this is little more than what we do in reading a good adventure novel or love story. Consider this book a little of each—an adventure novel traveling through the realms of your own consciousness, and a love story between your inner self and the universe that surrounds you.

HOW THE CHAKRAS WORK

Now that we have examined the history of the Chakra System, let's take a deeper look at the chakras themselves, and examine how they might work their powerful influence on mind and body.

As mentioned before, the word *chakra* is a Sanskrit word meaning "wheel" or "disk" and denotes a point of intersection where mind and body meet. Chakras are also called lotuses, symbolizing the unfolding of flower petals, which metaphorically describe the opening of a chakra. The beautiful lotus flowers are sacred in India. Growing from mud, they symbolize a path of development from a primitive being to a fully blossoming consciousness, mirroring the base chakra rooted in Earth, which evolves into the "thousand-petaled lotus" at the crown of the head. Like lotuses, chakras have "petals," which vary in number from chakra to chakra. Beginning at the bottom with the first chakra, the petals number four, six, ten, twelve, sixteen, two, and 1,000 petals. (See Figure 1.5, page 18.) Like flowers, chakras can be open or closed, dying or budding, depending on the state of consciousness within.

The chakras are gateways between various dimensions—centers where activity of one dimension, such as emotion and thought, connects and plays on another dimension, such as our physical bodies. This interaction, in turn, plays on our our interactions with others and thus influences another dimension—our activities in the outside world.

Take, for example, the emotional experience of fear, related to the first chakra. Fear affects our body in certain ways. We feel butterflies in our stomach, our breath is short, and our voice and hands may shake. These physical characteristics betray our lack of confidence in dealing with the world, and may lead others to treat us in a negative way, perpetuating our fear. This fear may have its roots in an unresolved childhood experience, yet still rules our behavior. To work with the chakras is to heal ourselves of old constricting patterns lodged in the body or the mind, or habitual behavior.

The sum total of the chakras forms a vertical column in our bodies called *sushumna*. This column is a central integrating channel for connecting the chakras and their various dimensions. (See Figure 1.6, page 19.) It can be thought of as a "super highway" on which these energies travel, just as our asphalt highways are channels through which physical items travel from the manufacturer to the consumer. We could say that the sushumna brings psychic energy from the "manufacturer" as pure consciousness (Divine Mind, God, Goddess, The Force, Nature, etc.) to the consumer, which is the mental and physical individual here on the Earth plane. One could view the chakras as being major cities located along the highway, each responsible for producing their own kind of goods. Rather than cities, however, I view them as sacred chambers in the temple of the body, where the vital force of consciousness can pool together on different levels.

Traveling beside, around, and through the sushumna, there are also many back roads, such as the Chinese acupuncture meridians, and the thousands of other *nadis*, subtle energy conduits, which Hindus have found within the subtle body. (See Figure 1.7, page 21.) Nadis can be thought of as alternate channels, such as the telephone network, gas lines, or stream beds, where we have special channels for moving certain kinds of energy, all passing through the same vortex.

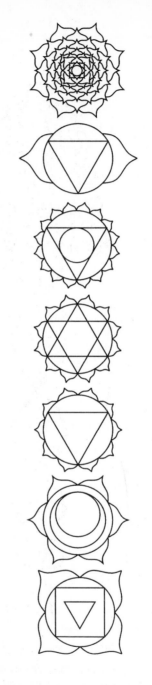

Chakra Seven

Chakra Six

Chakra Five

Chakra Four

Chakra Three

Chakra Two

Chakra One

FIGURE 1.5
Seven lotuses representing the seven chakras.

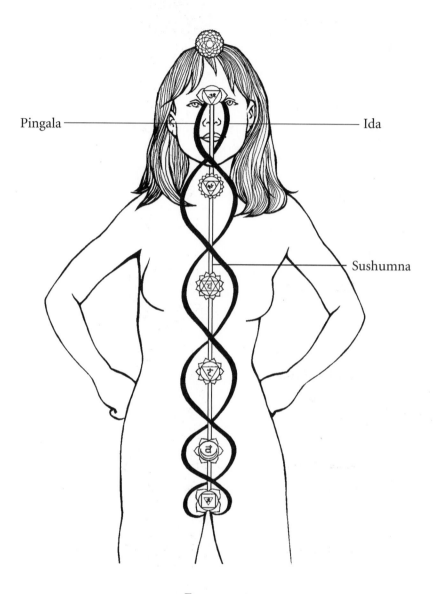

Pingala — — Ida

Sushumna

FIGURE 1.6
Sushumna, Ida, and Pingala.
(Author's Note: Some texts show Ida and Pingala crossing between the
chakras, while others show them crossing at the chakras. Others describe
the currents ending—or beginning—at the left and right nostril.)

If you would like to experience what a chakra feels like, the following is a simple exercise for opening the hand chakras and experiencing their energy:

> Extend both arms out in front of you, parallel to the floor with elbows straight.
>
> Turn one hand up and one hand down. Now quickly open and close your hands a dozen times or so.
>
> Reverse your palms and repeat. This opens the hand chakras.
>
> To feel their energy, open your hands and slowly bring your palms together, starting about two feet apart.
>
> When your hands are about four inches apart you should be able to feel a subtle ball of energy, like a magnetic field, floating between your palms. If you tune in closely, you may even be able to feel it spinning.
>
> After a few moments the sensation will subside, but it can be repeated by opening and closing the palms again, as above.

On a physical level, chakras correspond to nerve ganglia, where there is a high degree of nervous activity, and also to glands in the endocrine system (see Figure 1.8, page 22). While chakras are interdependent with the nervous and endocrine systems, they are not synonymous with any portion of the physical body, but exist within the subtle body.

Yet their effect upon the physical body is strong, as witnessed by anyone undergoing a Kundalini experience. I believe that the chakras generate the shape and behavior of the physical body, much as the mind influences our emotions. An excessive third chakra would exhibit a big, tight belly; a constricted fifth chakra results in tight shoulders or a sore throat; a poor connection through the first chakra may show up in skinny legs or bad knees. The alignment of one's spinal vertebrae also correlates to the openness of the chakras. For example, if our chest

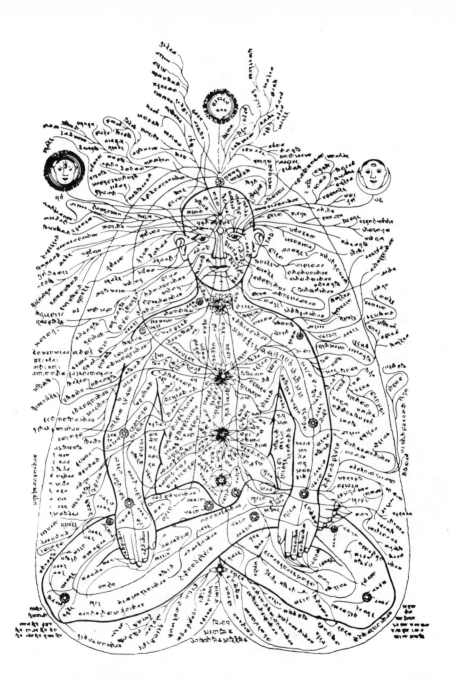

Figure 1.7
Ancient Hindu drawing of the nadis and chakras.
(Courtesy of University of the Trees Press)

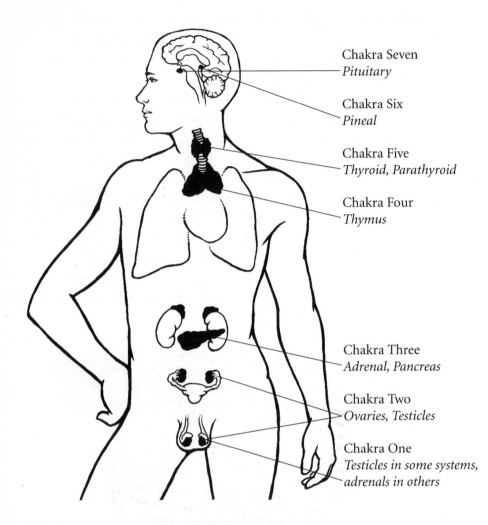

Chakra Seven
Pituitary

Chakra Six
Pineal

Chakra Five
Thyroid, Parathyroid

Chakra Four
Thymus

Chakra Three
Adrenal, Pancreas

Chakra Two
Ovaries, Testicles

Chakra One
*Testicles in some systems,
adrenals in others*

FIGURE 1.8
Common associations between the chakras
and the glands of the endocrine system.
(Some systems reverse chakras six and seven, making pineal a seventh
chakra gland and the pituitary related to the sixth.)

is collapsed, due to spinal curvature or somatic/emotional holding, the heart chakra may be impeded. The shape of our physical body may even be determined by our development from former lives, to be picked up and continued again in this life.

In metaphysical terminology, a chakra is a vortex. (See Figure 1.9.) Chakras spin in a wheel-like manner, attracting or repelling activity on their particular plane by patterns analogous to a whirlpool. Anything the chakra encounters on its particular vibrational level gets drawn into the chakra, processed, and passed out again.

Instead of fluid, chakras are made of symbolic patterns of our own mental and physical programming. This programming governs the way we behave. Like programming in a computer, it channels the way energy flows through the system and gives us different kinds of information. Each chakra—which literally means "disk"—can be thought of as programming on a floppy disk that runs certain elements of our

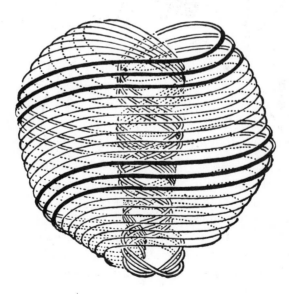

FIGURE 1.9
Metaphysical illustration of a vortex.
(Courtesy of Theosophical Publishing House)

lives, from our survival programs, to our sexual programs, to the way we think and feel.

Chakras send energy out from the core of the body, and they assimilate energy from outside that enters the core. In this way, once again, I define a chakra as *an organizational center for the reception, assimilation, and transmission of life energy*. What we generate determines much of what we receive, and in this way it behooves us to work on our chakras and clean up outdated, dysfunctional, or negative programming that may be getting in our way.

The content of the chakras is formed largely by repeated patterns from our actions in day-to-day life, as we are always the center point of these actions. Repeated movements and habits create fields in the world around us. Programming from our parents and culture, our physical body shape, situations we are born into, and information from previous lives are also important factors. These patterns can often be seen by clairvoyants when viewing the chakras. Their interpretations give us valuable insight into our behavior. Like an astrological chart, they show us *tendencies* of the personality, but are not by any means unchangeable. Knowing our tendencies tells us what to watch out for and what to enhance.

Through involvement with the outside world, patterns within the chakras tend to perpetuate themselves; hence the idea of *karma*—patterns formed through action, or the laws of cause and effect. Thus it is common to become trapped in any one of these patterns. This is called being "stuck" in a chakra. We are caught in a cycle that keeps us at a particular level. This could be a relationship, a job, a habit, but most often, simply a way of thinking. Being stuck can be a function of either overemphasis or underdevelopment of a chakra. The object of our work is to clean the chakras of old, nonbeneficial patterns so that their self-perpetuating actions have a positive influence, and our life energy can continue to expand to higher planes.

Chakras are associated with seven basic levels of consciousness. As we experience the opening of a chakra, we also experience a deeper understanding of the state of consciousness associated with that level.

These states can be summarized with the following keywords, though it must be remembered that these words are a gross oversimplification of the complexity of each level. (See Table of Correspondences, pages 42 and 43.) The chapters that follow will explain each chakra more fully. Their associated elements are given because the elements are of such crucial significance to understanding the quality of the chakra.

Chakra One: Located at the base of the spine, is associated with *survival*. Its element is *earth*.

Chakra Two: Located in the lower abdomen is associated with *emotions and sexuality*. Its element is *water*.

Chakra Three: Located in the solar plexus, is associated with *personal power, will, and self-esteem*. Its element is *fire*.

Chakra Four: Located over the sternum, is associated with *love*. Its element is *air*.

Chakra Five: Located in the throat, is associated with *communication and creativity*. Its element is *sound*.[16]

Chakra Six: Located in the center of the forehead, is associated with *clairvoyance, intuition and imagination*. Its element is *light*.

Chakra Seven: Located at the top of the head, is associated with *knowledge, understanding and transcendent consciousness*. Its element is *thought*.

Chakras can be open or closed, excessive or deficient,[17] or any of the various stages in between. These states may be basic aspects of someone's personality throughout most of their life, or something that changes from moment to moment in response to a situation. An ailing chakra may be unable to change its state easily, being stuck in either an open or a closed state. The chakra then needs healing by uncovering and removing whatever is blocking it. If a chakra is blocked in a closed state, then it is unable to generate or receive energy on that particular plane, such as love energy or communication. If a chakra is blocked in an open or excessive state, that means it tends to channel all energies through that particular plane, such as using all situations to further one's power or meet sexual needs, when other forms of behavior might be more appropriate. A closed chakra is a chronic avoidance of certain energies, while an excessively open chakra is a chronic fixation.

The quality and quantity of energy that one encounters on a particular plane has to do with how open or closed their respective chakra is, or how able they are to control this opening and closing at appropriate times. This governs the amount of activity and complexity we can effectively handle at any given level.

For example, someone with a tightly closed third chakra (personal power) would be terrified of confrontation, while another who is more open, may thrive on it. Someone with an open second chakra (sexuality) may juggle many sexual partners, while someone who is closed may avoid even feeling sexual. Someone whose throat chakra is excessive may talk too much and not really listen, while another may be scarcely able to get their words out.

There are specific exercises that are designed to facilitate the opening, discharging, or strengthening of each center, but one must first be able to understand the system as a whole. Once the system is understood, individual levels can be approached in various ways. One can:

- Focus attention on that area of the body, taking careful note of how it feels and behaves.

- Understand the philosophical working of that chakra and apply it.

- Examine the interactions in one's day-to-day life that level corresponding to that chakra.

In this work, any of the correlations to a particular level can be used to access the chakra and change the energy within.

For example, you can understand what condition your second chakra (sexuality) is in by first *tuning in to that area of the body* (abdomen, genitals). Is it fluid, alive, painful, tense, relaxed? The physical state gives us many clues about the internal processes. The next step is to *examine the meaning and function* of that particular chakra. What meaning do you ascribe to emotions and sexuality? What values do they hold for you? What kind of programming did you receive about those issues? Then you might examine the quality and quantity of emotional and sexual interaction in your life. Is it what you want it to be? Is it balanced between give and take? Is it an effortless flow of energy or a subject of fear and anxiety?

You can then work on improving the health of the second chakra by doing any of the following:

- Doing physical exercises that pertain to relaxing, opening, or stimulating the sacral area of the body.

- Working with its associated images, colors, sounds, deities, or elements, such as its constant movement and flow of water or its cleansing properties by: drinking lots of water, visiting a river, going swimming—all as a means to connect with its associated water element.

- Working through your feelings and values about sexuality and emotions, and bringing those new insights into your behavior with others.

Any or all of these processes may affect changes in your emotional or sexual nature.

The body and mind are inseparably interrelated. Each governs and affects the other, and each is accessible through the other. The seven major chakras are also inseparably interrelated. A block in the functioning of one chakra may affect the activity of the one above or below it. For example, you may have trouble with your personal power (third chakra) because of a block in communication (fifth chakra) or vice versa. Or perhaps the real problem may lie in your heart (fourth chakra) and only manifests in these other areas because it is buried so deeply. In examining the theoretical System as a whole (which will henceforth be capitalized) and applying it to your personal chakra system (lowercase) as it occurs uniquely within you, you learn to sort out these subtleties and patterns and make self-improvements according to your goals. This process will be explained in greater detail as we explore each chakra in depth.

Chakras exist in many dimensions simultaneously, and thus provide points of entry into those dimensions. In the physical realm, they correspond to particular areas of the body and may be experienced as butterflies in our stomach, frogs in our throat, pounding in our heart, or the experience of an orgasm. Working with the physical associations allows us to use the Chakra System to diagnose and, in some cases, heal illnesses.

Chakras also correspond to various types of activity. Work is a first chakra activity, as it relates to survival. Music, relating to sound and communication, corresponds to the fifth chakra. Dreaming, as a function of inner sight, is a sixth chakra activity.

In the dimension of time, chakras describe stages in personal and cultural life cycles. In childhood, the chakras open sequentially, starting with the first chakra, which is dominant during the first year of life, and moving upward toward the crown as we mature into adulthood.[18] As adults, we may focus on certain chakras more than others at various stages—creating prosperity, exploring sexuality, developing personal power, relationships, creativity, or spiritual exploration.

In terms of evolution, chakras are paradigms of consciousness that prevail in the world at a given time. Primitive humans existed primarily in the first chakra, where survival was the main focus of culture. Agriculture and ship travel marked the beginning of the second chakra era. At this millennial time, I believe we are passing from the third chakra era, where the primary focus has been power and energy, to the fourth chakra realm of the heart, where the focus is on love and compassion. While none of these transitions are smooth or sudden, certain phases can be clearly seen over the course of history. (See chapter 12.)

In the mind, chakras are patterns of consciousness—belief systems through which we experience and create our personal world. In this way, the chakras really are programs that run our lives. Our lower chakra programs contain information about the body in terms of survival, sexuality, and action. The higher chakras bring us to more universal states of consciousness and work with our deeper belief systems about spirituality and meaning. Sometimes we get locked into a program and it becomes our habitual way of interacting with the world around us. The man who sees every situation as a challenge to his power orients from his third chakra. The one who perpetually struggles with survival issues, such as health and money, has difficulty with chakra one. Someone who lives in his fantasies may be stuck in chakra six.

As you can see, the chakras have many complexities. As metaphors for the manifestation of consciousness on various planes of activity, they are invaluable. Yet, as a complete System, they offer even more understanding to the energetic dynamics of a human being.

SHIVA AND SHAKTI

There is no power-holder without power. No power without power-holder. The power-holder is Shiva. Power is Shakti, the Great Mother of the universe. There is no Shiva without Shakti, or Shakti without Shiva. [19]

In Hindu mythology, the universe is created by the combination of the deities Shiva and Shakti. The male principle, Shiva, is identified with pure unmanifest consciousness. He represents bliss and is depicted as a formless being, deep in meditation. Shiva is the inactivated divine potential equal to pure consciousness—separate from its manifestations. He is sometimes seen as the "destroyer" because he is consciousness without form—often destroying form to reveal consciousness. Shiva is believed to have the strongest presence at the crown chakra.[20]

Shakti, the female counterpart to this inactive consciousness, is the life giver. She is the entire creation and mother of the universe. Shakti, in her creation of the world, is the inventor of *maya*, commonly thought of as illusion. Early in the Sanskrit language, maya had the meaning of magic, art, wisdom, and extraordinary power.[21] Maya is the substance of the manifested universe, the mistress of divine creation. Maya is a projection of consciousness, but not consciousness itself. It is said that when "karma ripens, Shakti becomes desirous of creation and covers herself with her own maya."[22]

The root word *shak* means "to have power" or "to be able."[23] Shakti is the vital energy that gives power to the forming of life. It is through union with Shakti that the consciousness of Shiva descends and endows the universe (Shakti) with Divine Consciousness. Among mortals, the woman produces the child, but only with the man's seed. So, too, Shakti produces the universe, but only with the "seed" of consciousness that comes from Shiva.

Each of these deities has a tendency to move toward the other. Shakti, as she pushes up from the Earth, is described as the "divine aspiration of the human soul," while Shiva, descending from above, is the "irresistible attraction of divine grace" or manifestation.[24] They exist in an eternal embrace and are constantly making love, neither able to exist without the other. Their eternal relationship creates both the phenomenal and spiritual worlds.

Shiva and Shakti reside within each one of us. We have only to practice certain principles to allow these forces to join together bringing us enlightenment from the veil of maya, or realization of the consciousness buried within so-called illusion. When this occurs we will have, as the old meanings hint—art, wisdom, and the powers of creation within our very grasp.

LIBERATION AND MANIFESTATION

Consciousness thus has a twin aspect; its liberation (mukti) *or formless aspect, in which it is as mere Consciousness-Bliss; and a universe or form aspect, in which it becomes the world of enjoyment* (bhukti). *One of the cardinal principles [of spiritual practice] is to secure both liberation and enjoyment.*[25]

Shiva and Shakti can also be seen as representing two currents of energy through the chakras—one downward and one upward.[26] (See Figure 1.10, page 33.) The downward current, which I call the *current of manifestation*, begins in pure consciousness and descends through the chakras into the manifested plane, gradually becoming denser and denser at each step. To produce a theatrical play, for example, we must begin with an idea or concept (chakra seven). The idea then becomes a set of images (chakra six), which can be communicated to others in the form of a story (chakra five). As the idea further develops, and others get involved with it, we enter a set of relationships that help bring it about (chakra four). We give it our will and energy (chakra three), rehearsing the movements, and bringing its conceptual and physical elements together (chakra two) and finally, manifest the play on the physical plane (chakra one) in front of an audience. Thus we have taken our abstract conception which began in thought down through the chakras into manifestation. It is this path of manifestation that is said to be pulled by the enjoyment of life, or *bhukti*.

The other current, called the *current of liberation*, takes us out of the limitations of the manifested plane into freer and thus more expansive and inclusive states of being. In this path, the energy in matter is released to become lighter and lighter, as it moves up through the elements, expanding and transforming to a limitless state of pure being. Thus solid earth loses its rigidity and becomes water, then the energy of fire, the expansion of air, the vibration of sound, the radiation of light, and the abstraction of thought.

The liberating current is the pathway usually emphasized in the study of chakras, for it brings personal liberation. It is the pathway through which slow-moving, constricted energy gradually gains new degrees of freedom. It liberates us from outdated or constricting habits, from the veil of maya. It is the pathway through which we disentangle ourselves from the limitations of the physical world and find broader scope in the more abstract and symbolic levels. Each step along the liberating pathway is a rearrangement of matter and of consciousness, to produce more efficient, energy-rich combinations, a dissolution into our primary source. As this current originates below, it is fueled by the lower chakras—our roots, our guts, our needs, and desires.

While suffering from much prejudice, the downward current is equally important for it enables us to manifest. Each step downward is a creative act, an act of consciousness making choices, taking a step toward limitation, allowing constriction of freedom. Through this constriction, the abstract expanse of consciousness has a container that allows it to condense and become solid. In the downward current, each of the chakras can be seen as "condensers" of cosmic energy.

To manifest, we must limit. This requires creating boundaries, being specific, defining structure and form. To write this book, I must have structure to my life and limit my other activities long enough to complete it. To hold a job, raise a child, finish school, or to create anything tangible, we must be willing to accept limitation.

The liberating current brings us excitement, energy, and novelty, while the descending current brings peace, grace, and stability. In order for either of these pathways to really be complete, all of the chakras need to be open and active. Liberation without limitation leaves us vague, scattered, and confused. We may have wonderful ideas and lots of knowledge, but we are unable to bring these fruits to any tangible completion. On the other hand, limitation without liberation is dull and stifling. We become caught in repetitive patterns, clinging to security and fearing change. In order for us to be truly whole, both currents must be open and active.

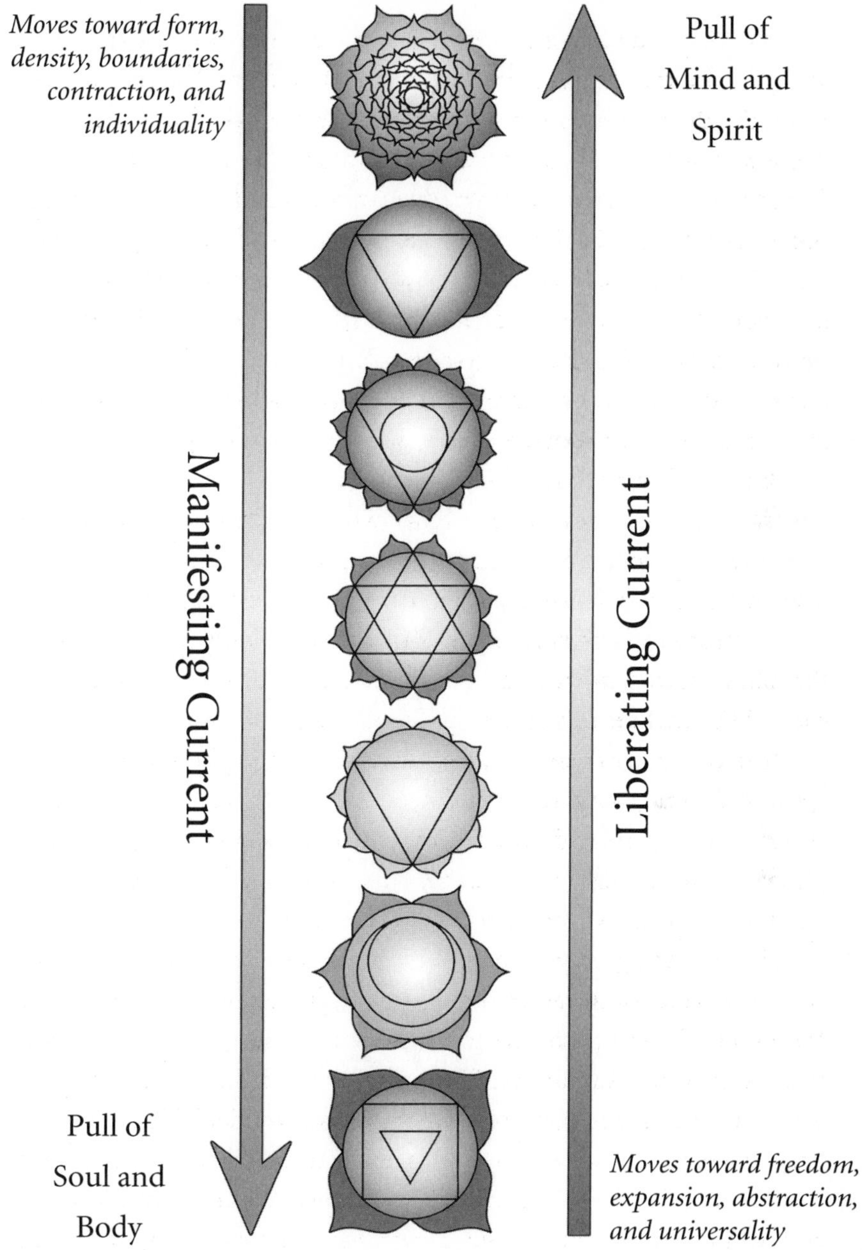

Moves toward form, density, boundaries, contraction, and individuality

Pull of Mind and Spirit

Manifesting Current

Liberating Current

Pull of Soul and Body

Moves toward freedom, expansion, abstraction, and universality

FIGURE 1.10
The current of manifestation and the current of liberation.

The chakras may be thought of as chambers in the body where these two forces mix together in different combinations. Each chakra has a different balance of liberation and manifestation. The lower we go in the system, the stronger the momentum of the manifesting current. The higher we go, the more the chakras are influenced by the liberating current. This basic polarity is an essential element to understanding how the system works as a whole.

THE THREE GUNAS

In Hindu mythology, the cosmos is believed to have evolved out of a primordial ground called *prakrti*, similar to the Western alchemical concept of *prima materia*. Prakrti is woven from three threads called *gunas*, or qualities, which create all that we experience. These qualities correspond, in our terms, to matter, energy, and consciousness.

The first of the gunas is called *tamas*, and it represents matter, mass, or the heavy stillness of inertia. It is prakrti in its densest form. The second guna is called *rajas*, representing energy in the form of motion, force, and the overcoming of inertia. This is prakrti in its energetic, changing form. The third is called *sattva*, meaning mind, intelligence, or consciousness. This is prakrti in its abstract form. The gunas can also be described as tamas, the magnetic force, rajas, the kinetic force, and sattva, the balancing force between these two. Sattva rules the causal plane, rajas rules the subtle plane, and tamas, the gross or physical plane.

In the continuous creation of the cosmos, the three gunas intertwine to form the various states or planes of existence that we experience. Arising from a basic state of equilibrium, the gunas maintain this equilibrium through constant flux. Other times tamas may dominate, giving us matter. At times rajas may dominate, giving us energy. When sattva is predominant, the experience is primarily mental or spiritual. However, the three gunas always retain their own essence, much as the three strands of a braid remain distinct, yet weave together to make one braid.

The totality of the gunas is believed to remain constant, mirroring the principles of energy conservation accepted by physics today. Within our braid, we may alter the number of strands in each section, yet the total size of the braid remains constant.

The chakras are comprised of varying proportions of the three gunas. These three qualities are the essence of a basic, unified primordial substance. Together they compose the dance of the universe, yet separately they are quite distinct. The gunas describe the steps in a cosmic dance and, by studying their interrelationship, we may learn the steps and join in the dance ourselves.

In the following pages, the terms matter, energy, and consciousness will be used quite freely. These terms describe qualities inherent in all aspects of life—the qualities of the three gunas. These terms are not three separate entities and are never found alone without varying proportions of their counterparts. In fact, it is impossible to actually separate them except under an intellectual framework. Energy, matter, and consciousness intertwine to form all that we experience in the same way as the gunas join together to form the cosmos.

The chakras are all comprised of these ingredients in various degrees. Matter (tamas) rules the lower chakras, energy (rajas) rules the middle chakras, and consciousness (sattva) rules the upper chakras. Yet some proportion of each thread is found at every level and in each and every living thing. To balance the weaving of these three basic threads is to bring balance to ourselves, in mind, body, and spirit.

CHAKRAS AND KUNDALINI

Her lustre is that of a strong flash of young lightning. Her sweet murmur is like the indistinct hum of swarms of love-mad bees. She produces melodious poetry . . . It is She who maintains all the beings of the world by means of inspiration and expiration, and shines in the cavity of the root lotus like a chain of brilliant lights.

—Sat-Chakra-Nirupana[27]

When Shakti resides in the base chakra, she rests. Here she becomes the coiled serpent, Kundalini-Shakti, wrapped three and one-half times around the *Shiva lingam* in the Muladhara. In this form she is the inherent potential in matter, the primordial feminine force of creation, and the evolutionary force in human consciousness. In most people she remains dormant, peacefully sleeping in her coiled abode at the base of the spine. Her name comes from the word *kundala*, which means "coiled."

When awakened, this Goddess unfolds from her coils and climbs upward, chakra by chakra, reaching for the crown chakra at the top of the head where she hopes to find Shiva descending to meet her. As she pierces each chakra, she brings that chakra's awakening to her subject. In fact, some believe it is only Kundalini-Shakti who can open the chakras. If she is able to reach the crown chakra and complete her journey, she is united with her counterpart, Shiva, Divine Consciousness, and the result is enlightenment or bliss.

Kundalini yoga is an ancient and esoteric discipline designed to arouse the Kundalini-Shakti force and raise it up the spine. It often involves initiation by a trained guru and years of specific yoga and meditation practices. However, there are many people on and off the spiritual path who are having spontaneous spiritual emergence experiences, some with genuine Kundalini awakenings, so it is worthwhile to examine this mysterious and powerful force.

The paths Kundalini takes are quite varied. Most commonly Kundalini begins at the feet or the base of the spine and travels up toward the head. This movement can be accompanied by shaking spasms or feelings of intense heat. Accounts of Kundalini, however, also include similar intense activity traveling from the head downward or from the middle outward. Sometimes Kundalini symptoms happen within a matter of seconds and then vanish, occurring at intervals of hours or years. At other times, the symptoms may last for weeks, months, or years.

Kundalini is generally a unique and powerful experience that results in a profound consciousness change. This change may be experienced as increased alertness, sudden insight, visions, voices, a feeling of weightlessness, a sense of purity within the body, or transcendent bliss. There is some evidence that Kundalini sets up a wave-like movement of the cerebrospinal fluid, which triggers the pleasure centers of the brain, giving us the "blissful state" so often described by mystics.

A Kundalini experience is not always pleasant, however. Many people have extreme difficulty functioning in their mundane lives while Kundalini is thrashing about through their chakras. While Kundalini pushes her way through your blocks, you may find difficulty sleeping or a dislike for energies associated with the lower chakras, such as eating or sex. (Yet some people become highly sexual after a Kundalini awakening.) There may also be some profound depression or fear as you look at your life through the eyes of this serpent Goddess. She is a healing force, though not always gentle, as the veils of illusion are drawn away from your normal reality. For those who experience spontaneous Kundalini awakenings and do not have a spiritual teacher to work with, there are some referral agencies that can provide you with experienced therapists who understand this spiritual energy and will not necessarily judge it as crazy or psychotic.[28]

The serpent is an archetypal symbol throughout the world representing enlightenment, immortality, and a path to the Gods. In Genesis, the serpent led Adam and Eve to taste the fruit from the Tree of Knowledge. This symbolizes the beginning of Kundalini, creating the unceasing desire for understanding, yet grounded in the material world (the apple). In Egypt, the pharaohs wore crowns with serpent symbols over their third eye to represent their godly stature. Did this represent ascended Kundalini? Even today the double serpent wraps itself around the staff of healing, forming the modern medical symbol, the caduceus. (See Figure 1.11, page 39.) The caduceus clearly imitates the winding of Ida and Pingala, the central nadis crossing between the chakras, surrounding the sushumna. (See Figure 1.6, page 19.) The entwined serpents are also symbolic of the double helix pattern of our DNA—the basic information-carrier of life.

Kundalini is a universal concept for a very powerful enlightening force. It is also a very tricky and unpredictable force to play around with; one which may be loaded with intense pain, confusion and frequently may be interpreted by the world as insanity. This may or may not be accompanied by the more positive aspects listed above. It opens the chakras, but like opening each cell in a jail, Kundalini may release whatever is lodged within the chakras. This may be expanded insights or experiences, or it may be old traumas or abuses that caused the chakra to shut down originally.

Kundalini does produce a profound state of consciousness, and this resulting state of consciousness may make it very difficult to get along in a world so predominantly "unenlightened." It may not support our current paradigm or be harmonious to the circumstances in our lives or the physical state of purity within the body. These discrepancies may make for a great deal of discomfort, but are not always to be avoided. Kundalini is basically a healing force, and pain is felt only when it encounters tension and impurities we are not quite ready to release. Learning to open the chakras allows a clear path for Kundalini that is less apt to be painful.

Theoretically, Kundalini produces a force that helps open the crown chakra, located at the top of the head. Because blocks in the chakras may trap our spinal energy, this chakra is often the hardest to reach. Classically, the crown chakra is considered the seat of enlightenment; however, I believe that it is the combined presence and connection of all the chakras together, given conscious attention, that brings enlightenment. With many people, their more enlightening moments come from bringing upper chakra consciousness down to tangible recognition, rather than the other way around.

The raising of energy to higher chakras occurs naturally and spontaneously when we relax deeply and pay attention to all of our chakras. Attempts to force the energy to rise often results in strain, tension, and a feeling of being "spaced out" or irritable to all those around us who are not doing the same thing. The latter produces an alienation that I

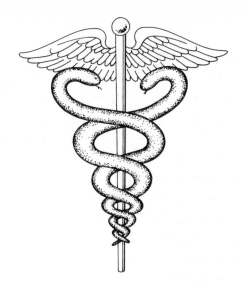

FIGURE 1.11
The caduceus, the modern symbol for healing, traces the
path of the chakras and nadis, emanating from the base
to the two winged petals at the top.

have found to be symptomatic of a lack of enlightenment. (Many people have come up to me at conferences to excitedly tell me of their
enlightened seventh chakra experiences, while not having the slightest
sensitivity to the fact that they were rudely interrupting a conversation, or were living in bodies that seemed horribly neglected.)

It is impossible to talk about chakras without mentioning Kundalini,
however, the raising of Kundalini is not the focus of this book. Kundalini
is not necessarily the best or easiest way to achieve realization any more
than driving through a stone wall is the easiest way to get to the house
on the next street. There are times when a strong force is needed to get
through a particularly stubborn block, but I prefer methods that are
natural, safe, and pleasant. When we take the scenic route, we can enjoy
the journey as much as the destination.

This book neither supports nor condemns disciplines designed to
arouse Kundalini. The drug LSD is a quick way to catch glimpses of the

higher worlds of superconsciousness, and it doesn't necessarily leave you there but may still effect some permanent change in a positive direction. Kundalini is even less predictable, generally more profound, and much more difficult to obtain. However, Kundalini is not the result of a drug, but a reorganization of our own life energy. It is a unique and valuable experience available to any sincere seeker of higher awareness.

What pain we encounter is only from our own resistance and the impurities Kundalini must burn away before she can reach her goal.

There is a great deal of research that is presently being done on Kundalini, and many theories have been formed about what it really is and how it is triggered. The theories listed below are the ones most pertinent to this book.

- **Kundalini is triggered by a guru.** Any interaction we have with other people takes place on a chakra level as well. (See Figure 1.12, page 45.) If we interact with people who are predominantly lower chakra, our own centers respond accordingly. We may be pulled down by such an interaction. Likewise, if an interaction occurs that stimulates the upper chakras, such as contact with a guru who has awakened his or her own Kundalini, this new influx of energy may awaken the disciple. When Kundalini is triggered by a guru, the experience is called *Shaktipat*. It awakens the centers and gets the Kundalini energy flowing, leaving its recipient free to experience both the wonderful effects as well as deal with the consequences it may affect in their lives and body.

- **Kundalini is sexual.** The practice of Tantra sometimes includes elaborate yogic sexual practices, designed to arouse Kundalini and achieve transcendence. Such techniques may vary from prolonged orgasm to total abstinence. Some say Kundalini and sexuality are mutually exclusive, while others believe they are inextricably linked. This will be discussed more fully in the chapter on chakra two.

- **Kundalini is chemical.** The sixth chakra is generally associated with the pineal gland. Melatonin, a chemical produced by this gland, is known to produce increased psychic ability, dream recall, visions, and hallucinogenic effects.[29] Some believe that the visions induced by Kundalini are a cycling of neurotransmitters. In some cases, Kundalini may be triggered by drugs such as coffee, marijuana, or hallucinogenic drugs.

- **Kundalini is the result of vibrational rhythm entrainment in the body.**[30] Undulations of the spine set off rhythms, which entrain with the heartbeat, brain waves and breathing patterns, stimulating various centers in the brain. These may be triggered by meditation, breathing rates, or pure chance, as in the cases of spontaneous awakening. This will be discussed further when we explore vibrations in the realm of the fifth chakra.

- **Kundalini is naturally produced when there is a clear, unblocked channel connecting all of the chakras.** This last is my own theory, which I see as an addition, rather than a contradiction to those above. If the chakras are seen as gears, then Kundalini is the serpentine motion that energy takes as it moves along those gears. In fact the chakras may serve as inhibitors of Kundalini, slowing it down so that it can be reasonably channeled and kept from burning up the mortal organism in which it occurs. At our present state of existence, the chakras themselves are not blocks, but stepping stones; at times, however, the unresolved patterns within the chakras may unnecessarily block this life force. Through a thorough understanding of our personal chakra system, we may be able to use Kundalini energy in a safe and predictable manner.

Table of Correspondences

Chakra	One	Two
Sanskrit Name	Muladhara	Swadhisthana
Meaning	Root Support	Sweetness
Location	Perineum	Sacrum
Element	Earth	Water
Energy State	Solid	Liquid
Psychological Function	Survival	Desire
Resulting in:	Grounding	Sexuality
Identity	Physical identity	Emotional identity
Orientation to Self	Self-preservation	Self-gratification
Demon	Fear	Guilt
Developmental Stage	Womb–12 mos.	6–24 mos.
Glands	Adrenal	Gonads
Other Body Parts	Legs, feet, bones, large intestine	Womb, genitals, kidney, bladder, low back
Malfunction	Obesity, anorexia, Sciatica, constipation	Sexual problems, urinary trouble
Color	Red	Orange
Seed Sound	Lam	Vam
Vowel Sound	*Oh* as in rope	*Oo* as in pool
Sephiroth	Malkuth	Yesod
Planets	Earth, Saturn	Moon
Metals	Lead	Tin
Foods	Protein	Liquid
Gemstones	Ruby, garnet, hematite	Coral, carnelian, yellow zircon
Incense	Cedar	Damiana
Yoga Path	Hatha	Tantra
Rights	to have	to feel
Gunas	Tamas	Tamas

Three	Four	Five
Manipura	Anahata	Vissudha
Lustrous gem	Unstruck	Purification
Solar Plexus	Heart	Throat
Fire	Air	Sound, ether
Plasma	Gas	Vibration
Will	Love	Communication
Power	Peace	Creativity
Ego identity	Social identity	Creative identity
Self-definition	Self-acceptance	Self-expression
Shame	Grief	Lies
18–42 mos.	3.5–7 years	7–12 years
Pancreas, adrenals	Thymus	Thyroid, parathyroid
Digestive system, liver, gall bladder	Lungs, heart, circulatory system, arms, hands	Throat, ears, mouth shoulders, neck
Digestive troubles, chronic fatigue, hypertension	Asthma, coronary disease, lung disease	Sore throats, neck and shoulder pain, thyroid troubles
Yellow	Green	Bright blue
Ram	Yam	Ham
Ah as in father	*Ay* as in play	*Ee* as in sleep
Hod, Netsach	Tiphareth	Geburah, Chesed
Mars (also Sun)	Venus	Mercury
Iron	Copper	Mercury
Starches	Vegetables	Fruits
Amber, topaz apetite	Emerald, tourmaline, jade	Turquoise
Ginger, woodruff	Lavender	Frankinscense, benzoin
Karma	Bhakti	Mantra
to act	to love	to speak and be heard
Rajas	Rajas/Sattva	Rajas/Sattva

Table of Correspondences

Chakra	Six	Seven
Sanskrit Name	Ajna	Sahasrara
Meaning	Command center	Thousand fold
Location	Brow	Top of Head
Element	Light	Thought
Energy State	Luminescence	Consciousness
Psychological Function	Intuition	Understanding
Resulting in:	Imagination	Bliss
Identity	Archetypal identity	Universal identity
Orientation to Self	Self-reflection	Self-knowledge
Demon	Illusion	Attachment
Developmental Stage	Puberty	Throughout life
Glands	Pineal	Pituitary
Other Body Parts	Eyes, base of skull, brow	CNS, cerebral cortex
Malfunction	Vision problems, headaches, nightmares	Depression, alienation, confusion
Color	Indigo	Violet, white
Seed Sound	Om	None
Vowel Sound	*Mmmm*	*Ng* as in sing
Sephiroth	Binah, Chokmah	Kether
Planets	Jupiter, Neptune	Uranus
Metals	Silver	Gold
Foods	Entheogens	Fasting
Gemstones	Lapis, quartz	Diamond, amethyst
Incense	Mugwort	Myrrh, gotu kola
Yoga Path	Yantra	Jnana
Rights	to see	to know
Gunas	Sattva	Sattva

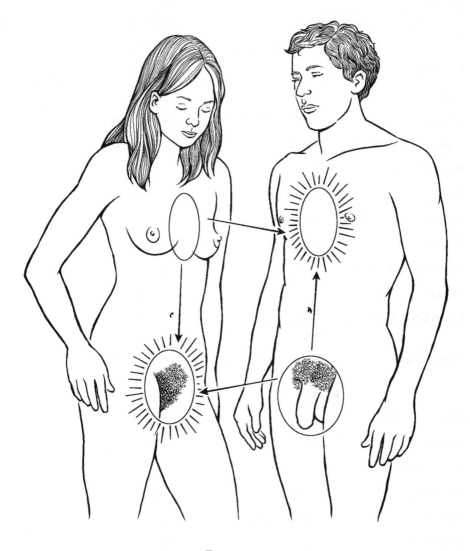

FIGURE 1.12
While he may be acting from a lower chakra physical/sexual level,
bringing her attention to this area, she may in turn stimulate his
heart chakra by emanating at this level.

INTRODUCTORY CONCLUSIONS

It is at this point that some of the basic theories and biases of this book need to be presented. There is much that corresponds to standard systems (if one can find enough agreement to even say what those are), yet many things differ. The theories in the following pages are the result of making connections between the beliefs of the past, present, and projected future of researched information on the Chakra System, as well as numerous other relevant metaphysical and psychological systems.

This is meant to be presented as theory, not dogma; the presentation of an idea, not a religion. Hopefully, it is something valuable to the expansion of one's consciousness regardless of religious or philosophic orientation. The theses are as follows:

- There are seven major and several minor chakras in the subtle body which act as gateways to dimensions spanning from matter to consciousness.

- In the human being, these seven planes correspond to archetypal levels of consciousness as well as various physical attributes.

- The chakras are created by the interpenetration of two major vertical currents.

- The lower chakras are of equal value and importance to the upper chakras for human beings at our present level of development.

- The Chakra System describes a pattern of evolution, and the human race is presently going from the third level to the fourth.

- The chakras also correspond to colors, sounds, deities, dimensions, and other subtle phenomenon.

- The System has immense value for personal growth and use in diagnosis and healing.

- These seven levels are proportional to the possible number of planes in a similar ratio to the seven colors of the rainbow and the spectrum of electromagnetic waves. The seven basic chakras are merely the vibrations that we can perceive with our present "equipment," just as the colors of the rainbow are all that we can perceive with the naked eye.

- The chakras are in constant interplay and can only be separated intellectually.

- The chakras can be opened through various physical exercises, tasks, meditations, healing methods, life experiences, and general understanding, leading to more profound states of consciousness.

PRELIMINARY EXERCISES

Alignment

In order for the chakras to work smoothly, they need to be aligned with each other. The most direct alignment is with the spine relatively straight (a spine too straight is rigid and tense, blocking the opening of the chakras).

> Standing with feet shoulder-width apart, stretch your hands up high over your head, reaching with your whole body, stretching out each of your chakras. Feel how this elongated position encourages the chakras to align.

> When you return to a normal standing position, try to maintain that sense of height, aligning your body so that the central core of each major section (pelvis, solar plexus, chest, throat, head) feels in direct alignment with the central axis of your body. Allow your feet to connect solidly below you and feel the central core (*sushumna*) that connects all the chakras.

Practice the same alignment from a seated position, either in a chair or cross-legged on the floor. Try slouching and returning to an erect spine, feeling the difference in your body's energy and your mind's clarity.

Establishing the Currents

The Manifesting Current

Stand or sit comfortably, spine straight, feet planted firmly on the floor, shoes off. Tune into the vertical axis of your body. Allow yourself to find a comfortable position of balance where this vertical axis is calm, centered, and effortless to maintain. Breathe slowly and deeply.

Mentally reach out through the top of your head and allow yourself to experience the infinite vastness of the sky and space above you. Breathe into this vastness and imagine yourself drinking it in through the top of your head, pulling it down into your head, letting it cascade across your face, your ears, the back of your head, and down across your shoulders and arms.

Allow your head to fill again with this "cosmic" energy, this time letting it tumble into your neck, down into your chest, filling it as you breathe in . . . and out . . . in . . . and out. As the chest fills, let your belly release, allowing this energy to fill your solar plexus, your abdomen, your genitals and down into your buttocks, through your legs, into your feet and out. Let it go deep into the Earth.

Go back to the top of your head and repeat. As you begin the process again, you may choose to think of this energy in a more concrete form: as light, a particular color, a form of divinity, a column of bubbles or stream of wind, or just simply movement. Repeat the process until you feel that your image comes easily and flows smoothly from above your crown to the Earth below your feet.

The Liberating Current

When the above exercise is comfortable, you can begin working with the upward current in a similar manner.

> Through your feet and legs, imagine energy from the Earth (red, brown, or green; solid, yet vibrant) coming up through your legs into your first chakra, filling up there and flowing on into your genitals, abdomen, and solar plexus. Filling again into your heart and chest, neck and shoulders, face and head, and out through the top of your head, releasing any tension it encounters outward and above. Work with this current until it, too, flows smoothly.

> When these two currents are smooth, try running both of them at once. See them mixing and combining together at each of the chakra levels. (If you would like to work with colors, see the meditations at the end of chapter 7, "Chakra Six.")

As you go through your day, be aware of these two currents running through you. Make observations as to which one is stronger and at what times of the day or during what activities. Perhaps your body needs to develop one current more than the other in order to balance your energies. Notice where a current may get hung up on a particular block of tension. Play with the two currents and see which one is more effective in pushing through the block.

ENDNOTES

1. From a song by Rick Hamouris, recorded on *Welcome to Annwfn*, available from Nemeton, P.O. Box 8247, Toledo, Ohio.

2. Chakras and energy currents are mentioned in the Atharva Veda, (10.2.31), (15.15.2–9).

3. Georg Feurstein, in *The Shambhala Encyclopedia of Yoga*, refutes the Aryan invasion theory and pushes the date of the Vedas back into the third or fourth millennium BCE. He counters that the lighter-skinned Aryans were native to India, due to similarities in the ancient Indus-Sarasvati civilization.

4. Troy Wilson Organ, *Hinduism*, 183.

5. The eightfold path consists of the *yamas* (restraints), *niyamas* (observances), *asana* (postures), *pranayama* (breathing), *pratyahara* (withdrawal of senses), *dharana* (concentration), *dhyana* (absorption), and *samadhi* (enlightenment).

6. Arthur Avalon, *The Serpent Power: The Secrets of Tantric and Shaktic Yoga*.

7. *The Serpent Power* actually lists six centers, plus the Sahasrara (thousand-petaled lotus of the crown).

8. The five Koshas are: *annamayakosha*, or physical sheath, *pranamayakosha*, or energy sheath, *manamayakosha*, or mind sheath, *vijnanamayakosha*, or wisdom sheath, and *anandamayakosha*, or bliss body.

9. See Georg Feurstein, *The Shambhala Encyclopedia of Yoga*, 68–69. Nine chakras are described in Pandit Rajmani Tigunait, Ph.D. *Sakti: The Power in Tantra, A Scholarly Approach* (Honesdale, PA: Himalayan Institute, 1998), 111.

10. Chakras one and two are combined as one center, as are chakras six and seven, giving five in all.

11. Caroline Myss, *Anatomy of the Spirit*.

12. For more detail on comparing the chakra system and the ten sephiroth, see endnote 11.

13. Arthur Young, *The Reflexive Universe*.

14. See Rosalyn L. Bruyere, *Wheels of Light: A Study of the Chakras*.

15. For more active suggestions on ways to experience the chakras, including yoga postures, journal exercises, meditations, tasks, and rituals, see Judith and Vega, *The Sevenfold Journey: Reclaiming Mind, Body, and Spirit through the Chakras.*

16 . Classically, there are only five elements associated with the chakras—earth, water, fire, air, and ether, respectively from bottom to top. Chakra five is associated with *sabda*, or sound. It is my modernization that links the "elements" of light and thought to the upper two chakras.

17. For more explanation of excess and deficiency see my book *Eastern Body, Western Mind.*

18. For more details on chakras and childhood developmental stages, see my book *Eastern Body, Western Mind.*

19. Avalon, *Serpent Power*, 23.

20. The first chakra, however, contains the Shiva lingam, which is the form of Shiva invigorated by the presence of Kundalini-Shakti, who resides there in her sleeping form.

21. Sir Monier Monier-Williams, *Sanskrit-English Dictionary*, 811.

22. Lizelle Raymond, *Shakti—A Spiritual Experience.*

23. Swami Rama, "The Awakening of Kundalini," *Kundalini, Evolution, and Enlightenment*, ed. John White (Anchor Books, 1979), 27.

24. Haridas Chaudhuri, "The Psychophysiology of Kundalini," Ibid., 61.

25. Avalon, *Serpent Power*, 38.

26. Sri Aurobindo also describes ascending and descending currents in many of his writings.

27. Verses 10 and 11 of the *Sat-Chakra-Nirupana*, as translated by Arthur Avalon in *Serpent Power.*

28. Spiritual Emergence Network, run by California Institute of Integral Studies (415) 648-2610, or Kundalini Research Network, P.O. Box 45102, 2483 Younge St., Toronto, Ontario, Canada, M4P 3E3.

29. Philip Lansky, "Neurochemistry and the Awakening of Kundalini," *Kundalini, Evolution, and Enlightenment*, ed. John White (Anchor Books, 1979), 296.

30. Lee Sannella, M.D. *Kundalini: Psychosis or Transcendence?* Also see Itzhak Bentov, *Micromotion of the Body as a Factor in the Development of the Nervous System*, 77 ff.

PART TWO

JOURNEY THROUGH THE CHAKRAS

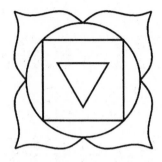

CHAKRA ONE

Earth

Roots

Grounding

Survival

Body

Food

Matter

Beginning

Chapter 2

CHAKRA ONE: EARTH

OPENING MEDITATION

YOU ARE ABOUT TO GO ON A JOURNEY. IT is a journey through the layers of your own self. It is a journey through your life, through the worlds within and around you. It begins here, in your own body. It begins now, wherever you are. It is your own personal quest.

Make yourself comfortable, for the journey is not short. It could take months, years, or lifetimes, but you have already chosen to go. You began long, long ago.

You have been provided a vehicle in which to take this journey. It is your body. It is equipped with everything you might need. One of your challenges on this journey is to keep your vehicle nourished, happy, and in good repair. It is the only one you will be given.

So, we begin our journey by exploring our vehicle. Take a moment to feel your body. Feel it breathing in . . . and out . . . Feel your heart beating inside, the moisture in your mouth, the food in your belly, the sensation of cloth on your skin. Explore the space your body occupies— height, width, weight. Find the front and back, top, bottom, and sides. Begin a dialogue with your body, so that you may learn its language. Ask your body how it feels. See if it is tired or tense. Listen to the answer. How does it feel about going on this journey?

You have been given a vehicle for this journey, but it is not something you have—it's some thing you are. You are your body. You are a body living a life in this physical world—getting up in the morning, eating, going to work, touching, sleeping, bathing. Feel your body going through its daily routines. See the number of interactions it has with the outside world in a day—notice the interchange of hands touching doors, steering wheels, other hands, papers, dishes, children, food, your lover. Think about how your body has grown and learned and changed over the years. What has it become to you? Do you ever thank it for taking care of you?

What is the world like that your body interacts with? Feel the textures, smells, colors, and sounds around you. Be your body feeling them—all the sensations your mind might miss—but your body experiences. Feel the hardness of the earth in wood, cement, and metal. Feel its straight lines, its solidity, its permanence. Feel the soft firmness of the Earth in its natural state—with its trees and grasses, lakes, streams, and mountains. Feel its curving gentleness, its protection, and abundance. Feel the richness of this planet with its infinity of forms. Feel its immensity, its solidity, and how it supports you as you sit in your place on it, reading this book.

This planet is a vehicle, too. It takes us through time and through space. Feel the Earth as a central unified entity—a living body, just like you—with an infinity of cells, working together as a whole. You are a cell in this great body, part of Mother Earth, one of Her children.

We begin our journey here, on this great body of Earth. Our long climb upward begins by going down. We go down into this body, as we go down into our own bodies—into our flesh, into our guts, into our legs and feet—digging our roots deep into the Earth, which supports and nourishes us. We move deep into her rocks and soil, deep into her guts of red-hot lava, seething deep below, into her source of life and movement and power.

When we sink deeply, we come to the base of our spine and find a red glowing ball of energy, glowing like the core of the Earth. Feel this molten energy running down your legs, through your knees, into your feet. Feel it running through your feet, into the floor beneath you, through the floor and down into the Earth, burrowing between rocks and roots, finding nourishment, support, and stability. Feel this cord of energy as an anchor, settling you, calming you, grounding you.

You are here. You are connected. You are solid, but you are molten inside. Deep within your roots you find your past, your memories, your primal self. Your connection here is simple, direct. You remember your heritage, your ancient self as a child of the Earth. She is your teacher.

What is this matter that comes from the Earth? Think of the chair you are sitting in—the tree it once was, the cotton in the field, the cloth on the loom, the workers that transported it, sold it, sat on it before. Think of the things you have—the complexity in each one of them, their abundance.

Think of the financial abundance you may have. However large or small it may be, think of it as a gift from the Earth. How does it come to you? What does your body do to get it? What do you use it for? Think of this money as a stream of life running into you and out of you, through your hands, your feet, your heart, and your mind. As it flows through you, feel yourself in constant exchange with the Earth. Let the feeling of abundance come up from the Earth, into your feet, your legs, your pelvis, stomach, heart, and hands. Feel its expression in your throat, its recognition in your vision, its imprint in your mind. Take a deep breath and let it go down again, through your body, through your head, neck, shoulders, arms, chest, belly, genitals, legs and feet, and down into the Earth, down below the surface of the Earth, finding stability, finding nourishment finding peace.

Your body is the journey, and it is where you begin. It is your connection to the physical world, your foundation, the home of your dance. You are the place from which all action and understanding will arise, and to which it will return. You are the testing ground of truth.

You are the ground on which all things rest. You are the Earth from which all things grow. You are here, you are solid, you are alive.

You are the point from which all things begin.

CHAKRA ONE SYMBOLS AND CORRESPONDENCES

Sanskrit Name:	*Muladhara*
Meaning:	Root support
Location:	Perineum, base of spine, coccygeal plexus
Element:	Earth
Function:	Survival, grounding
Inner State:	Stillness, security, stability
Rights:	Right to be here, right to have
Outer Manifestation:	Solid
Glands:	Adrenals
Other Body Parts:	Legs, feet, bones, large intestine, teeth
Malfunction:	Weight problems, hemorrhoids, constipation, sciatica, degenerative arthritis, knee troubles
Color:	Red
Sense:	Smell

Seed Sound:	Lam
Vowel Sound:	O as in rope
Petals:	Four—vam, sam, sam, sam
Tarot Suit:	Pentacles
Sephira:	Malkuth
Planets:	Saturn, Earth
Metal:	Lead
Foods:	Proteins, meats
Corresponding Verb:	I have
Yoga Path:	Hatha yoga
Herbs for Incense:	Cedar
Minerals:	Lodestone, ruby, garnet, bloodstone
Guna:	Tamas
Animals:	Elephant, ox, bull
Lotus Symbols:	Four red petals, yellow square, downward pointing triangle, Shiva lingam, around which Kundalini is coiled three and one-half times, white elephant, eight arrows outward. Above the *bija* (seed syllable) is the Child Brahma and the Shakti Dakini.
Hindu Deities:	Brahma, Dakini, Ganesha, Kubera, Uma, Lakshmi, Prisni
Other Pantheons:	Gaia, Demeter/Persephone, Erda, Ereshkigal, Anat, Ceridwen, Geb, Hades, Pwyll, Dumuzi, Tammuz, Atlas
Archangel:	Auriel
Chief Operating Force:	Gravity

MULADHARA—THE ROOT CHAKRA

*By energism of consciousness, Brahman is massed; from
that matter is born and from matter Life and Mind and
the worlds.*

—Mundaka Upanishad 1.1.8[1]

Our journey up the spinal column begins at the base of the spine,
home of the first chakra. This is the foundation of our entire system—
the building block on which all the other chakras must rest—so this
chakra is of crucial importance. It relates to the element *earth*, and all
solid, earthly things, such as our bodies, our health, our survival, our
material and monetary existence, and our ability to focus and manifest
our needs. It is the manifestation of consciousness in its final form—
solid and tangible. It is our need to stay alive and be healthy, and the
acceptance of limitation and discipline so crucial to manifestation.

In this system, earth represents form and solidity, our most condensed state of matter and the "lowest" end of our chakra spectrum.
It is visualized as a deep, vibrant red, the color of beginning, and
the color with the longest wavelength and slowest vibration in the
visible spectrum.

The Sanskrit name for this chakra is *Muladhara,* which means "root
support." The sciatic nerve, traveling from the sacral plexus down
through the legs, is the largest peripheral nerve in the body (about as
thick as your thumb) and functions much like a root for the nervous
system. (See Figure 2.1, page 61.) The feet and legs, which provide loco-
motion, enable us to perform tasks necessary to obtain life sustenance
from the earth and its environment. Our legs touch the ground below
us and connect our nervous system with the earth, our first chakra element. We respond then, kinesthetically, to gravity—the basic underlying force of the earth—constantly pulling us downward. This force
keeps us connected to our planet, rooted in material existence.

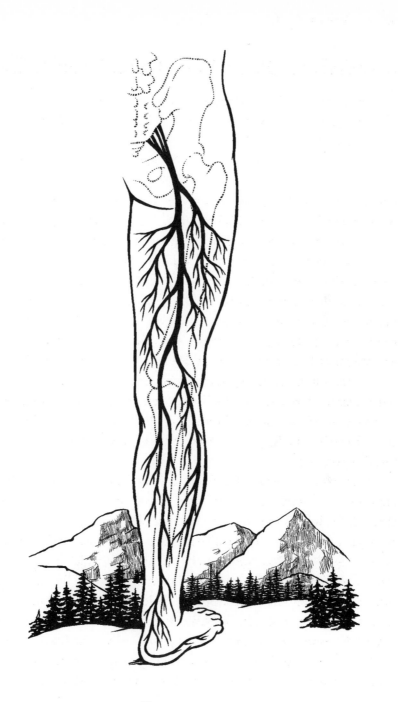

Figure 2.1
Sciatic nerve as a root.

This center is depicted as a lotus of four petals within which is a square. (See Figure 2.2, page 63.) This can be seen as representing the four directions and the firm foundation of the material world, which in many systems has come to be symbolized by a square. As the first chakra relates to Malkuth, the base sphere in the Kabbalistic Tree of Life, these four petals also reflect the four elements of the material kingdom.

Within this square is a small triangle pointing downward from a column of energy representing the sushumna. This represents the earth-oriented downward force of the chakra. Within the triangle is the Kundalini serpent wrapped around the Shiva lingam, which points upward. This chakra is the home and resting place of Kundalini. Below the triangle is a seven-trunked elephant, named *Airavata*, representing the heavy, matter-like quality of this chakra and the seven pathways out of it, which correspond to the seven chakras. We may also associate the elephant-headed God, *Ganesha*, Lord of Obstacles, with this center, as he is grounded, full-bellied, and happy with his physicality. Other deities depicted in the square are the five-faced *Child Brahma*, dispelling fears, and the female *Dakini*, the manifestation of Shakti at this level, with spear, sword, cup, and skull. In the center of the square is the symbol for the seed sound, believed to contain the essence of the chakra, which is *lam*. These images and sounds are all symbols that can be used in meditation on this chakra.

In the body, the first chakra is located at the base of the spine, or more accurately, the perineum, midway between the anus and the genitals. It corresponds to the section of the spine called the coccyx, as well as the coccygeal spinal ganglion and the lower lumbar vertebrae from which this ganglion sprouts. (See Figure 2.3, page 65.) In keeping with the correlation to solid matter, this chakra relates to the solid part of the body, especially the bones, the large intestine (which passes solid substances), and the fleshy body as a whole. There are minor chakras in the knees and feet that transmit sensations from the ground below to our spinal column for information concerning motor activity. These are sub-chakras to the first and second chakras—grounding outlets for the body as a whole.

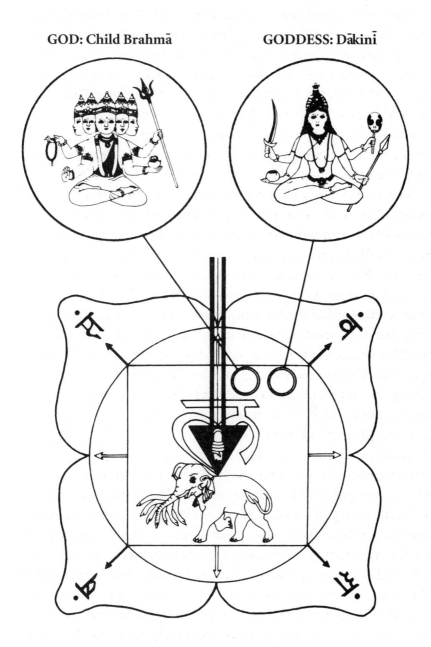

GOD: Child Brahmā   GODDESS: Dākinī

FIGURE 2.2
Mūlādhāra chakra.
(Courtesy Timeless Books)

We have described chakras as vortices of energy. At the level of the first chakra, our vortex is the most dense of any chakra level. It is tamas at its essence: at rest, inert.

If you were to cross a stream with a very strong current, you would find it difficult to walk through the force of the water rushing upon you. If many such forces came from all directions, focusing on a central point, you could not pass through it at all. The meeting of these forces produces a field that is so dense it seems solid. Chakra one has this kind of density.

This solidity is valid from the point of view of the body, which cannot pass through it, but not of the higher nonmaterial activities of our intelligence. We know that atoms are mostly empty space. We can see through glass, even though it is solid; we can hear through walls, and we can use our intelligence to make apparatuses that allow us to see through the illusion of matter as a solid entity.

And yet, it is this solid matter that provides the basis of our consensus reality. It is this matter that is our constant, and without its relatively changeless solidity, our lives would be quite difficult. Imagine if every time you came home your house was in a different shape or in a different place; or if your children changed beyond recognition from day to day. How confusing it would be!

At our present level of evolution, matter is an undeniable reality and necessity. We cannot separate ourselves from it, for we are made up of it. Without a body we die, and to deny our body is to die prematurely. Likewise, we cannot deny our connection to the Earth we live on, and the vital part it plays in supporting our future. To deny attention to our foundation is to build on shaky ground. The purpose of this chakra is to solidify this ground.

Consciousness in the Muladhara chakra is primarily concerned with physical survival. It is our instinctual fight or flight response. To ignore this chakra or its earthy element is to threaten our very survival, both personally and collectively. If we do not balance this chakra before we progress to others, our growth will be without roots, ungrounded, and will lack the stability necessary for true growth.

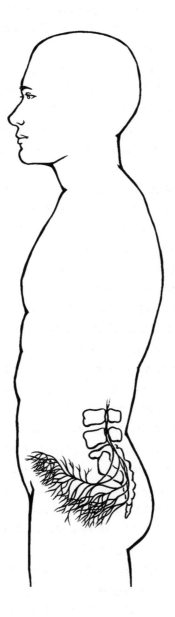

Figure 2.3
Coccygeal spinal ganglion and the lower lumbar vertebrae.

When our survival is threatened, we experience fear. Fear is a demon of the first chakra—it counteracts the sense of safety and security that the first chakra ideally brings. Inappropriate levels of fear can be a sign that the first chakra foundation is damaged. Facing our fear can help the first chakra wake up.

There is a common belief within various spiritual philosophies that we are "trapped" in physical bodies, awaiting release from this bondage. This belief supports the denigration of the body and perpetrates a mind/body split. This denies access to the vast beauty and intelligence that our bodies store in their trillions of cells.

The physical world is only a trap if we see it as such and quickly becomes a friend to anyone who understands its part in the greater structure. As we travel up the spinal column, we will come to understand more about these other levels and manifestations. We will also come to appreciate the sanctity and security that comes from substance and matter.

GROUNDING

The liberating current, ever moving toward higher consciousness, is the pathway most commonly associated with the Chakra System. Until recently there has been less said about sending our energy downward, into the Earth, along the current of manifestation. This is often seen as less spiritual and, therefore, less worthy of our time and attention. Too many spiritual paths ignore the importance of *grounding*.

Grounding is a process of dynamic contact with the Earth, with its edges, boundaries, and limitations. It allows us to become solidly real—present in the here and now—and dynamically alive with the vitality that comes from the Earth. While mechanically our feet may touch the ground with every step, this contact is empty if we are cut off from the feelings in our legs and feet. Grounding involves opening the lower chakras, merging with gravity, and descending deeply into the vehicle of the body.

Without grounding, we are unstable; we lose our center, fly off the handle, get swept off our feet, or daydream in a fantasy world. We lose our ability to contain, to have, or to hold. Natural excitement, or charge, becomes dissipated, diluted, and ineffectual. When we lose our ground, our attention wanders from the present moment, and we appear to be "not all here." In this state, we feel powerless and, like a vicious circle, may no longer want to be here.

Our ground anchors the very roots for which this chakra is named. Through our roots, we gain nourishment, power, stability, and growth. Without this connection we are separated from nature, separated from our biological source. Cut off from our source, we lose our path. Many people who cannot find their true path in life have simply not yet found their ground. Sometimes they are busy looking up instead of down, where the feet meet the path.

Our roots are made from our guts—the instinctual feelings that get programmed from the memories of our past, our racial and cultural heritage, and the indestructible fabric of our being. C. J. Jung describes this instinctual base as the realm of the collective unconscious —a vast and powerful realm of inherited instincts and evolutionary trends. When we reclaim these roots, we strengthen who we are, and draw on the vast wisdom of this instinctual realm.

When we are grounded, we are humble and close to the Earth. We live simply, in a state of grace. We can embrace stillness, solidity, and clarity, "grounding out" the stresses of everyday life, and increasing the vitality of our basic life force.

Resting on the ground, we cannot fall, which provides a sense of inner security. It is through grounding that our consciousness completes the manifesting current. It is at the first chakra plane that ideas become reality. From the great diversity of imagination to the intricate requirements of the physical world, the Earth plane is the testing ground of our beliefs. That which has ground, substance, and validity will find its way to manifestation. That which has roots will endure.

In today's urban world, there are few people who are naturally grounded. Our language and cultural values reflect the superiority of the high at the expense of the low, i.e., to be highly regarded, to hold one thing *above* another, to get high, to have things look up. Socially and economically, intellectual work is better rewarded than physical labor. Our natural bodily processes such as waste elimination, sexuality, birth, breastfeeding, or nudity are considered dirty, to be done only in private and often with much guilt. Control of our health is put in the hands of an elite class, denying us the sense of our own innate healing potential. Our power structures in business, government, and organized religion flow hierarchically, from the top down, controlling and often trampling that which is below in order to serve the "higher cause" of that which is above.

By losing touch with our ground we have lost the sense of our intricate connection with all life. We become ruled by a part instead of the whole—and, furthermore, a part that is isolated, fragmented, and out of touch. Ignoring our ground, it is no wonder that we face a health care crisis and ecological destruction.

In an alienated and "ungrounded" culture, where most values do not favor the body or its pleasures, we develop pain. Our bodies hurt after a day at the computer or a day of driving. The stress of competition and fast living do not give us a chance to rest and renew, or to process that hurt, to release it. As we develop pain, we become, ironically, more resistant to grounding, for to ground is to be "in touch." Getting in touch means feeling that pain. Yet this is the first step in making ourselves whole so that we begin to heal.

As we become more mechanized and urbanized, our contact with the Earth and nature becomes more tenuous, and with it our health and self-worth. Our power is transferred to the upper body where it, too, is tenuous and must be constantly guarded. Because we see ourselves as separate, power becomes an act of manipulation rather than connection. We lose touch with our animal nature, and with it our sense of instinctual power, grace, and peace. When we have a sense of self that comes from the body, we have less need to affirm ourselves through ego inflation. Ground is home—it's familiar, safe, and secure. It has a power of its own.

Grounding implies limitation. While the mental energy of the upper chakras is boundless, the lower chakras are far narrower in their scope. Language limits and, therefore, specifies our thoughts. Yet I could name a thousand things I could not fit in a large house, for the physical world has even more limitation. Each step down through the chakras becomes simpler, more definitive, and more constricted.

While frightening to some people, this limitation is an essential creative principle. If we didn't limit our activities, we would accomplish nothing. If I didn't limit my thoughts as I typed this manuscript, I couldn't write. Far from being a negative, limitation creates a container that allows energy to build and gel into substance. *To manifest, we must be willing to accept limitation.* Grounding is a harmonious acceptance of natural limitation. It is just as crucial to the development of consciousness as any meditation or raising of energy. In the words of the immortal *I Ching*:

> *Limitation has success . . . . Unlimited possibilities are not suited to man; if they existed, his life would only dissolve in the boundless. To become strong a man's life needs the limitations ordained by duty and voluntarily accepted.*

> —Hexagram 60: Wilhelm Baynes version

Grounding is a simplifying force. We are bringing our consciousness into the body which, for all practical purposes, exists in one space and one time only—the here and now. Our thoughts, by contrast, are much more versatile, extending outside of space and time. We can fantasize about being in the mountains for our next summer vacation, and perhaps even see and feel the warmth of the sunshine. But our body remains where we are—at our desk with snow outside the window and bills piled in front of us. If we spend too much time fantasizing, we may never get enough work done to even take the vacation. Then it is time to get back to the Earth plane, do some grounding, and take care of survival needs.

The human organism is a finely tuned instrument capable of receiving and transmitting an enormous variety of energies. Like any stereo receiver, we need to plug it in before we can receive the various frequencies. Grounding is the process of plugging ourselves into the Earth and the world around us, completing the circuit that makes us a channel for the great diversity of life energies around us.

Just as a lightning rod protects a building by sending excess voltage into the ground, so, too, our grounding protects the body from becoming "overloaded" by the tensions of everyday life. Through grounding we send the impact of stressful vibrations into a larger body that can handle them. A small child, for example, buries his head in his mother's shoulder on hearing a loud noise. He is, in a sense, grounding that vibration in her body.

Measurements have shown that when the human body is standing on the ground, it is electrically grounded as well. There is an electrostatic field surrounding the Earth with a resonant frequency of about 7.5 cycles per second.[2] The late Itzhak Bentov discussed a micromotion of the body that consists of the constant vibration of the heart, cells, and bodily fluids. He determined that this micromotion vibrates at a frequency of 6.8 to 7.5 cycles per second. Therefore, the body's natural frequency resonates with the Earth's ionosphere. Connecting physically to this great body, as in walking or lying on the Earth, our own bodies enter into this resonance more deeply.

Grounding is a way of coping with stress. The downward channel gives us an outgoing circuit and protects us from psychic overload. The physical world is safe and stable. We can always return to our favorite chair, a good meal, and familiar surroundings when we need to feel calm and secure. This stability makes it easier to work on higher planes. When the body feels secure, well-fed, and healthy, our consciousness can flow to other levels.

Chakras filter energy from the environment. Their spinning pattern vibrates at a certain rate allowing only matching vibrations to enter into the internal core of consciousness. The rest recedes into the background, soon to be completely forgotten by the conscious mind (although the subconscious mind may often remember quite well). When too much abrasive energy is found in our surroundings, the chakras will close down to protect the subtle body from this caustic invasion. Overloaded chakras are difficult to open. Grounding is a way to discharge this excess tension.

Grounding brings clarity through stillness. Every action causes a reaction. If we can "still" our reactions to some aspect of a vicious cycle, we are "stepping out of the world of karma." We are then able to stop the cycle. This is analogous to letting dirty water sit in a glass long enough for the mud to settle to the bottom, clearing the water.

Many people experience difficulty because their upper chakras are too open, while their lower chakras are not stable enough to support the barrage of psychic energy they pick up around them. At its extreme, this creates serious mental disorders, such as psychosis. A psychotic individual has lost touch with his ground and with consensus reality. Through techniques of grounding, psychic overload can be discharged, giving patients stability to match their sensitivity. Even simple physical touch can help to ground someone in intense pain. Physical exercises or making something with one's hands is also useful, as well as any of the grounding exercises described at the end of this chapter or in *The Sevenfold Journey*.[3]

Grounding is like focusing a camera lens, where the object is to get two images to merge into one. As our astral body becomes firmly connected with our physical body, our senses of the physical world around us becomes sharp and clear. If another person were to look at us when we were particularly grounded, they would also experience a dynamic clarity about us—a presence in the eyes and body—whether or not that person had ever seen an "aura."

In this state of "groundedness," decisions are more easily made, worries about the future are more easily assailed, and enjoyment of the present moment takes on a new luster and challenge. This is not a state that is detrimental to expanded consciousness, but one that enhances it.

Grounding forms a foundation. A person desiring to study medicine "grounds" themselves in the physical sciences as an undergraduate. In opening a new business, one first gets "grounding" from someone more experienced in the field and finds financial support. Our first chakras are the foundations on which everything we do rests. Our bodies are a microcosm of the world we create around us. The work we do and the foundations we build are of utmost importance to the success of whatever follows.

For many people, work itself is a grounding activity. Aside from providing our basic tool of survival—money—the routine of working a job according to a regular schedule can provide a basic structure that supports the life around it. This routine, while it may be drudgery at times, can actually be beneficial in its limitations. It builds a foundation. Through focus and repetition, energies become dense enough to manifest. If we are involved with constant change, we are like a rolling stone that gathers no moss. We're kept at a survival level because we are constantly building new foundations. Only through focus and repetition can we achieve expertise in an area leading to larger manifestation of goals, be they physical or ideological.

Chakras, however, must be balanced. While the stability of grounding is a necessary state to achieve, undue attachment to this security can be detrimental. The physical world is not the goal, but only a tool. It is possible to dominate our consciousness with addictions to material comforts, and the acquisition of more and more of them becomes the basis of many people's lives. It is this that is seen as a detriment to the growth of consciousness and one that makes material existence a trap. Once again, it is only undue *attachment* to this security that becomes a trap, not the basic satisfaction of this need.

Grounding is not dull and lifeless, but dynamic and vibrant. Generally it is our tension that makes us lethargic, and tension results from alienation between various parts of ourselves. As these parts are simplified and integrated, we experience increased vitality.

Intellectually, it is easy for people to understand the need for grounding. But the experience cannot really be explained in words. It is a cumulative skill; one session of grounding meditations may produce some effect, but it is only over time that the real benefits may be achieved. As grounding is the foundation for all else we may do, it is well worth it to take the time. (See the grounding exercises at the end of this chapter.)

SURVIVAL

First chakra consciousness is oriented toward survival. This is the maintenance program that protects the health of our bodies and our day-to-day mundane needs. Here we function from an instinctual level, concerned with hunger, fear, the need for rest, warmth, and shelter.

Survival demands awaken our consciousness. Threats to survival stimulate the adrenal glands for that burst of extra energy needed for fight or flight. As the body gets energized, awareness is heightened. The challenge of survival requires us to think and act quickly, and to innovate new solutions. Our consciousness is spontaneously focused on our situation in a way that rarely occurs at other times.

In order to consolidate our energy in the first chakra, we must first see that our survival needs are met in a healthy and direct way, so that our consciousness is not dominated by them. To ignore these demands is to be constantly pulled back into survival consciousness, making us unable to "get off the ground."

In the primal roots of our collective unconscious lie the memories of a time when we were more connected to the Earth, the sky, the seasons, and the animals—a connection that was integral to our survival, and one that was the foundation for our first developments of intelligence. We, too, were hunted like the animals we ate. What we lived on, we were also a part of. Survival was a full-time concern.

Currently, the situation is quite different. Now our survival is indirect. Our food comes from a store, our heat from a button on the wall. No longer do we need to lie awake at night guarding our food from a wild and hungry beast (unless it's a family member!). No longer do we need to keep the fire alive out of ignorance about how to relight it. Instead we need to worry about our car breaking down on the way to work, that we have enough money to pay the utilities, or that our home isn't burglarized when we go out of town.

Still, the survival instinct remains, and losing a job, coming down with an illness, or being evicted from an apartment can trigger our first chakras into working overtime. When this happens we experience panic. Survival energies flood our system, but we may not know what to do with them. The answer may not be running or fighting, which is what the body is preparing us to do, but claiming our roots in a more conscious way.

When Muladhara is activated by danger or pressing circumstances, the response is similar to a computer searching for information on a floppy disk. The first chakra disk stores all our survival information. The "operating system" of the body then "boots" that information into the attention of the conscious mind.

The body reacts instantaneously. The spine makes contact to the Earth, via the legs, adrenaline rushes through the bloodstream, the heartbeat accelerates, increasing blood supply, and the senses are sharpened dramatically. Our sleepy consciousness awakens. It is the beginning of heightened awareness where Kundalini, who lies coiled around the Muladhara, may begin her ascent.

When survival information is not needed immediately, the chakra goes on automatic. It routinely checks internal and external environments to see that all things remain in order, and that they are conducive to the ongoing existence of the organism. When there is a threat, pre-programming in the first chakra takes over and our consciousness is dominated by the needs of the body.

There is very little we can do to interfere with this process without harming the body once the first chakra takes over. If we don't take a rest, our illness advances until we have no choice. If our income is threatened, or if we are suddenly evicted from our home, our attention is dominated by these situations until they are resolved. Like the force of gravity, we can only accept its pull and learn to work with it.

One who is perpetually plagued by health problems or constantly struggling with financial crisis is caught on this first chakra level. Some unresolved conflict, whether it be physical, circumstantial, or psychological, is keeping their consciousness trapped at this level. There is usually an insecure, panicky feeling—one which may pervade other areas of life, even when there is no need for it. As long as these situations remain unresolved, the person will have difficulty raising any appreciable amount of consciousness to higher levels. Exercises for dealing with such problems involve grounding and working with the first chakra, and some of these are listed at the end of the chapter. But first it is important to understand the ramifications of consciousness at this root level, namely, *the right to be here.*

If this is your experience, ask yourself, what keeps you from wanting to be here? From whom do you need permission to take care of yourself? What is the fear of grounding, of becoming stable, of standing on your own two feet? Who is responsible for your survival? How much of your thinking is unrealistic dreaming, not grounded in the world around you? How was your survival provided for in your childhood, by whom, and at what cost? Are you connecting with your body, listening to it, administering to its needs? Do you have the *right* to be here, to take up space, to have what you need in order to survive?

An important aspect of the ability to maintain survival at a comfortable level has to do with the ability *to have* things—to contain, to keep, to magnetize materiality into our own sphere. To be and to have—these are the rights of the first chakra.

The ability to have is an acquired skill. Some, born wealthy, are raised to expect abundance in their lives. To buy the best brand in the store, to order the most expensive meal in a restaurant—these come more naturally to those raised to it, and it's easier for them to maintain that level, even when finances are not provided. Expecting prosperity makes it easier to create.

Most of us were not so lucky. Raised with concepts of scarcity, we chew our nails over buying a new dress, we panic over whether to take a pleasant job that pays less, and we're nervous when we take a day off.

We make do with what we have whenever possible, rather than risk extravagance. We don't allow ourselves luxuries, and if we do, it is often with guilt or worry. This is an inability to "have"—a first chakra programmed on a foundation of scarcity rather than abundance.

Developing our ability to have things begins with increasing *self-worth*. Paradoxically, allowing ourselves to have more also increases our self-worth, both literally and figuratively. It helps to look objectively at what we allow ourselves to have, in terms of money, love, time to ourselves, rest, or pleasure. A teacher I knew once told me she could never allow herself to buy a new pair of socks, but could buy them for her husband, and then take one of his old pairs for herself! Obviously, she could spend the money, but she herself couldn't have the benefit. Some people find it easy to spend money on extravagance, but hard to take time for their own relaxation. Others have a hard time accepting love or pleasure. When we look closely at what we allow ourselves to have, we get a chance to laugh at ourselves—to see the discrepancies between what we could have and what we allow ourselves to have. Somehow, taking care of ourselves has been depicted as selfish or evil. Yet, not taking care of ourselves results in a need to compensate in some other area, or have others provide for us.

In order to fully be here, we must be able to assert ourselves, to claim our own place in the world, and to secure our survival. We need to raise our ability "to have" high enough to fit our needs. If our unconscious says, "No, I don't deserve it," our conscious minds are given an extra obstacle to overcome.

Our ultimate foundation for our survival is the Earth itself. Unfortunately, the Earth is also in a state of survival at this time. The threat of ecological collapse, nuclear holocaust, and the scarcity of clean air and water—all affect our own feelings of survival, either consciously or unconsciously. To pass into a new era does not mean we leave behind the old, but instead incorporate it. As we ignore the Earth, She pulls us back again to ground, to the here and now, to bring into balance that which is threatened.

Culturally, this puts us all in a state of survival. As we tune into the Earth, as we get more deeply in touch, we can't help but touch a feeling of planetary panic about our future existence. Just as a threat to our personal survival heightens our own awareness, so do ecological threats heighten planetary awareness. It is often a crisis that wakes people up.

If we are to reach the spiritual levels of the upper chakras, we must see the spiritual side of our material existence. The planet we live on is one of the finest examples of beauty, harmony, and spirituality that matter can express. By understanding this, we can better develop and express the beauty within our own material existence.

Being in survival is a cue to "wake-up"—to heighten our awareness, to examine our foundation: our ground, our body, and the Earth. This is the purpose of the first chakra. It is where we begin, and where we rest at the end of the journey.

THE BODY

Here in this body are the sacred rivers, here are the sun and moon, as well as all the pilgrimage places. I have not encountered another temple as blissful as my own body.

—Saraha Doha

Just as our houses are homes for our bodies, our body is home for our spirit. While attention may wander to distant places, we still return to the same bundle of flesh and bones throughout the entirety of our lives. Our bundle may change dramatically in the course of a lifetime, yet it is still the one and only home we will have throughout life. As our body interacts with the world, it becomes our personal microcosm of that world.

The task of mastering the first chakra is ultimately to understand and heal the body. Learning to accept our body, feel it, validate it, love it—these are the challenges that await us here. The language of the first chakra is *form*, and our body is the physical expression of our personal form. As we examine the form—by look, touch, movement, or inner sensation—we learn the language our body speaks and discover ever deeper parts of ourselves.

Each chakra brings us a level of information. The body is the hardware through which the information is received, as well as the "hard copy" of all the data and programming within us. Etched in the flesh and posture of the bones are our pains and our joys. Coded within our nerve impulses are our needs and habits, memories and talents. Within our genes is our ancestry, within our cells the chemistry of the food we eat, and as our heart beats out our rhythm, our muscles mirror our daily activities.

To understand the body, we have to *be* the body. We have to be its pain, its pleasure, its fear, and its joy. To see the spiritual being as separate is to cut ourselves off from our ground, our root, our home. We become less than whole, split, out of touch with the information our bodies can communicate.

This is not to deny the philosophies that state "you are not your body, but something more" but to enhance them. We are our bodies, and through that understanding we become something more. We become grounded, all here, in touch with all that goes on inside us. We more fully experience the spiritual and emotional parts of ourselves, for which the body is a vehicle.

Our body is made up of trillions of tiny cells, which by some miracle hang together into one composite whole. Like a gravitational field, the first chakra draws matter and energy toward itself, while various levels of consciousness organize them into a working whole. Accepting the body is accepting the central integrating structure that unites our many divergent parts. It is the container for the soul.

Our body expresses our life. If our shoulders feel burdened and heavy, our body is telling us we carry too many burdens. If our knees don't want to support us, our body is telling us that we don't have adequate support in our life, or perhaps that we lack flexibility. If our stomach has chronic pain, there is something in our life that we can't stomach.

An exercise I often do with clients who are beginning bodywork is to write a statement for each part of their body, beginning with the words "I am ... or I feel ...." If they are speaking for their neck, and their neck is cramped, they write "I am cramped." If their knees feel weak, they write, "I feel weak." I then read back all the statements from the body as a whole, without defining what part it came from. These turn out to be statements about how they feel about themselves as a whole in their life at that time.[4]

To validate the body is to identify with it. If my chest is hurting, I admit that my emotional heart is hurting. To consolidate ourselves at this level, we must make peace *with* our body so that we can then be at peace *in* our body. It is through the first chakra that we gain our physical identity, which gives us solidity as human beings.

Self-nurturance is a key to taking care of the body. Resting when we need to rest, eating well, exercising, and giving the body pleasure all help to keep the first chakra happy. Massages, hot baths, good food, and pleasant exercise are all ways of nurturing ourselves and healing the mind/body split that results from the mind over matter paradigm. We cannot be integrated and whole if the two polarities are pitted against each other. Instead, through the body, we can have an experience of mind *within* matter.

Eating—the ingestion of solid matter into our bodies—is a first chakra activity. It grounds us, nourishes us, and maintains our physical structure. Through food, we take into ourselves the fruits of the Earth—the first chakra element. If we are going to study the material part of our existence, it is necessary to look at what it is that makes up that material body. The food we digest is the matter we transform to energy, and it follows that what we eat affects our energy output. Eating clean and nourishing food is a first step for establishing a healthy foundation in the first chakra.

For some this means eating nothing that is not the purest and freshest of foods from the local farm. For most, this is not practical. A need for that much purity would leave us starving in a typical urban environment. The most we can hope for is to be conscious of what we eat. Avoiding heavily processed foods, foods that are rich in refined sugars, and "empty foods" without nutritional benefits are a beginning for anyone who wishes to strengthen the health of their body and their first chakra. One can still be malnourished while eating entirely out of health food stores. Natural foods do not always imply a balanced diet. Balance is of even greater importance than purity.

The intricacy of human nutritional needs is far too complex to include here. It is a service to your first chakra to read a book about nutrition. It is surprising how many people do not consider this a necessity when eating is such a basic function in our lives. If we use our bodies for ninety years without reference to the owner's manual, no wonder they break down!

FOOD AND THE CHAKRAS

As culture and consciousness continue their inevitable evolution, it is only natural that our physical state is changing too. As our physical state changes, so must our eating habits. However, those who think they can eat their way to enlightenment may find the path slow and arduous.

The proper diet for expanding consciousness cannot be prescribed as a generalization for anyone. The diet one chooses should fit his or her needs, goals, and body types. If you weigh 220 pounds and labor all day on the construction site, you have different needs than the ninety-nine-pound secretary who sits in an office. Most commonly, a vegetarian diet is recommended for developing sensitivity and raising consciousness to "higher" states. Yet this diet is not for everyone, and can even be harmful if nutritional balance is not maintained.

Food has basic vibrational qualities, which are above and beyond their nutritional makeup. Food prepared lovingly by a family member is far more beneficial than food prepared by someone who hates her job in a fast food restaurant. Various types of food have different vibrational qualities as well and can be roughly corresponded to the various chakra levels as follows:

Chakra One: Meats and Proteins

From flesh to flesh, meat is probably the most physically oriented food you can eat. Meat takes longer to digest than most other foods and, therefore, stays in the digestive tract longer. For this reason it occupies energy in the lower part of the body, often limiting or dominating energy that might otherwise flow toward the upper chakras. Meats and proteins are good foods for grounding. Too much of them, however, leaves the body sluggish and overly *tamasic*. If, on the other hand, one feels weak, disoriented, or out of touch with his body and the physical world, a good meal of fleshy foods can do much to ground him.

It is not necessary to eat meat to be grounded. It is the protein that is most important for the structural tissue associated with the first chakra. A vegetarian diet with proper protein can provide enough "foundation food" to keep the first chakra happy. It is then important to eat such foods as tofu, beans, nuts, eggs, and dairy products.[5]

Chakra Two: Liquids

Chakra two is associated with water, therefore, pointing to liquids. Liquids pass through the body more quickly than solids and help cleanse the body and keep the kidneys from becoming overloaded with toxins. Juices and herbal teas can aid this cleansing process. We must have enough liquid to remain healthy.

Chakra Three: Starches

Starches are an easily converted energy food, relating to the fire element of the third chakra. Starches that come from whole grains rather than processed flours are assimilated by the body more slowly and more thoroughly. More quickly absorbed foods, such as simple sugars or stimulants, also provide energy, but prolonged use of them depletes the general health of the third chakra. Addiction to "energy foods" shows an imbalance in the third chakra. Sugar addiction can point to (as well as cause) third chakra imbalance.

Chakra Four: Vegetables

Vegetables are a product of photosynthesis, something that our bodies are incapable of producing. Vegetables trap the vital energy of the sunlight, as well as a good balance from the earth, air, fire (sun), and water. Vegetables are a product of cosmic and Earth processes in natural balance, reflecting the balanced nature of the heart chakra. In the Chinese system, they are neither yin nor yang, also representing the balance and neutrality characteristic of this chakra.

Chakra Five: Fruits

Fruits are said to be highest on the food chain because when ripe, they drop to the ground and do not require the killing of plants or animals to harvest them. Fruits are rich in vitamin C and high in natural sugars. They pass through the system the most quickly of all solid foods, and leave the energy free to travel to the upper chakras.

Chakras Six and Seven

It is more difficult to recommend foods for these higher chakras as they are not linked with bodily processes, but with mental states. Certain mind-altering substances such as marijuana or psychedelic drugs are known to affect these centers, sometimes beneficially and sometimes not. In relation to food, fasting is most relevant to the upper chakras.

Note: It must be understood that mere ingestion of meat will not make someone automatically grounded, nor will a diet of pure vegetables open a heart chakra that is otherwise closed. The objective is to obtain a balance among the chakras, and a balance within a person's diet helps to bring this about. The previous listings are merely offered as a guideline for correcting existing imbalances. A person who eats few vegetables is not courting the vibrational aspects of the heart chakra with diet. A person who lacks protein may feel flighty and ungrounded.

The body runs on energy, not food. While much of that energy is obtained from food, we will find that energy from other chakras, such as love, power, or higher states of consciousness, often decreases our need for food.

MATTER

The material world may be nothing but illusion—but ah . . .
such an exquisitely well-ordered illusion!

—Anodea Judith

We have described each of the chakras as being a kind of vortex—a swirling intersection of forces. These forces begin as straight movements (linear vectors) moving through the frictionless void. In the context of the Chakra System, we have described them as the downward movement of manifestation and the upward movement of liberation, much like condensation and expansion. One is centripetal—moving inward, toward a center and toward itself—and the other centrifugal—moving away from the center. When these two forces encounter each other, they encounter opposition and polarity, and assume secondary, circular movements or vortices, that create the chakras.

Consider twirling a ball on a string. The string represents limitation—a centripetal force similar to gravity. If you shorten the string as you spin, the orbit gets faster and smaller—more tightly bound around the center. The field created by the revolving ball appears more dense, until it seems solid, just like a moving propeller blade. Shortening the string is analogous to increasing the gravitational field. The greater the mass of a body, the stronger its field of gravity, and the more it will attract other bodies.

Materialization occurs when there are enough forces of similar nature and direction to reach a critical mass, resulting in manifestation. This can be seen in anything from streams of water running into the sea, to like-minded people bonding around a common cause. As the focus of energy increases, the manifestation becomes more pronounced, and then draws more energy toward itself—a vortex of positive feedback. The center of this focus is analogous to what the Hindus call *bindu*, a dimensionless source-point that acts as a seed for manifestation.

At the bottom of our chakra column the forces coming down from the top have gone through six levels, gaining density with each one, so they are the most solid at chakra one. The upward forces of dispersal, however, are relatively undeveloped in the first chakra. With a heavy emphasis inward and little movement outward, we have many centripetal forces that lock into place with each other and create the material world we see around us.

Materialization, then, *is a cohesion of similarity created by the indrawing of the center.* This core structure draws toward itself those forms that are responsive toward its particular cohesive force. Money attracts money—the more we have, the easier it is to create—especially when a critical mass is reached. Squares attract squares because they fit in with the central structure, as in the design of a house or a grid of streets.

Gravitation is a basic first chakra principle, as it condenses consciousness and energy into materialization. Whether we're talking about mass or money, the more we have of something, the easier it is to attract more of the same. This principle can both ground us, giving us security and manifestation, or trap us, keeping our consciousness bound to limited forms. As something becomes larger and more dense, it also becomes more inert, or tamasic. This means it is less able to change. If you have a big house with lots of possessions, it is more difficult to move.

The physical realm appears relatively solid and unchanging. In reality, however, the atoms that make up our perception of solidity are almost entirely empty space! If we enlarge one of the smaller atoms 100 billion times, its height and width become as large as a football field. The atom's nucleus would then be large enough for us to work with—about the size of a tomato seed. Electrons, traveling around the nucleus, are far smaller still—about the size of a virus. Imagine these electron/viruses occupying a space as big as a football field with a tomato seed in the center. Between the nucleus and the electrons there is nothing but empty space through which they move, yet we have the illusion of solidity.

In fact, electrons (and photons) are described by physicists as diffuse fields of energy, and only "exist" as discrete particles when observed with the proper apparatus. It is consciousness itself, in the act of observation, that causes the diffuse field to collapse into discrete particles. In the words of Albert Einstein:

> *We may therefore regard matter as being constituted by the regions of space in which the field is extremely intense . . . There is no place in this new kind of physics both for the field and matter, for the field is the only reality.* [6]

Einstein proved that matter is condensed energy. When energy becomes highly concentrated, it warps the structure of space-time, creating what physicists call a gravity well. The larger the mass of an object, the deeper the gravity well, and the stronger it pulls in other objects.

The Hindus talk about the material world as being made up of maya, or illusion. In this century, research in physics has managed to pierce through the veil of illusion that upholds the solidity of matter. Through the use of huge particle accelerators, physicists have been able to probe the subatomic realm, discovering truths that shake our Newtonian perceptions of the physical world. (Even the apparent solidity of particles in the atom's nucleus is an illusion, because they are made up of point-like entities called quarks, which are about the size of an electron.) Strangely enough, these discoveries, while making earlier science sorely inadequate, have correlated many beliefs of Eastern religions. Now both science and religion are pointing to the conclusion that the universe is a dynamic interplay of varying aspects of energy and consciousness. If there is a unifying field behind the world we experience, it is the very consciousness with which we perceive it.[7]

FIRST CHAKRA EXERCISES

Grounding Meditation

Find a comfortable chair, and sit with your back straight and both feet planted firmly on the floor. Take a deep breath. Feel your body expand and contract as you breathe. Feel your legs, your feet, and the floor they are placed on. Feel the solidity of that contact. Feel the chair beneath you. Feel the weight of your body in it, and how the force of gravity naturally pulls you downward, easily, soothingly.

Bring your attention to your feet. Ever so slightly press your feet into the floor and feel your legs engage with the Earth plane. Do not let this pressure become tension so that the muscles in your legs tighten, but feel a subtle current of energy running from your first chakra down into the Earth. Try to keep this current going as we move on to grounding the upper body.

As you tune into the weight of your body, you will gradually become aware of a center of gravity at the base of your spine. Feel how your body is now resting on that point, and focus on it as if it were an anchor, holding you down. When you feel anchored at this spot, you can begin to integrate the rest of your body into your grounding.

Tune into your torso, focusing your attention on the central channel of your body. This is not the spine, which is closer to the back of the body, but that part of our internal core that is aligned over our center of gravity.

Take a moment to align the top of your head, your throat, heart, stomach, and abdomen—all the other chakras—with the base chakra on which they rest. Take a deep breath and allow this alignment to gently settle in and balance over the first chakra.

We have now established a vertical column of energy. Imagine this column as a great cord—preferably of a deep red color—running from far above your head, through the center of your body, and down into the ground, passing directly through the empty space between your seat and the floor. Take special time to make sure this cord runs through your anchor point in the first chakra and continues not only to the ground, but deep down into it. If you can, visualize it going all the way to the center of the Earth—with the Earth's gravitational field pulling it down to its core.

Spend some time at this point checking to keep all the parts going—the feet slightly pressing into the floor, the chakras aligned directly over each other, the red column of energy pulling us downward, the harmonious feel of gravity rooting us, anchoring our physical and subtle bodies together.

Gradually let your torso sway forward and back, side to side, and then in a circular motion over this first chakra point. Notice how the point at the base of your spine does not move—yet the body moves around it. We want to be able to keep our grounding even in movement, and this allows the body to practice this skill.

Allow excess tension to drain off into the ground, still keeping the feet slightly pressed into the floor. Then return to stillness once again.

Yoga Postures

The following hatha yoga exercises work on stimulating and releasing energy from the Muladhara chakra itself:

Knee to Chest (**Apanasana**)

The simplest version of this posture is to lie flat on your back with both knees bent, placing your feet on the floor approximately two feet from the buttocks.

Leaving one foot on the floor, bend the other knee toward the chest, lacing your arms around the shin bone just below the knee. (See Figure 2.4, page 89.)

Take a deep breath, and on the exhale, allow yourself to pull the knee in even tighter. Imagine the root ball at the base of your spine opening and expanding. Allow your groin to deeply relax, and feel the first chakra expand all along the place where your leg meets your torso. Keep the shoulders relaxed and the entire spine on the floor.

Repeat on the other side.

After doing each leg, you may wish to grab both legs at once, bending them into your chest.

Bridge Pose (**Setu Bhandasana**)
This pose allows the legs to make firm contact with the ground while making dynamic contact with the spine.

Begin lying flat on your back with your arms straight at your sides, palms down. Bend your knees, placing your feet parallel to each other, hip-width apart, so that your heels come just to the tips of your fingers.

Press into the feet (without raising your body), and feel the earth energy bring solidity to your legs.

Next, press your feet even more firmly into the floor so that your spine is lifted, vertebrae by vertebrae, much as you might lift a strand of pearls one pearl at a time, until you are resting on your feet and upper vertebrae. (If possible, clasp the hands together under the back, pressing the chest upward and the shoulders together behind you.) Ideally, the line from your knees to your shoulders should form a straight plane. (See Figure 2.5, page 89.)

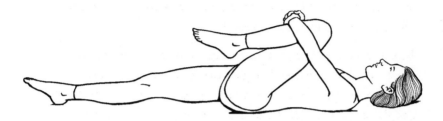

Figure 2.4
Knee to Chest.

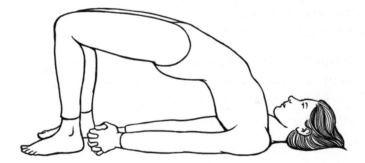

Figure 2.5
Bridge Pose.

Feel the support of your legs and feet in this position. Feel the spine connected and energized by this support. Breathe deeply and hold for at least three complete breaths.

Return the spine to floor, again one vertebrae at a time, at last relaxing the buttocks and allowing the feet and legs to relax. You may keep the knees bent in preparation for repeating the pose, or allow your legs to lie flat on the floor and feel the relaxation coming into your lower chakras.

Half Locust and Full Locust (Shalabhasana)

Lie face down on the floor with your arms beneath your body, palms touching the front of your thighs.

Keeping the knee straight, point the right leg out along the floor, making it as long as possible. As you continue to push *down* toward the right foot, begin to lift the right leg a few inches off the floor. (See Figure 2.6, page 91.) Feel the first chakra working to make this pose happen.

After a few moments (depending on your strength) lower the leg and repeat on the other side.

If this was easy for you, do the Full Locust, lifting both legs at once in the same fashion as described above. (See Figure 2.7, page 91.)

Head-to-Knee Pose (Janus Sirsasana)

Sit up straight with your legs extended out in front of you. (*Dandasana*) Bend the right knee and bring the right foot in to your groin.

Lift the pelvis up out of the groin, lifting the chest and turning the sternum directly out over your extended left leg. Inhale. (See Figure 2.8, page 92.)

With an exhale, bend the hips and trunk downward and stretch the arms forward, reaching for your left foot, keeping

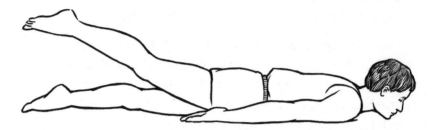

FIGURE 2.6
Half Locust.

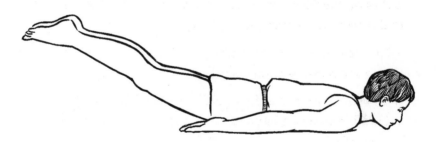

FIGURE 2.7
Full Locust.

the back as flat as possible. This will stretch your hamstrings and the back of your knee, as well as extending the spine.

Go to the edge between what is comfortable and what is tight, and stop at the edge and breathe deeply, sinking ever so slightly deeper into the pose with each exhalation. Stay for fifteen to twenty seconds or as long as you can comfortably hold the pose.

Sit up on an inhale. Lift the back. Then change legs and repeat on the other side.

Deep Relaxation

This hatha yoga practice is also called conscious relaxation. It essentially involves grounding and relaxing each part of the body, one at a time. It is nice to record on audio tape or have someone read the instructions in a smooth, hypnotic voice, but it is also easy to do at your own rhythm without any commands.

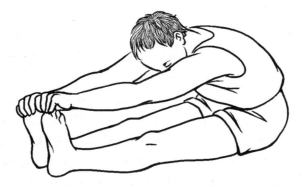

FIGURE 2.8
Head-to-Knee Pose.

Lie flat on your back and get comfortable. Make sure you are warm enough, for the body gets so relaxed in this exercise that it often gets cold. You may need a light blanket.

Begin breathing deeply, and keep the breath going in a comfortable, steady rhythm throughout the whole meditation.

Raise your left leg a few inches off the floor. Hold your breath for a few seconds and tighten each muscle in your leg. Then, with a gush of released breath, let all the muscles relax and let the leg fall into the floor like a dead weight. Give it a small shake, ground it, and let it be. Repeat for the right leg, tightening, holding, then letting it go.

Move on to your right arm, making a fist and tightening all the muscles as hard as you possibly can. Release. Now tighten the left arm: lift . . . tighten . . . hold . . . release.

Roll your head from side to side, stretching all the muscles in your neck. Raise the head slightly off the floor, hold, tighten, release.

Curl up your nose, purse your lips, and scrunch your eyes together. Hold, tighten, release. Repeat with your mouth open, tongue out, and face stretched. Hold, tighten, release.

Mentally go over each part of your body, one at a time and check to see if the parts are really relaxed. Begin with the toes, the feet, the ankles, the calves, knees, and thighs. Check to see that your buttocks are relaxed, your stomach, and your chest, breathing in and out, in and out, slowly and deeply. Check to see that your neck is relaxed, your mouth, tongue, cheeks, forehead.

Now allow yourself to observe your body, peacefully breathing in and out, in and out, deeply relaxing. Observe your thoughts, letting them come and go effortlessly. If you wish to make changes in your body, now is a good time to make silent commands or affirmations. Keep them positive, such as "I will be strong," rather than "I won't be weak."

When you are ready to return, begin flexing your fingers and toes, and wiggling your legs and arms. Open your eyes and return to the world refreshed.

Movement Exercises

Nearly anything that makes contact with the Earth is grounding. Moving the energy into the feet is the first step. The following bioenergetic exercise is excellent for this purpose:

Stand comfortably, arms at your sides. Rise up on your toes and come down hard on your heels, bending your knees as you do. Pretend you are sinking into the floor. Raising and lowering your hands with the rise and fall of your body can help to emphasize the downward flow. Repeat this several times for a good warmup.

Basic Grounding Stance

Stand upright with your feet hip-width apart or slightly wider. Allow your feet to be just slightly pigeon-toed, with the heels wider than the toes. Bend your knees out over the feet just slightly.

Press into the floor as if you were trying to push two rugs apart from each other with your feet. Feel the solidity and strength it gives you in your lower body.

Hold this pose a few moments and imagine holding your ground in a difficult situation.

If you wish to get even more charge into your legs, breathe

in and bend the knees, breathe out and straighten them slowly, but not completely. Repeat for several minutes. Never allow yourself to "lock" your knees, as it cuts off the grounding circuit.

The Elephant

This is designed to bring even more energy into the legs.

> With feet parallel and hip-width apart or wider, bend over with your knees slightly bent and touch your palms to the floor. Move your hands forward if this is difficult. (See Figure 2.9A, page 96.)
>
> Inhale and bend your knees to about forty-five degrees. Exhale and straighten your knees until they are almost straight, but never locked. (See Figure 2.9B, page 96.)
>
> Repeat until you feel a shaking or streaming of energy in your legs—usually within a few minutes if done correctly.
>
> Slowly come back up, spine curved and belly relaxed, until you are standing. Be sure to keep your breathing full and deep during this exercise, and let out any sound that feels natural.
>
> Flex your knees a few times, shake your legs out, and stand comfortably, feeling the effects.
>
> Repeat as often as necessary.

Pushing the Feet

Also a bio-energetic exercise.

> Lie on your back and raise your legs, with knees relatively straight, but not completely straight.
>
> Push your legs into the air with your feet flexed, your toes pointing toward your head. Push into your heels. (See Figure 2.10, page 96.)

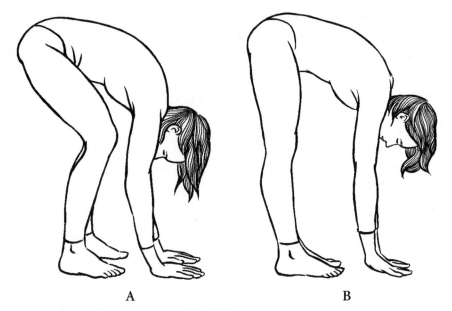

A   B

FIGURE 2.9
The Elephant.

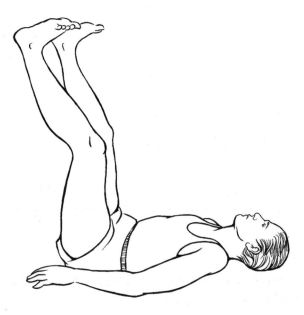

FIGURE 2.10
Pushing the Feet.

If you find a place that makes your legs vibrate, stay at that point and let the vibration continue as it energizes your legs and hips.

Common Sense Grounding Exercises

Stamping

This is excellent to do after getting out of bed in the morning, and is nicely followed by a foot massage from a "footsie roller," tennis ball, or lover, when possible.

> Stamp one foot several times and then the other. This helps to open the foot chakras and make contact with the solidity beneath us.

Jumping Up and Down

This helps us make contact to the Earth plane, both by pushing against gravity and by sinking into it. This exercise also helps to energize the legs. It is best done on an earthy surface rather than pavement or a hard floor, due to the impact on the legs.

> Pretend you are a little child and jump up and down, letting everything relax and become very loose. Each jump down should be accompanied by a bending of the knees and a sinking into the Earth.

Kicking

Kicking removes tension from the legs, as long as it is not kicking into anything solid.

> Lie on a bed and kick your legs rhythmically. Try it with knees bent and with legs straight, experiencing the results of both.

Jogging

Jogging energizes the feet, legs, and torso, steps up the metabolism, and increases the breathing rate.

> Jog on dirt outdoors for a wonderful grounding exercise.

Riding

This is an interesting grounding exercise for the urban environment.

> Ride a bus or train, standing up, without hanging on to anything. Bend your knees and keep your weight low to maintain your balance. Learn where your center of gravity is.

Resting

Very little is ever said about the extreme benefits of just slowing down, sitting in a chair, relaxing, and doing nothing. This is the most common grounding practice in America today.

Massage

Massage of any kind helps to relieve tension and reconnect the psyche to the body. A foot massage is especially helpful in grounding.

Eating

Many people eat to ground themselves. This is because it works. Overeating, however, puts one out of touch with the body and can unground them.

Sleeping

Sleeping is bringing the body to rest and to stillness. It is the grounding at the end of each day that regenerates us for the following day. Pleasant dreams!

ENDNOTES

1. Some say the related first chakra gland is the gonads because they are physically closer to chakra one, but the adrenals are the glands that get triggered in the "fight or flight" syndrome when survival is threatened. Adrenals also relate to the third chakra in that they flood the body with energy.

2. Itzhak Bentov, *Stalking the Wild Pendulum*, 53.

3. See Judith and Vega, *The Sevenfold Journey: Reclaiming Mind, Body, and Spirit through the Chakras*. A book of exercises and practices for chakra development.

4. For a more thorough description of this exercise, see Judith and Vega, *The Sevenfold Journey*, 71, 72.

5. Vegans, who eschew eggs and dairy as animal by-products, would deny that these foods are necessary. The argument here is not whether one can survive without them, but whether a diet supports grounding. A vegan diet practiced for more than a brief period is not a grounding diet, even though it may be very good for purification purposes.

6. Quoted in M. Capek, *The Philosophical Impact of Contemporary Physics*, 319.

7. For a deeper discussion of Eastern mysticism and Western science, see Fritjof Capra, *The Tao of Physics*.

RECOMMENDED SUPPLEMENTAL READING FOR CHAKRA ONE

Anodea Judith and Selene Vega. *The Sevenfold Journey: Reclaiming Mind, Body, and Spirit through the Chakras*. Freedom, CA: The Crossing Press, 1993.

Capra, Fritjof. *The Tao of Physics*. New York, NY: Bantam Books, 1975.

Couch, Jean. *The Runner's Yoga Book*. Berkeley, CA: Rodmell Press, 1992.

Haas, Elson. *Staying Healthy with Nutrition*. Berkeley, CA: Celestial Arts, 1992.

Keleman, Stanley. *The Human Ground: Sexuality, Self, and Survival*. Berkeley, CA: Center Press, 1975.

Keleman, Stanley. *Your Body Speaks its Mind*. Berkeley. CA: Center Press, 1975.

Myers, Dr. Norman, ed. *Gaia: An Atlas of Planet Management*. New York, NY: Anchor Books, 1984.

Sessions, George. *Deep Ecology*. Salt Lake City, UT: Peregrine Smith Books, 1985.

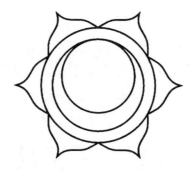

CHAKRA TWO

Water

Change

Polarities

Movement

Pleasure

Emotions

Sexuality

Nurturance

Clairsentience

Chapter 3

CHAKRA TWO: WATER

OPENING MEDITATION

QUIETLY YOU LIE AT PEACE, ALIVE against the Earth. The Earth that is still, solid, unmoving. You are still, yet for every ebb and flow of breath there is movement in your body. There is change. From inner to outer and outer to inner, the path between the worlds is woven through you. The path of change.

As your chest rises, the breath moves through your nose, throat, and lungs. It ebbs and flows, as evenly and gracefully as waves upon a shore. Back and forth . . . empty and full . . . in and out.

Inside, your heart beats, your blood pulsates, a river of life connects each and every cell within you. Blood flows outward . . . blood flows in toward the center again. Your cells expand and contract, ever reproducing, dying. Wiggle a finger back and forth. Impulses of nerves run down your arms. Your breathing continues . . . in . . . out . . . in . . . out.

Deep in your belly you become aware of a warm glow of orange, pulsing through your pelvis, through your abdomen, through your genitals. Pulsations of orange light move in rivulets down your legs, up again through your thighs, flowing through your belly, and up through your back to nourish all of you.

You are alive. You are a wave of motion. Nothing within you is truly still. Nothing around you is still. Everything is constantly changing at each and every moment. Every sound, every ray of light, every breath is an oscillation, back and forth, constantly moving, swaying, flowing. A flow of constant change, changing every moment from the last. By the time you finish this meditation, both you and the world will be different.

Within your body is a river of change. Find the subtle inner flows of movement and thought, moving up, down, around, and through. Find them and follow them. Allow them to gain momentum—removing obstacles by easing any tension you may find. Exaggerate their flow with outward movements: sway in your chair, rock back and forth, creating a rhythmic motion. Let the rhythm build until you feel like getting up— even with this book in your hand—get up and move around, swaying on your feet, circling with your hips, bending your knees, always keeping the flow even and steady . . . remembering roots below. You sway, back and forth . . . up and down . . . in and out . . . expanding, yet ever returning to your core self once again.

You move with the flow of water, sometimes slow like a great river, sometimes quickly like a spring stream, sometimes languishing like a quiet lake, sometimes passionate like the waves of the sea. Raise an arm and imagine water flowing down through it. Feel the wet fluid run down your back, your buttocks, your toes.

Think of the water as it flows from the sky, caressing the mountains, running in rivulets to its various pools. Imagine water raining down on you, caressing your body, running in rivulets down your pelvis and legs, down to soften the Earth below. You are the rain as you fall effortlessly from Heaven to Earth.

You are many droplets as your thoughts fall from your mind. In tiny movements, the tides within you grow and move—faster as they plunge downward, cascading over pinnacles of earth—then slowly as they slither serpentine across great valleys of your fertile fields.

Until, as one, you ebb and flow with the tides of the sea, pulled by the moon in its dance of dark and light. Your oceans, vast and deep, abound with life. Your passion reaches outward, spills onto the shore, and returns again within you. You drink in all the change around you, pulling its movement through you as your life ebbs and flows. In . . . and out . . . you breathe.

From the vast depths of ebb and flow, you reach. You touch. You find your body. Sensation flows into your hand across your skin. Sensation known to none but you. Your hand moves across curves of flesh and follows lines of movement You sway to the sensuality of your touch. Inside you rise emotions—churning, yearning, flowing, bubbling. They reach and touch and rise, becoming movements, waves change, the water flows, within, without.

You are alone, yet others are around you. They, too, ebb and flow, and change and touch and yearn. Your movements flow to join them, desiring to unite, to merge, to move toward something new. Your hands long to touch, to pull the oceans closer, to feel the flow of other tides mixing with your own.

Your belly heaves, your sex awakes, you thirst for touch, and reach beyond yourself. You find your "other"—different yet the same. Exploring, you begin to merge. The movements build within you, exalting you, expressing you, caressing you. Your passions swell in ocean waves to crash upon the shore and satisfy your needs. The waters ebb and flow, nurture, cleanse and heal, as they flow with each yearning, each movement, each breath. Ecstatic in uniting, you merge, complete within yourself and completed once again within another. You dance, and rise and fall . . . and rest.

You are water—the essence of all forms, yet formless. You are the point from which each direction flows, and you are the flow. You are the one that feels, you are the one that moves. You are the one that embraces the other.

Shall we flow together and join our souls in this journey down the river of life? Shall we flow together to the sea?

CHAKRA TWO
SYMBOLS AND CORRESPONDENCES

Sanskrit Name:	*Svadhisthana*
Meaning:	Sweetness
Location:	Lower abdomen, genitals, womb
Element:	Water
Function:	Desire, pleasure, sexuality, procreation
Inner State:	Feelings
Outer State:	Liquid
Glands:	Ovaries, testicles
Other Body Parts:	Womb, genitals, kidney, bladder, circulatory system
Malfunction:	Impotence, frigidity, uterine, bladder or kidney trouble, stiff lower back
Color:	Orange
Sense:	Taste
Seed Sound:	Vam

Vowel Sound:	Oo as in "due"
Guna:	Tamas
Tarot Suit:	Cups
Sephira:	Yesod
Celestial Body:	Moon
Metal:	Tin
Food:	Liquids
Corresponding Verb:	I feel
Yoga Path:	Tantra
Incense:	Orris root, gardenia, damiana
Minerals:	Carnelian, moonstone, coral
Petals:	Six
Animals:	Makara, fish, sea creatures
Hindu Deities:	Indra, Varuna, Vishnu, Rakini (name of Shakti at Svadisthana level)
Other Pantheons:	Diana, Jemaya, Tiamat, Mari, Conventina, Poseidon, Lir, Ganymede, Dionysius, Pan
Archangel:	Gabriel
Chief Operating Force:	Attraction of opposites

CHANGING LEVELS

*We often think that when we have completed our study of
one we know all about two because two is one and one. We
forget that we still have to make a study of "and."*[1]

—A. Eddington

We began our upward journey through the chakras by going down—
into the Earth, into stillness and solidity. We gained an understanding

of our bodies, our grounding, and things associated with one. We are now ready to introduce a new dimension: that which comes about when one meets another and becomes two.

It is here that our initial unity becomes duality. Our point becomes a line, giving it direction, dividing one side from another. We move from the element of earth to that of water, where solid becomes liquid, stillness becomes movement, form becomes formless. We have gained a degree of freedom but also more complexity.

Our consciousness moves from a feeling of unity to the realization of difference. Our understanding of self now includes an awareness of the other. Connecting with another, desire arises, and with it our emotions and sexuality. We long to unite, to overcome our separateness, to reach out and grow. These are all aspects of consciousness at the second chakra—all of which induce *change*.

Change is a fundamental element of consciousness. It is what commands our attention, awakens it, makes us question. A sudden noise awakens us from slumber. Changes in the length of the days caused us to study the Earth's movement in the heavens. Without change, our minds become dull. Without change, there is no growth, no movement, and no life. *Consciousness thrives on change.*

In Chinese philosophy, the *I Ching* ("Book of Changes") is a system of wisdom and divination based on the concept of change as the result of two polaric forces, yin and yang. They represent, respectively, feminine and masculine, earth and heaven, receptive and creative. Change is produced by the constant interaction of these forces, fluctuating around a state of balance. (See Figure 3.1, page 109.)

Consciousness in the second chakra, like the I Ching, is stimulated by the dance of polarities. In the upper chakras we reach levels of consciousness that transcend dualism, but in the second chakra, duality becomes the motivating force for movement and change. Duality, rising out of our initial unity, seeks to return to unity. Hence, opposites attract. Polarities, by their mutual attraction, create movement. If we are to begin in solid earth and transform all the way to infinite consciousness, there must be some movement to get the process started.

This movement is the essence of the second chakra's purpose in the overall Chakra System. It is the opposite of the first chakra's stillness. Where the first chakra seeks *to hold on and create structure*, the second chakra's purpose is to *let go and create flow*. Flow allows one thing to connect energetically with another. It is the difference between a point and a line.

Motion exists within every known part of the cosmos and is an essential characteristic of all energy, matter and consciousness. Without movement the universe is static, fixed, and time ceases to exist. There is no field to create the illusion of solid matter and we would instead experience its emptiness. To quote Dion Fortune:

> *It is pure movement in the abstract which gave rise to the Cosmos. This movement gave rise eventually to the locked up nodes of opposing forces which are the prime atoms. It is movement of these atoms which forms the basis of all manifestation.*[2]

We are all part of this constant process of movement, moving through many dimensions simultaneously. We move through physical

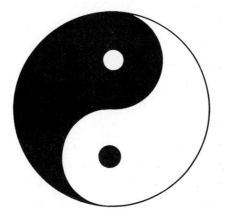

FIGURE 3.1
Yin-Yang symbol, showing how each is balanced and contained by the other.

space, as well as through feelings, through time (from one moment to the next), and through consciousness (from one thought to the next). We move through a world in motion, a world in constant change. Movement is an essential part of the life force—the essence of what separates life from death, the animate from the inanimate. Rocks don't move—people do. Let us flow then through the element of water in this second wheel of life—discovering how it brings us movement, pleasure, change, and growth.

SVADHISTHANA— THE WATER CHAKRA

We may affirm absolutely that nothing great in the world has been accomplished without passion.
—Georg Wilhelm Friedrich Hegel[3]

The second chakra is located in the lower abdomen centered between the navel and the genitals, although it encompasses the whole section of the body between these two points. (See Figure 3.2, page 111.) It corresponds to the nerve ganglion called the *sacral plexus*. This plexus hooks into the sciatic nerve and is a center of motion for the body. Because of this it is often called the "seat of life." (Some people associate this chakra with the Hara point in martial arts, though I believe this area to be midway between the second and third chakras.)

The second chakra is also described by some to be located over the spleen. This pushes the chakra out of alignment with the rest, and theoretically, I find no conclusive evidence that the energy some clairvoyants perceive at the spleen is one of the major chakras. In male anatomy the genitals are very close to the first chakra, and the differences between the first two chakras are very subtle, allowing for possible confusion. But in female anatomy the womb is a definite second chakra, and is easier to perceive as a separate center than the male second chakra. It is possible that these theories (largely from the

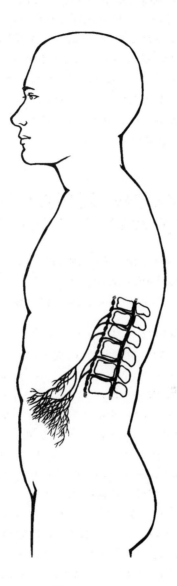

FIGURE 3.2
Sacral plexus and nerve ganglion.

Theosophists at the beginning of this century) were based on male bodies, and that they were further influenced by the sexually repressive values of that time, thus subduing the second chakra. The spleen does seem to be sensitive to emotional changes, yet it is not to be confused with the second chakra in the System presented here.

The element of this chakra is water, therefore, the chakra corresponds to bodily functions having to do with liquid: circulation of blood, urinary elimination, sexuality, and reproduction, as well as all the qualities of water, such as flow, formlessness, fluidity, and surrender.

This chakra is the center of *sexuality* as well as *emotions, sensation, pleasure, movement,* and *nurturance.* In the Tree of Life, the second chakra corresponds to Yesod, the sphere of water and the moon. Its associated celestial body is the moon which pulls the oceans of water to and fro in a dualistic rhythmic motion.

In Sanskrit, the chakra is called *Svadhisthana,* usually translated as "one's own abode," from the root *sva* meaning "one's own."[4] We also find in it the root *svad* which means "to taste sweet" or "to taste with pleasure, to enjoy or take delight."[5] When the plant has deep roots and is well-watered, then the fruit is sweet. To open the second chakra is to drink with delight in the sweet waters of pleasure.

The Tantric symbol for Svadhisthana has six petals, generally of a red (vermilion) color, but also contains two more lotuses within the chakra. (See Figure 3.3, page 113.) At the base of the middle lotus, shines a crescent moon, which contains an animal called a *makara,* an alligator-like creature with a coiled tail, reminiscent of the coil of Kundalini. He is a water creature believed to represent consuming desire and passions which must be harnessed in order to pass onward. I think of him as the animal instincts that lurk in the vast depths of the personal unconscious.

As mentioned in chapter 1, the chakras are connected by a non-physical channel running straight up the center of the body called the sushumna. Two alternate channels control the yin and yang energies, Ida and Pingala, twisting in figure-eight patterns around each chakra

God: Viṣṇu   Goddess: Shakti Rākinī

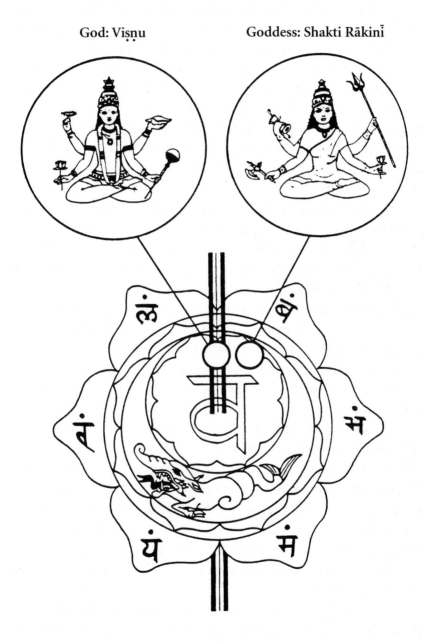

FIGURE 3.3
Svādhiṣṭhāna chakra.
(Courtesy Timeless Books)

and running alongside the sushumna. (See Figure 1.6, page 19.) These channels are among thousands of subtle energy channels called nadis, Sanskrit for "flowing water."[6] Ida and Pingala represent the lunar and solar aspects, respectively.

In terms of the brain, specific stimulation of these channels, such as in alternate nostril breathing (*nadi shodhana*), would alternately stimulate the right and left hemispheres of the cortex (see page 217 for instructions). Research shows that these two halves of the brain are responsible for vastly different kinds of thinking and that both halves are quite necessary for balanced understanding. The right side of the body is run by the left half of the brain, responsible for speech and rational thinking. The left half of the body is run by the right half of the brain, the more intuitive, creative side.

The two nadis, Ida and Pingala, meet in the first chakra and again in the sixth. Balance between the two halves of the brain constitutes a necessary condition for the clairvoyance characteristic of the sixth chakra. In the second chakra, the nadis cross above and below, surrounding the chakra on either side. (See Figure 3.4, page 115.) In order to benefit equally from both these energies, it is important to exalt in the dance of dualities, without getting caught in extremes and losing our center.

Movement and flow along these nadis contribute to the spinning of the chakras. (See Figure 3.5, page 116.) As energy flows upward to the right nostril through the Pingala, for example, we have a directional flow around each chakra complemented by its opposite, a downward energy on the other side of the chakra, flowing through the Ida. The two movements, turning in opposite directions around each side of the center, causes the chakras to spin. The crossing of the nadis between the chakras makes each center spin in an opposite direction to the one above and below. As each chakra spins in opposite direction to the one above and below, the chakras can then act like gears that mesh together and form a sinuous movement of subtle energy up and down the spine.

The concepts of yin and yang also apply to the chakras themselves. Chakra one is yang, as it is our beginning, our foundation, and an odd

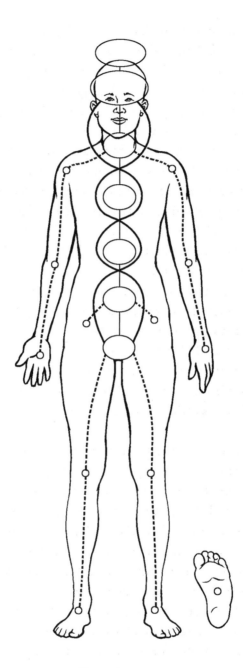

FIGURE 3.4
The major and minor chakras and their chief pathways.

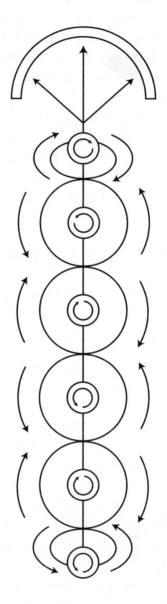

FIGURE 3.5
The spinning of the chakras as a result of polaric currents,
Ida and Pingala.

number. Chakra two is yin, thus encompassing more of the "feminine" qualities associated with receptivity, emotions, and nurturance. The bearing of new life, centered in the area of Svadhisthana (the womb) is distinctly feminine. Water is receptive, adopting the shapes of that which it encounters, following the path of least resistance, yet gaining power and momentum as it flows.

The second chakra is related to the moon. Like the moon's pull on the tides, our desires and passions can move great oceans of energy. The moon rules the unconscious, the mysterious, the unseen, the dark, and the feminine. This gives the center a very distinct power of its own as we move from our depths outward to create change in the world.

THE PLEASURE PRINCIPLE

Every perfect action is accompanied by pleasure. By that you can tell that you ought to do it.

—Andre Gide[7]

The human organism, as well as other living creatures, has a natural inclination to move toward pleasure and away from pain. Freud called this the pleasure principle. Like the instinct to survive, it is an innate biological pattern, closely related to the survival instinct of the first chakra. Pain is an indication that something is threatening the organism, while pleasure generally indicates that the situation is safe, freeing our attention for other things.

The pleasure principle extends far beyond the realm of mere survival, however. Many things are pleasurable that do not directly assist our survival at all. In some cases, they may actually be detrimental to it, such as spending money on frivolous items or activities or ingesting harmful drugs. These activities may deplete our resources, both in the body and the checkbook. In other cases, pleasure enables us to move more deeply into the temple of the body and, feeling fulfilled, have a foundation for power, love, creativity, and meditative concentration, which are all aspects of the chakras above.

Pleasure, as befits the duality of the second chakra, is a two-edged sword. It's an easy chakra to get trapped in, yet the trap can result from avoiding pleasure as much as indulging in it. The balancing of any chakra requires opening to its particular energy, *without becoming excessively attached.*

Pleasure and emotional sensations are processed in a lower section of the brain called the *limbic system.* The limbic system controls the hypothalamus, which in turn controls the hormonal levels and the regulation of the autonomic (involuntary) nervous system functions, such as heart rate, blood pressure, and breathing. Therefore, soothing stimulation to this part of the brain actually helps regulate and relax these hormones and processes,[8] and there is some indication that it actually helps us live longer and stay healthier.[9]

It has been suggested that the segregation in humans between the cerebral cortex (conscious thought centers) and the limbic system has resulted in self-destructive and violent tendencies in modern humans.[10] The connection between the cortex and limbic system is conducive to grace of movement, as there is no separation of mind and body to "check" movements and impulses, which can make them overly controlled or awkward. This segregation is nonexistent in other animals.

Pleasure invites us to expand, while pain generally makes us contract. If we are to expand from the fixed form of the material world into limitless consciousness, pleasure may be one of the first steps along that path, inviting consciousness to travel through the entire nervous system as well as to reach out toward others. In addition, pleasure invites surrender, which is a necessary process for spiritual awakening.

Pleasure helps the mind and body establish better communication. Through pleasure, we learn to relax and release tension. Impulses then flow freely throughout the whole organism, without fear of suppression. Gradually these impulses create rhythmic, coherent patterns soothing to the whole nervous system.

Pleasure allows us to tune into our senses. It is emphasized in some Buddhist and Hindu belief systems that both pleasure and the senses are misleading—that through sensation we deprive ourselves of knowing the true nature of reality. Yet the senses are the very extension of that consciousness that seeks to know. If our senses truly deprived us of reality,, would we not all be better off blind, deaf, and tasteless? Is this not *senseless* instead of *sensible*? Our subtler senses may allow us to see the inner planes, but the dulling or repression of the gross senses is no way to achieve this! Extrasensory perception is only sensation in its most refined aspect. How else do we become *sensitive*? As Alan Watts wrote: "Ascetic spirituality is a symptom of the very disease which it intends to cure."[11]

Sensation is a valuable information source for all levels of consciousness. It provides the raw data that eventually becomes information, stored and analyzed by the brain. Ignoring bodily sensations cuts us off from the valuable feelings and emotions that play a part in transferring information to the brain and in moving psychic and physiological energy through the body. Sensations are the building blocks of our feelings and emotions. Without them we are lifeless and disconnected.

Pleasure and sensation are essential features of the second chakra. If desire is the seed of movement, then pleasure is the root of desire, and sensation is the medium of pleasure. Pleasure is essential for the health of the body, the rejuvenation of spirit, and the healing of our personal and cultural relationships.

Unfortunately, we are taught to beware of pleasure, that it's a dangerous temptress waiting to lure us away from our true path. We are taught to repress our need for pleasure, and in so doing, repress our natural bodily impulses, and once again, segregate mind and body. We don't easily allow ourselves enjoyment of even the simple pleasures—time for a little extra sleep, a leisurely walk, or comfortable clothing. These stringent measures arise from the mind, but seldom from the body. We then may experience a backlash in our emotions.

EMOTIONS

Emotions (from the Latin *movere* "to move" and *e* meaning "out") promote the evolution of consciousness through the body. When we emote, we are moving energy out of the unconsciousness, through the body, and into the conscious mind. This flow of consciousness charges the body, cleanses it, and heals it. It is a movement of our life force through which we achieve change. We are back to the basic elements of the second chakra: movement and change.

In a preverbal child, emotional expression is the only language spoken or understood—the only means for a child to express his inner state. When emotions are appropriately mirrored by adult caretakers, a child forms a reasonable *emotional identity*. This emotional identity enables us to identify different emotional states later in life, both in ourselves and others.

Emotions are inherently tied in with movement. We repress feelings by restricting movement, and conversely, movement can free the emotional holding that causes chronic tension. We can think of the basis of emotion as wanting to move away from that which is painful, and toward that which is pleasurable. Emotions are a complex, instinctual reaction to pleasure and pain. They begin in the unconscious and, through movement, are allowed to come into consciousness. To block an emotion, we restrict movement. Then the emotion may remain in the unconscious—meaning we are unaware of it—yet still wreak havoc on our lives. It is acting from *unconscious* motivations that so often gets people in trouble.

It takes energy to repress emotion, so releasing emotions releases tension (if done appropriately). Absence of tension creates a harmonic flow within the body/mind. This creates pleasure of an even deeper level, allowing deeper connections with others.

The suppression of primary pleasures creates a need for overindulgence, turning pleasure into pain. Pain is an indication that we are going in the wrong direction. The suppression of pleasure creates a deprivation in the body that demands more of our consciousness than it deserves. Only through satisfaction and resolution can our awareness evolve safely to broader levels. It is said of Kama, the Hindu God equivalent to Eros: "Kama is worshipped by the yogis, for he alone, when pleased, can free the mind from desire."[12]

Pleasure and emotions are the root of desire. Through desire we create movement. Through movement we create change. Consciousness thrives on change. This is the essence and function of the second chakra.

SEXUALITY

Lust, the primal seed and germ of the spirits, existed first . . .
The seers, looking into their hearts, discovered the kinship of
the existent and the nonexistent.

—Rg Veda 10.129.4

Desire, which is known as Kama or "love," is dangerous when
it is considered as the end. In truth, Kama is only the begin-
ning. When the mind is satisfied with the culture of Kama,
then only can the right knowledge of love arise.

—Rasakadamvakalika[13]

Sexuality is a sacred ritual of union through the celebration of difference. An expansive movement of the life force, it is the dance that balances, restores, renews, reproduces. It is the production ground of all new life—and in that sense—of the future. Mover and healer of the life force within us, sexuality is a profound rhythm pulsing through all biological life.

Sexuality is a life force. Yet we live in a culture where this element of our lives is either repressed or exploited. Television screens allow our children to watch countless murders and crime shows but censor any scenes that involve nudity or lovemaking. Hard work and upward mobility are stressed (and stressful), while those who engage in life's simple pleasures are called lazy, weak, or self-indulgent. Still, the need for pleasure pushes onward, and people instead seek negative outlets in the form of alcohol and drugs (to loosen cultural inhibitions), sexual addiction, violence, rape, and crude pornography, while millions of dollars' worth of advertising play on the repressed sexuality in all of us. When something vital and natural is taken away, the resulting gap can be used as an implement for control. What's taken away is sold back to us, piecemeal, and we are less than whole because of it.

James Prescott has made studies of cultures comparing sexual repression to the incidence of violence. The more stringent the taboos are about sex, the more violent the culture. Conversely, the more sexually permissive the culture, the lower the crime rate.[14] For the health of our bodies and for the health of our culture, sexuality is an important essence to understand and preserve.

Sexuality is also an important consideration in terms of the chakras and Kundalini. There is a great deal of indication that higher consciousness and sexuality are closely related, although theories about how are many and divergent.

In yoga philosophy, one hundred drops of *bindu* (the dimensionless points of focus that comprise physical matter, sometimes also correlated to semen), when sublimated, distill into one drop of *ojas* (divine consciousness). As a result, many serious yoga disciplines, and most preconceptions about the chakras, prescribe celibacy as a way to transform bindu to ojas. Since this belief is pervasive throughout many mystical paths, it is worth taking the time to examine its pros and cons.

As in the history of most religions, early Hinduism was primarily a magical system for obtaining better material comforts such as larger crops and better animals. This system grew in its rituals to eventually include huge sacrificial slaughterings. It is likely that this produced a reactionary swing in the opposite direction, which commonly occurs with cultural mores. The Jains, among others, founded a heterodox system that believed that one should not kill anything—even vegetables—and because life was not possible without this, they became a "celibate order of itinerant monks, noted for extreme asceticism," some renouncing even clothes and/or food.[15] The purpose of these renunciations was to become free of karma in order to further liberation. Other subsects of Hinduism adopted asceticism as a way of internalizing the sacrifices that were previously expressed in the fire rituals, thus raising one's *tapas* or internal fires. This internal heat was felt to be a sign of "magicoreligious power" and more valuable than the pleasures given up.[16] The sacrifice of pleasure became the replacement for human or animal sacrifice.

In India, where one's household life and one's spiritual life are usually assigned to different chronological stages, the act of sexual union, which could result in children to raise, altered the course of one's spiritual path—sending it through a householder stage. While this wasn't frowned on for the average person, it was certainly a deterrent to the person who had already chosen a monk's life. Therefore, sex was to be avoided.

Celibacy, as a road to enlightenment, is also based on male physiology, where the retention of semen may have had a physiological basis of preserving bodily strength in a purely vegetarian and often sparse diet. The reality for women may be entirely different.

In Hindu mythology sexuality is everywhere. Shiva is often worshiped and represented by his phallus, the Shiva lingam, a symbol which appears abundantly throughout India. Krishna was known for his frequent amorous adventures, and erotic images are carved on temples everywhere in India. Shiva and Shakti are eternally making love. Among the Gods, sexuality was sacred. Why not then for mortals?

There is some research that shows there are chemical reactions involving sexuality, which may affect the raising of Kundalini and the opening up of psychic faculties. The pineal gland, often associated with the sixth chakra (clairvoyance), is rich in a derivative of serotonin, called melatonin. This chemical may easily transform into a compound called *10 methoxyharmalan*, which is potentially hallucinogenic, giving inner visions.[17] The pineal gland contains photo-receptors, and as we discuss the sixth chakra in further chapters, we will see that light and visionary experiences play a large part in this level of consciousness.

Evidence suggests that melatonin and the pineal gland in general exhibit an inhibitory effect on the female and male gonads in mammals. The reverse is also true: sexual hormones, such as testosterone, estrogen, and progesterone inhibit the production of melatonin as well.[18] Therefore, stimulating these hormones through increased sexual activity could adversely affect the opening of this third-eye chakra, and too much activity in the higher centers could adversely affect the sex drive.

Unfortunately, research on Kundalini and psychism is still limited and there is not enough evidence to establish firm conclusions. What causes this chemical change? Is the state of "hallucination" possibly caused by the catabolism of melatonin, necessarily a beneficial state to be in? Are there other ways of triggering it? Is it that undue emphasis in one part of the chakra spectrum would decrease energy in its opposite end? While evidence is not yet conclusive, the implications are still worth noting.

Celibacy, under the right conditions, can help open the doorway to altered states of awareness, and raise energy up the sushumna. However, it must be stressed that without training in the techniques of channeling this energy, whether it be yoga, martial arts, or simply meditation, it may do the practitioner little benefit, instead creating nervousness and anxiety. If these techniques are unfamiliar, find a teacher with whom you can study who has already been through some of these experiences.

Celibacy can help one to break away from old, nonbeneficial patterns and habits. Sexual force that is not permitted expression as sexuality will find an outlet in another way. Yogis believe that bypassing this center will send this energy up the spine to higher centers. This is generally true for those who practice Hatha or Kundalini yoga and have the channels open and ready to handle this energy. However, among the numerous clients and students I have encountered over the years, I have not found any celibates who struck me as any higher, happier, or better adjusted than those who include healthy sexuality as part of their lives.[19] Repressing sexuality often decreases the life force itself, and deprives us of the incredible pleasure and learning experience that comes from a relationship.

If celibacy is used to open previously blocked channels, it is not necessary to remain celibate all the time. Once these channels are open, they may remain clear, whether or not sex is engaged in. Often it is merely a matter of breaking old patterns, much like fasting is a way of breaking poor eating habits.

It is not always the case that celibacy will be beneficial to the growth of an individual, even under the proper circumstances. Some people, for example, habitually wall themselves off from others. For them, a sexual relationship could be one of the most enlightening things they could engage in. A relationship (which by necessity involves more than just the second chakra) can be a profound impetus for growth. We extend our experience by uniting with another. Within our bodies we are quite individual, but as we climb up the chakra column, the boundaries become more and more diffuse, and the realization that we are all one becomes more apparent. The path to enlightenment is often a matter of breaking through these illusions of separateness. Celibacy can enforce separateness, and sexuality can open the way for dissolving boundaries.

The drawbacks to celibacy can be as plentiful as the rewards. The sacrum is the center of our emotional feelings and the initiator of movement within the body, giving us a feeling of vitality and well-being. Frustrated sexuality can lead to lower back pain, leg cramps, kidney troubles, poor circulation, and stiffness through the hips.[20] Stiffness in the sacrum may result in knee trouble as well, for it throws the body weight off from the central line of gravity. This stiffness gradually works its way through the body, and a feeling of lifelessness may ensue. Changing this pattern is often difficult, for opening the center may involve encountering emotional pain, hitherto kept in check.

Chakras open and close gradually because they are the result of patterns from actual interactions. Just as we can't dribble a basketball that's resting on the floor, people with closed second chakras often have a hard time finding sexual partners to help open the chakra, while a chakra that is already open may attract more partners than it can handle. The only way to combat this is to open and close the chakras gradually and gently.

Denying the body intimacy and sexual release is denying some of the greatest pleasure the body can have. This goes against our biological pleasure principle. Denying this pleasure also cuts us off from the subtler feelings and emotions housed in the lower chakras. We become cut off from our ground, our wholeness, our sense of inner satisfaction and peace.

Wilhelm Reich, in his research into the bioelectric currents of the body, found that sexuality was crucial in the healthy flow of this energy through the body. Reich felt that only through orgasm could we achieve a "complete circuit" of bioelectric flow through the body, essential to mental and physical health. "The complete flowing back of the excitation toward the whole body is what constitutes gratification."[21] He further found that dammed-up sexual energy resulted in anxiety, centered mainly around the cardiac and diaphragmatic region.

The same excitation which appears in the genitals as pleasure, manifests itself as anxiety if it stimulates the cardiovascular system . . . sexuality and anxiety present two opposite directions of vegetative excitation.[22]

It is likely that this anxiety produced in the "cardiac and diaphragmatic region" is similar to the early sensations of Kundalini, as it rushes into the third and fourth chakras located in those areas. Whether one considers this feeling to be a manifestation of anxiety or the force of Kundalini pushing through the chakras is a matter of opinion. This can only be based on personal experience. One's spiritual maturity, or readiness to handle psychic energy, has a great deal to do with the effects produced by sexuality *or* celibacy, and the consciousness-expanding effects that either of these experiences can bring.

In keeping with the theory of this book, each chakra needs to be open and active for a healthy flow of energy through the whole body/mind. Sexuality is a resolution and celebration of our differences. Healer of the body, joiner of hearts, movement of life, sexuality is the water wheel of life that moves the earth below and tempers the fire above. We wouldn't be here without it.

TANTRA

Sexual union is an auspicious Yoga which, through involving enjoyment of all the sensual pleasures, gives release. It is a Path to Liberation.

—Kaularahasya[23]

It must be remembered that the Chakra System came out of Tantric philosophy. Tantrism, in reaction to the dualistic nature of Patanjali's *Yoga Sutras*, and other ascetic ideals, teaches that the body is sacred and the senses can bring enlightenment, ecstasy, and joy. It is for this reason that Westerners often equate Tantra with sexual practice, even though Tantric philosophy is far wider in scope, and embraces a combination of many yogic and Hindu philosophies, of which sexual union is only a minor part.

Among elements of Tantric philosophy is a polytheistic worship of deities, of which the union of Shiva and Shakti, mentioned earlier, are said to bring supreme bliss. Through weaving together complimentary threads, such as masculine and feminine, spirit and matter, light and darkness, self and other, we escape the separation of dualistic thinking and enter a more wholistic philosophy. Tantra seeks to embrace rather than deny, yet still has as its goal, the liberation of consciousness into supreme realization.

The word *tantra* comes from the Sanskrit root *tan* meaning "to stretch." Tantra literally means "a web or loom."[24] This Sanskrit term has also come to mean "essence," "underlying principle," or "doctrine." The same root also appears in words for family and birth in Sanskrit as in *tanaya*, "to continue a family," and *tanus*, "of the body."[25]

Tantra, therefore, symbolizes the weaving of the basic underlying fabric of existence. Through stretching and reaching out, we both encounter and create this divine fabric. Shiva and Shakti, in their constant interaction as pure consciousness and its manifestations, are the divine threads. The weaving is done when we allow these divinities to work through us.

The perception of duality is often considered to be a source of pain and alienation. Tantra is the sacred dance of reuniting duality—of restoring that which is separate into oneness again. The result of this is an ecstatic experience of unity—with ourselves, our partners, and the universe around us.

The passage of energy between the couple engaged in sexual activity is far more than an exchange between the genitals. A couple, face to face, have all their chakras aligned between them. Through the intensity of sexual excitement, each chakra vibrates more intensely, and passage of energy between one body and another is enhanced and woven together at all levels. Whether the couple then chooses to focus this energy at a physical, mental, or heart chakra level becomes a matter of mutual choice.

Sexual symbology is plentiful in Indian art and mythology, and the Shiva lingam, with or without a Goddess (yoni), was fervently worshiped by the ancients. While the female was highly regarded as a sacred tool for obtaining liberation, it was the male who was the target for this enlightenment.

Whether the female was considered to be enlightened already, or whether she was not considered at all is unclear. Even today, it's generally the males who go off to join the temples and lead a spiritual life, just as it's most often the males who become the "enlightened" masters and spiritual teachers of these students. It is often these male gurus who prescribe celibacy and austerities for pursuit of the spiritual path, and teach that liberation cannot happen without an approved teacher. Sometimes, however, the woman, or *Tantrika*, is considered the guru.

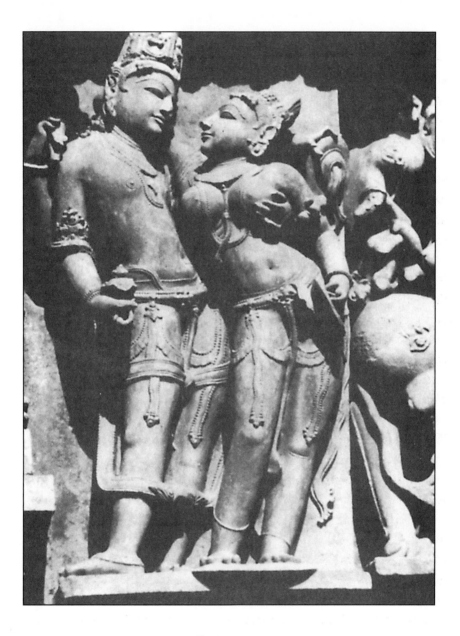

FIGURE 3.6
Tantra photo of Indian figures.

Yet, the Goddess was considered indispensable, if not supreme, where it is said: "Shakti performs all the physical needs of Shiva. The bodiless Shiva, being the nature of Pure Consciousness, must have the creative energy of Shakti for support." Another says: "Without Shakti, the lover is but a corpse."[26] As Shiva and Shakti live within each of us, partners practicing Tantra may elect to represent one or the other.

The purpose of Tantra is the same as any other aspect of yoga—to attain liberation from limited consciousness, most commonly by raising energy up the spinal column. The transcendental experience of union with another soul serves to bring one into an altered state of consciousness. In this state, entry into the higher worlds is more accessible.

Most Tantric practices attempt to use the force created by the arousal of sexual energy to awaken the Goddess Kundalini, and push Her up the spine. It is not believed that the untrained can achieve this liberation without previous instruction and practice in disciplines designed to open and arouse these centers, such as meditation or yoga. Like the use of celibacy, it is only through knowledge of psychic pathways that this experience can bring transcendence. Yet, there are many cases of spontaneous awakenings from tantric sexuality without gurus. Whether it's Kundalini that is triggered, or merely an ecstatic state of union, tantric sexuality is a religious experience—achievable by anyone.

In Tantra, it is believed that the body, both male and female, is a temple—a place of worship. This means keeping the body purified and healthy as well as bringing it sexual pleasure. Tantrics practice yoga *asanas* (postures) and breathing exercises regularly, maintain proper diet, and study the psychic pathways. It is also necessary that one's partner regard the body with the same respect, or true merging of the energies is unlikely.

Correct practice of the Tantric Arts leads to the creation of the mystic child, a vehicle of liberation through which one may attain magical powers (*siddhis*). This child is not a physical being, although conception of a child under these circumstances would certainly charge the fetus with the highest of our personal divine energy. The mystic child refers instead to a psychic "aura body," experienced as an added energy source of a higher dimension. This body of psychic energy can then be used in a particular circumstance, i.e., healing, performing some task, or self-protection. Western practices of sex magic are very similar in this regard, using deities as interpenetrating forces that, when combined, endow the receiver with paranormal power.

NURTURANCE

To be tender, loving, and caring, human beings must be tenderly loved and cared for in their earliest years, from the moment they are born.

—Ashley Montagu[27]

Nurturance is the final summation of sexuality and a fundamental need of the body, the mind, and the soul. Nurturance means caring for, feeding with energy, love, and touch. Nurturance is the essence of maternal qualities, our first experience of blissful transcendence, of warmth and security.

The simple act of touching is of extreme importance to the healthy functioning of the human organism. The skin can be considered the outer layer of the nervous system. The skin is the boundary of our bodies. Through touch, that boundary is gently broken down, permeated by another, and our whole internal system enhanced and stimulated.

In laboratory studies with rats, it has been shown that small mammals will choose being touched over eating when deprived of both. When all other conditions are equal, petted rats learn faster and grow faster than those treated coldly.[28]

In humans, those treated with adequate doses of touching and mothering grow to greater emotional stability than those who are deprived. Without touching, the important mind/body interface may remain seriously underdeveloped.[29]

Nurturance helps control the production of hormones responsible for growth by stimulating the limbic system of the brain. This also aids in relaxation of the heart and breathing rate, controlled by the autonomic nervous system.

Stimulation alone is a factor in increasing intelligence and developmental progress in infants. Pleasurable stimulation adds stability and trust to this development.

It is not only infants that are profoundly affected by the touch of other living creatures. Emotional satisfaction and fulfillment—be it nurturance, pleasure, or sexual release—is generally soothing to the whole organism.

The first step in learning to work with others is the mutual enhancement of our internal energy. Through these pathways we pave the way for further growth, harmony, and peace. The simple act of touch, of reaching out to soothe, is the healing aspect of the second chakra. We are saying to another, "We are here." We allow ourselves to transcend our separateness, get out of our egos, and feel the sense of connection so vital to our harmonious survival on this planet. The role of the second chakra is an important one indeed. Suppression of this chakra provokes vital imbalances that inhibit rather than enhance the flow of expanding consciousness.

Anyone can nurture. Everyone needs it. Like watering a thirsting plant, we respond to flow, to movement, to the dance of life in its infinite pleasures and mysteries. Through this act, life is renewed and preserved.

CLAIRSENTIENCE

Clairsentience is the psychic sense of the second chakra, the first stirrings of "higher" consciousness and the development of greater sensitivity toward others.

Clairsentience is the ability to sense other people's emotions, also called *empathy*. Like the feeling level discussed earlier, this "sensing" does not always become information recognized by the cognitive properties of the brain. It is experienced more as a subtle feeling, as if we were experiencing the feeling ourselves. Just as we can ignore some of our own emotions, many clairsentient people do not recognize the emotions they pick up from others, yet their body and ensuing actions still respond. Still others may recognize the emotions while not understanding that the source was outside of themselves.

Mothers psychically tuned to their children are the most common group of clairsentients. A child may be at school, away from the mother, and the mother will sense a difficulty in which the child has suddenly found him or herself. The mother may or may not consciously recognize the source of the disturbance, though it affects her nonetheless. Other people experience clairsentience by walking into a party and becoming immediately aware of the expectations and feelings of all their friends that are present. They may suddenly feel expected to act in a certain way. They may also experience abrupt mood changes as they involuntarily take on the moods of one friend or another. Often these people have an aversion to crowds and avoid parties.

Most people are clairsentient to some degree. The phenomenon usually occurs more strongly in people who have a proclivity for clairvoyance or telepathy, characteristic of the upper chakras. If the upper chakras are not open enough to be conscious of this psychism, the clairsentient is often unpleasantly influenced. Their attention is constantly whisked outside of their central column, and others' difficulties speak more loudly than their own voices. A confusion about the self ensues, especially confusion about the motivation for one's actions. "I don't know why I'm doing this—I don't really want to." "I feel so depressed since talking to Sally and I don't know why." These feelings can often be the result of someone else's moods or wishes.

Clairsentience is a valuable source of information and helpful in the development of psychism. With conscious attention, it is an aid rather than a detriment. Many people get psychically bombarded by the unconscious broadcasting of surrounding difficulties. For these people, grounding is of utmost importance for it brings our attention into the central line of our body, helping us sort out "whose energy is whose." Recognition of the phenomenon is the next step. Knowing the difference between your own and another's emotional needs helps to consciously tune out unwanted broadcasts. Many clairsentients feel compelled to respond to the needs they psychically pick up from others and, with recognition, this can become a choice rather than a duty.

Awareness of the other should be balanced by awareness of the self. The two should never be without a good dose of common sense. Only we, from inside ourselves, can judge.

CHAKRA TWO EXERCISES

Exercises for opening the second chakra involve working with movement in the hips and lower abdomen. Some are aimed merely at opening, while others are aimed at stimulating and moving energy in and through this area.

Exercises for the whole body involve touching and nurturance, such as massage and sexual activity. Simple self-nurturing activities such as long, hot baths, showers, or swimming (all having to do with water) should not be overlooked. Nurturing ourselves is the first step in receiving or giving nurturance to others.

Water Meditation

Step One

Water is cleansing, both internally and externally. Begin with a large glass of water, and sit quietly while you drink it. Feel it pouring down inside you. Feel the coolness of it, the wetness, and feel it as it hits your stomach. Imagine it passing all through your body—your veins, muscles, digestive system. Take a wet finger and rub it on your face, feeling the cool, refreshing quality.

Step Two

The next step is to clean yourself. This is a ritual water cleansing and should be both thorough and enjoyable. You can use a shower, a bath, a lake, stream, or even a hot tub. Make sure the area around you is clean; it is hard to feel clean in a dirty environment.

If it is a bath or shower you are choosing, pick your favorite towels, soaps, and lotions and have them nearby. If it is a stream, have a smooth, flat area where you can lie out to dry. If a hot tub, arrange for some privacy for yourself afterward.

As you soak yourself in water, go through each part of your body, saying: "Now my hands shall be clean; now my feet shall be clean; now my face shall be clean," etc. Become one with the water. When you are through, visualize the water taking away any negativity you don't want in your life. If you are in a natural environment, you could throw something (non-polluting) in the water to signify that negativity; if you are in an urban environment, some symbolic liquidcan be thrown in the toilet, or down the drain.

As you lounge in your bath with the water around you, think of the ebb and flow of cycles in your life. Look at yourself as an instrument of movement. If you were to stand back and look at yourself from another dimension, what patterns would you notice in your movements through life?

Think of the things you would like to get rid of in your life at this time—habits, tendencies, hurts, or fears. See them flowing out of you, through your grounding cord, like a river flowing out to the sea. Imagine the rain coming down and refilling the river with fresh water, replenishing it.

Then think of the things you would like to have come into your life—new patterns, people, or events. Imagine a waterfall over your head, pouring these blessings upon you. Feel yourself taking them in and letting them flow through your whole body.

Yemaya is the African Goddess of the sea, the great Mother. "She is envisioned as a large and beautiful woman, radiant and dark; nurturing and devouring; crystal clear and mysteriously deep."[30] She is the nurturer, the consoler, the healer, the maternal one whose belly is as big as all life. As you sit in your bath, imagine yourself being rocked and nurtured by this great sea-mother. Feel yourself in the womb of the Goddess, about to be born. Ask Her what purposes She has for you in this birth. Ask Her for help in making your birth smooth and easy. Accept Her nurturing. Take it into yourself, and imagine sharing it with others. Thank Her for your birth.

Dress yourself in clean clothes. Pour yourself another glass of water, and drink it silently, thinking about the cyclic nature of water, and how you fit into those cycles. If possible, visit a large body of water soon.

The Goddess Pose

Lie flat on your back and relax, especially in the legs, pelvis, and lower back. Bend your knees, bringing your feet in close to your buttocks.

Slowly allow your knees to part, allowing the weight of the legs to stretch the inner thighs. (See Figure 3.7, page 139.) Try to relax. Do not push your legs farther than is comfortable. Hold this position for two minutes or more.

Bring your knees together again. This should be done very slowly and smoothly, at all times breathe deeply and remember to relax. This puts you in touch with your sexual vulnerability, which paradoxically must be understood before you can fully open yourself up on this level.

From this pose you can then slowly open and close the legs, breathing in as you open and exhaling as you close. This may produce a kind of quivering vibration in the legs and pelvis.

Pelvic Rock I

Starting on your back with legs bent, slowly begin to rock your pelvis upward and downward with each breath. Inhale fully into your chest and belly (see Figure 3.8, page 139), then exhale fully. At the end of each exhale, push slightly with your feet so that your pelvis comes off the ground, pushing the small of your back into the floor beneath you. (See Figure 3.9, page 139.)

Pelvic Rock II

On a soft surface such as a mattress, do the Pelvic Rock I sequence, but this time moving the pelvis up and down more quickly and with as much force as possible. (See Figures 3.8 and 3.9, page 139.) Let yourself make any sounds that are natural. This helps to release blocked energy.

Hip Circles

From a standing position, bend your knees slightly, and drop your pelvis forward, so that it is directly in your central line of gravity.

Keeping the knees bent and flexible, rotate the pelvis in smaller, then larger, circles. (See Figure 3.10, page 140.) The head and feet should remain in the same place while the pelvis alone does the moving. Try to make the movement as smooth as possible.

Scissors Kicks

This exercise helps to move energy through the pelvis, often into the upper chakras. It is a classic, strong Kundalini-raiser with powerful results. It is important not to strain and to avoid sore muscles. Stay in tune with the body.

Lie on your back and relax. Lift your legs six to twelve inches off the floor and spread them apart.

Bring the legs together again and then kick apart again. (See Figure 3.11, page 140.) After about five of these, I'm sure you will want to rest.

After resting, bring your legs (knees straight) perpendicular to the floor and spread apart. Bring them together and down. Repeat until tired. Raising the legs should be accompanied by an inhale, while lowering the legs should be accompanied by an exhale.

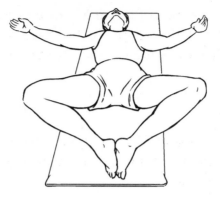

FIGURE 3.7
Goddess Pose.

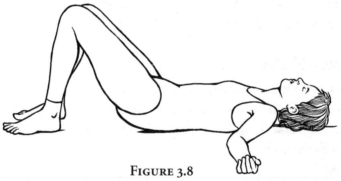

FIGURE 3.8
Pelvic Rock I.

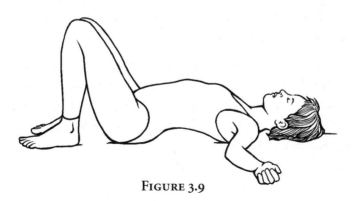

FIGURE 3.9

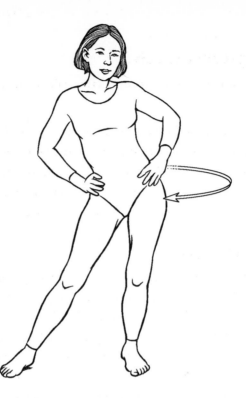

FIGURE 3.10
Hip Circles.

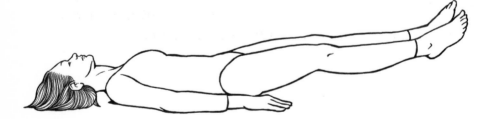

FIGURE 3.11
Scissors Kicks.

Walking from the Pelvis

Have you ever seen jazz dancers? This walk is like the movement of a jazz dance.

> While bending the knees and keeping the pelvis very flexible, walk with your weight low and swing your hips in an exaggerated motion. What does it feel like to move from this level? What does the motion feel like in your body? Allow your whole body to swing freely as you walk.

Emotional Release

There are many exercises using breathing, massage, and various postures that facilitate the expression and release of emotions. These are quite powerful and should be undertaken only with an experienced therapist. Reichian bodywork, bioenergetics, and rebirthing are three such disciplines. If you are interested, find books or therapists who can tell you more.

It is important to remember, however, that any emotions that arise during these exercises should be processed—that is, moved out. Crying, yelling, kicking, or merely asking someone to hold you are all acceptable and encouraged ways of working through the blocks that may reside in this (or any) chakra. It is good to find friends who can work with you and provide the nurturance that is needed.

ENDNOTES

1. A. Eddington, "The Nature of Physics," as quoted by Richard M. Restak, M.D. in *The Brain, The Final Frontier* (Warner Books, 1979), 35.

2. Dion Fortune, *The Cosmic Doctrine*, 55.

3. Georg Wilhelm Freidrich Hegel, as quoted by Jack Hofer in *Total Sensuality* (NY: Grosset & Dunlap, 1978), 87.

4. Monier-Williams, *Sanskrit-English Dictionary*, 1274, ff.

5. Ibid., 1279.

6. Ibid., 526.

7. Andre Gide as quoted by Jack Hofer, op. cit., 111.

8. Bloomfield, *Transcendental Meditation: Discovering Inner Awareness and Overcoming Stress*, 78-82.

9. Theresa Crenshaw, M.D., *The Alchemy of Love and Lust: How Our Sex Hormones Influence Our Relationships*, 276, ff.

10. Bloomfield, op. cit., 43–45.

11. Alan Watts, as quoted by John **Welwood**, *Challenge of the Heart*, 201.

12. Alain Danielou, *The Gods of India*, 313.

13. Douglas and Slinger, *Sexual Secrets*, 169.

14. James Prescott, "Body Pleasure and the Origins of Violence," *The Futurist*.

15. Margaret and James Stutley, *Harper's Dictionary of Hinduism*, 123.

16. Ibid., 300.

17. Philip Lansky, "Neurochemistry and the Awakening of Kundalini," *Kundalini, Evolution and Enlightenment*, John White, ed. (NY: Anchor Books, 1979), 296–7.

18. Ibid., 296.

19. This does not include gurus, who have entered an entirely different level of consciousness than the average Westerner, though many gurus have inappropriately transgressed sexual boundaries, indicating there was some kind of flaw in their practice of celibacy. See Kramer and Alstad, *The Guru Papers: Masks of Authoritarian Power*.

20. Twenty years of personal experience doing private and group therapy and teaching.

21. Wilhelm Reich, *The Function of the Orgasm*, 84.

22. Ibid., 110.

23. Douglas and Slinger, *Sexual Secrets*, opening quote.

24. Stutley, *Dictionary of Hinduism*, 298.

25. Monier-Williams, *Sanskrit English Dictionary*, 435.

26. Lizelle Raymond, *Shakti—A Spiritual Experience*.

27. Ashley Montagu, *Touching*, 208.

28. Ibid., 12 ff.

29. Ibid., 208.

30. Luisah Teish, *Jambalaya*, 118.

RECOMMENDED SUPPLEMENTAL READING FOR CHAKRA TWO

Anand, Margo. *The Art of Sexual Ecstasy: The Path of Sacred Sexuality for Western Lovers.* LA: J.P. Tarcher/Putnam, 1989.

Bass, Ellen and Laura Davis. *The Courage to Heal: A Guide for Women Survivors of Sexual Abuse.* NY: Harper & Row, 1988.

Douglas, Nik and Penny Slinger. *Sexual Secrets.* NY: Destiny Books, 1979.

Eisler, Riane. *Sacred Pleasure.* SF: Harper & Row, 1995.

Feuerstein, Georg. *Tantra: The Path of Ecstasy.* Boston, MA: Shambhala, 1998.

Goleman, Daniel. *Emotional Intelligence.* NY: Bantam, 1995.

Sanders, Timothy L. *Male Survivors: 12 Step Recovery Program for Survivors of Childhood Sexual Abuse.* Freedom, CA: The Crossing Press, 1991.

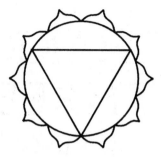

CHAKRA THREE

Fire

Power

Autonomy

Will

Energy

Metabolism

Technology

Transformation

Self-esteem

Chapter 4

CHAKRA THREE: FIRE

OPENING MEDITATION

We are still, yet we sense a growing warmth within us. We are alone, yet we sense others around us, longing to break free, longing for warmth and light. There is a form here, but it is empty. There is life here, but it is still. There is awareness here and it is awakening!

From a place of stillness, we call forth movement. Slowly reaching out, expanding, breathing, stretching, flowing. Into form, we invoke life. Its spark from the fire of the place between—between ourselves and others, between past and future, between the known and the unknown.

We move and dance, pleasure singing through us as the dance of life burns its way through our fears and our pains. Feel the warmth of pleasure melting tension, pulsating, growing—the rhythms lifting and moving, healing and soothing, warming and cooling.

From a place of infinite movement we call on the Self. We call on the Self to awaken to another part of the journey. We call upon the Self to awaken to the sun, the fire, the warmth, the transformation. We call upon the Self through our will, and it rises to our call.

We reach for the sun and call upon the yellow ray. The ray of life, the ray of creation, the ray of consciousness, the spark of fire . . . . We call upon the flame to burn within us and temper our passions into strength. With strength we fight the dark, pushing and straining, to realize it is part of ourselves, part of our strength, part of our fear. We laugh, and put down the fight, merging, becoming whole, becoming stronger. We pass between the pillars of light and dark, honoring both . . . and find ourselves in a new and glorious land. A land of bustling activity, teeming with life, sparkling like stars with shining rivers of light reflecting the sun.

The sparks catch our eyes, we turn toward their glow and they move and dance, connecting and igniting all that they touch. They touch something within, igniting strength, will, action. Sparks fly, igniting other threads, other fires . . . they explode, burn bright . . . and are gone.

We are lifted, we are lightened, we are laughing. We feel our bodies sway with the rising heat, hot tongues of fire moving within us, expanding, contracting, but growing ever wider, yet returning always to its source within us. Our bodies now burning, radiating heat and light and strength and will. Power pulsating through us, from above, below, around, and running through, transforming all that is within and without, our bellies bursting with joy.

Feel this energy deep within your body, burning with the fire of your own life. Feel it pushing deep into the Earth, down through the Earth, to the hot molten center of Earth. Feel it return from the Earth, rising up from the heat below, through your legs, your pelvis, your belly, moving up through your body, through each part of your body—your arms, your hands, your chest, neck, and head.

Feel it flowing out of you, connecting with other sparks, filaments of energy, other fires of life. Feel it connect with the thoughts inside you, your constant sparking of neurons, interconnecting filaments of energy, lines of thought, patterns in a web, ebbing and flowing in pulsing flames, burning with the glow of activity.

You are now a vital intersection of energy, merging, combining, exploding, radiating. Expend your awareness without and within, weaving a web of power, like a fire, growing higher and brighter. Power flows through you effortlessly, easily, calmly. You are one with the powers around you and within you.

Think of the times when you knew this power. Times when you felt this connection, vitality, importance, and strength. Think of the times power flowed through you, like warmth from the sun. Think of those times and feel them now. Feel your body radiate their purpose, dance with their majesty, sing with their strength.

In this fiery world of activity you are a channel for power around you. You open to it, you burn with it, you drink it in, and you pass it on . . . easily, effortlessly, willingly, joyfully.

Your power peaks and returns, feeding the fire within—a molten core, feeding your body, silently charging, ready to expand again when your next purpose calls.

The fire has burned high, and the coals now glow with warmth. Exhilarated, your body relaxes. A smile plays on your lips, your hands are at peace with the strength they have carried, and you again return to the gentle breathing . . . in . . . and out . . . in . . . and out . . . in . . . and out.

Satisfied, you rest.

CHAKRA THREE
SYMBOLS AND CORRESPONDENCES

Sanskrit Name:	*Manipura*
Meaning:	Lustrous gem
Location:	Navel to solar plexus
Element:	Fire
Outer Form:	Plasma
Function:	Will, power, assertiveness
Inner State:	Laughter, joy, anger
Glands:	Pancreas, adrenals
Other Body Parts:	Digestive system, muscles
Malfunction:	Ulcers, diabetes, hypoglycemia, digestive disorders
Color:	Yellow
Seed Sound:	Ram
Vowel Sound:	Ah as in "father"
Petals:	Ten
Tarot Suit:	Wands
Sephira:	Hod, Netzach
Planets:	Mars; also the Sun
Metal:	Iron
Foods:	Starches
Corresponding Verb:	I can
Herbs for Incense:	Dragon's blood, sandalwood, saffron, musk, cinnamon, ginger
Minerals:	Amber, topaz, yellow citrine, rutilated quartz
Animals:	Ram
Sense:	Sight

Guna:	Rajas
Lotus Symbols:	Ten petals of blue, downward triangle with Hindu solar crosses (svastikas). At the base is a running ram.
Hindu Deities:	Agni, Surya, Rudra, Lakini
Other Pantheons:	Brigit, Athene, Helios, Apollo, Amaterasu, Belenos, Apis, Ra
Archangel:	Michael
Chief Operating Force:	Combustion

AND THE WHEEL BURNS . . .

What is this life flowing in our bodies like fire? What is it?
Life is like a hot iron. Ready to pour. Choose the mold and
life will burn it.

—Mahabharata[1]

From earth to water to fire! Our dance grows, impassioned now as we reclaim our bodies and reach through emotion and desire to find will, purpose, and action. We grow in strength, we feel our power rising from our guts, descending from our visions, releasing joyously from our hearts. We now enter our third chakra, rising up from the combined levels of the first two chakras and embracing the growing current of consciousness that descends from the upper chakras.

Here the element *fire* ignites the light of consciousness, and we emerge from the unconscious, somatic levels to the exciting combination of psyche and soma that creates willed action. As we activate our power, we direct our activities toward a higher purpose.

Let's examine how the first two chakras combine to bring us this new level. The first chakra brought us solidity, stability, focus, and form. Here we experienced unity. From this ground, we moved to chakra two and experienced difference, change, and movement. Here we embraced polarities and discovered the passions of difference, choice, emotion, and desire. We expanded beyond mere survival instincts toward the desire for pleasure and merging with another.

As we put together matter and movement, we find that they create a third state: *energy*. If we rub two sticks together, we eventually get a spark that can ignite a fire. In the physical world, we call this combustion. In the body, it relates to metabolism. Psychologically, it relates to the spark of enthusiasm that ignites power and will; in our behavior, it is the realm of activity.

This is our third chakra. Its purpose is *transformation*. Just as fire transforms matter to heat and light, the third chakra transforms the passive elements of earth and water into dynamic energy and power. Earth and water are passive. They flow downward, subject to gravity, and follow the path of least resistance. Fire, by contrast, moves upward, destroying form, and takes the raw energy of matter to a new dimension—to heat and light.

If we are to rise upward through all seven chakras, it is the fire of our will that propels that movement. It is through our will that we liberate ourselves from fixed patterns and create new behavior. It is our will that steers us away from that path of least resistance, that addictive habit, or the expectations of others. It is through our will that we take actions that are difficult or challenging, moving toward something new. As we take these actions, we begin to transform, but the first step is breaking old patterns.

Thus, the initial task of the third chakra is to *overcome inertia*. In physics, inertia refers to the tendency of an object to remain in the state it is in—either in motion or at rest—unless acted upon by some other force. In the third chakra, the will combines the forces of stillness and movement, earth and water, each shaping the other. The momentum of a golf club hitting a stationary ball will get the ball moving. A catcher's mitt, held still, will stop a baseball in flight. Our will combines holding and moving in a way that directs action and shapes our world.

The hardest part is getting started. Once we get a fire going, it burns more easily, only needing to be stirred and fed. Once we get a business started, we then use its returns as fuel to keep it productive. Once we overcome inertia to the point where energy is produced easily, the third chakra "kicks in" and begins producing power with less effort and will. Doing something with ease and grace is the mark of true power.

A moving object, when it interacts with other objects, creates heat. Heat, in turn, stimulates movement, which allows new combinations to occur. Particles collide and combine; states of matter are changed; molecules may bond to other molecules; solids change to liquids; liquids change to gas; flour and eggs become cake. Fire is the transforming influence that can destroy form and release energy.

The sun is a primary example of transformational fire and could even be called a macrocosmic third chakra. The sun and other stars like it began as a diffuse cloud of hydrogen gas (with traces of heavier elements). Present theory states that a shock wave from a nearby supernova impacted the hydrogen cloud, causing it to collapse on itself. This created thousands of vortices, each with a gravitational field strong enough to draw in the necessary material to create a solar system. As the vortex of hydrogen that was to become our solar system collapsed, heat was generated through internal friction. Eventually the combination of heat and gravity triggered the process that makes our Sun shine.

The Sun produces heat and light through nuclear fusion. Its heat is so extreme that the hydrogen nuclei are propelled into each other with enough force to overcome their mutually repelling electrical charges, and fuse into slightly less massive helium nuclei. The difference in mass is converted to pure energy, which generates more heat and movement, thus perpetuating the whole process. Nuclear fusion requires a gravitational field strong enough to act as a container and create sufficient density for the process to be self-generating. Once again, we see how gravity, the force of chakra one, gives rise to movement, chakra two, resulting in energy, the force of chakra three. The energy then keeps the whole cycle running.

The chakras are all interdependent facets of a basic unified field of consciousness. They do not act separately and can only be separated intellectually. Likewise, we cannot separate energy from movement any more than we can separate it from mass. Mass, movement, and energy are three inseparable qualities of our physical world. The first three chakras represent a trinity of fundamental principles regulating our physical bodies and all matter. Together they form a dance of cause and effect, which gives us the energy for activity. Without a supply of energy, we have no power. But energy alone is not enough to constitute power. For that, the energy must be directed.

It is the descending current of consciousness that guides this energy into purpose. It is intelligence that forms the intention that shapes will and directs activity. In this way, the descending current brings us form, while the ascending current brings us energy. Only when the two combine do we have power.

To enter this chakra is to embrace the inner power that comes from the integration of bodily energy with conscious intelligence. In this way, we become effective agents of transformation.

MANIPURA—THE LUSTROUS GEM

The Manipura chakra is like the morning sun; meditating on it with gaze fixed on the tip of the nose one can stir up the world.

—Gorakshashatakam (tenth century)

In the body, the third chakra is located in the solar plexus, over the adrenal glands. This is where we get those "butterfly" feelings when we're nervous—when the third chakra isn't feeling confident and powerful. It's a flighty feeling that brings our energy up instead of down, yet stimulates and awakens us to heightened sensitivity. When we are grounded, this stimulation can be empowering and vitalizing. Without grounding, we may get a flurry of undirected energy.

As the name solar plexus implies, this is a fiery, solar chakra, bringing us light, warmth, energy, and power. It represents our "get up and go," our action, our will, our vitality. Extending from just below the sternum down to the navel, it is also called the "navel chakra." (See Figure 4.1, page 156.) One of its associations with power comes from the belief that all the major nadis (psychic currents) originate from the navel. As this is the source point for all prenatal nourishment and energy, it is not surprising that psychic pathways are originally established along these lines.

In correspondence with fire as combustion, the third chakra rules over metabolism, and is responsible for the regulation and distribution of metabolic energy throughout the body. This is done through the combustion of matter (food) into energy (action and heat). The digestive system is, therefore, an important part of this process, and a barometer for the health of this center. Problems such as diabetes, hypoglycemia, or stomach ulcers relate directly to this center.

Of crucial importance to metabolism is air, the element of chakra four. Without air, fire does not burn; cells do not metabolize.[2] When our breathing is constricted, our metabolism is hindered. When we have no room to breathe, our power is limited. Likewise, when we use power without compassion (chakra four), we risk perpetuating harm and oppression.

We can assess the health of this third chakra in many ways. Physically, we can examine the body structure in the solar plexus area. Tight hard stomachs, large pot bellies, or sunken diaphragms are all indications of third chakra imbalances. You can feel and look at your own body to explore this center. How does your physical body shape itself around this center? Does it expand or contract beyond its basic shape at this level? Large bellies may indicate an excessive need to be in power, to dominate and control, or simply an egotistical need to take up space. A weak, sunken chakra indicates a fear of taking power, a withdrawal into the self, a fear of standing out. Excess weight in general can be a third chakra malfunction, because it says the body is not properly metabolizing its solid matter (food) into energy.[3]

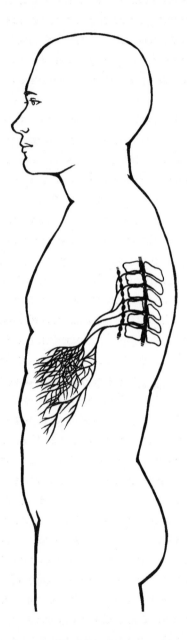

FIGURE 4.1
Chakra Three, the navel chakra (solar plexus).

You can also analyze yourself in terms of the element fire. Are you frequently cold? Do you prefer cold or hot drinks? Do you crave or avoid hot, spicy foods? Do you sweat easily, have fevers or chills? Is your temperament quick and energetic or slow and lethargic? These things give us an indication of whether we have excessive or deficient fire in our bodies.

In Sanskrit, this chakra is called *Manipura,* which means "lustrous gem," because it shines bright like the sun—a radiant, glowing center. Its symbol is a lotus with ten petals, within which is a downward-pointing triangle, surrounded by three T-shaped "svastikas" (Hindu symbols for fire, not to be confused with Nazi swastikas).[4] (See Figure 4.2, page 158.) The power to manipulate our surroundings is partially related to the ability of our hands, with ten fingers, extending out into the world around us. Ten is also the beginning of a new cycle, as our entry into rajas is the beginning of a new kind of awareness.

Within the lotus is a ram, a powerful and energetic animal, usually associated with Agni, Hindu god of fire. In the chakra itself, the deities depicted are the god Vishnu, and his partner, the Shakti Lakini, three-faced and four-armed, dispelling fear and granting boons. The letter inside the lotus is the seed sound *ram*. Meditating on this lotus is said to give the power to create and destroy the world.[5]

Fire is the spark of life that ignites will to action. Fire is the spark between Shiva and Shakti, the power that lies between polarity. Fire in our bodies keeps us warm, active, and energized so that we, too, may be transformers. Human beings need and give warmth. The power of the third chakra is the power of life, of vitality, and of connection—not the coldness of control and domination. The energy and fire in our bodies reflects our ability to combine with the elements around us, for fire is a process of combination and combustion.

Fire is radiant, so the third chakra is yang and active. When afraid or feeling powerless, we withdraw, and become passive and yin. We hold our movements in check and use one part of ourselves to control another. When we block our own power and expression, we are withdrawn and appear cold and controlled.

God: Vishnu   Goddess: Lākinī

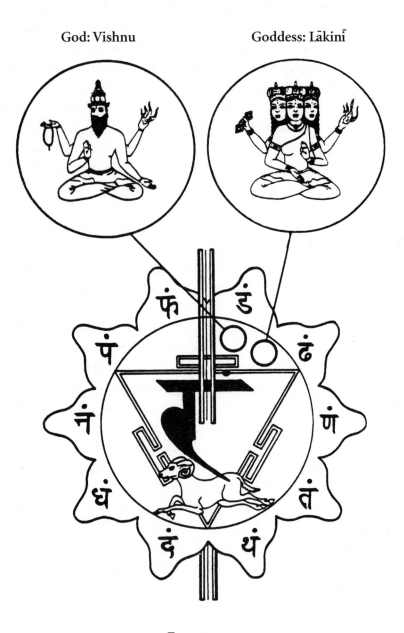

FIGURE 4.2
Manipūra chakra.
(Courtesy Timeless Books)

This control takes energy to maintain, yet it does not produce energy. Eventually we become depleted. Our natural enthusiasm for activities dwindles, and instead we have to "manufacture" energy for our projects, reaching for stimulants, such as coffee or sweets, which temporarily energize, but eventually deplete our vitality.

When we withdraw from life, we become a closed system. Our expression turns in on itself, often in anger and self-criticism, which wears us down further. Fire takes fuel to burn, and in a closed system, the fuel eventually burns up. Only in a dynamic state of interaction with the world can we keep up the movement and contact that feeds our fire and zest for life.

To break the cycle of fear and withdrawal takes a reconnection with the self in a loving and accepting way. If we are not in touch with the first two chakras—with our body and ground, our passions and pleasures—we have little fuel for our fire. Desire gives our will enthusiasm and makes it more dynamic.

If we are not loving with ourselves, giving ourselves room to breathe, to explore, to make mistakes, then we have no air for the fire to burn. If we are not connected to spirit, we have no spark for the fire, and all the fuel in the world is useless. If we are not centered within ourselves, we see the power as outside ourselves, rather than feeling it within.

The energy in our bodies is dependent on our ability to connect, to merge, to nourish ourselves from what surrounds us. It is dependent on our comfort with power, with our basic self-confidence. This chakra is also related to self-esteem, which brings strength to our will. When our will is effective, our self-esteem is enhanced. Then, we can better direct our lives toward that which we love, that which ignites us, challenges us, renews us. These are all elements that call for integration and development in the third chakra.

POWER

The power of open systems is not a property one can own, but a process one opens to.

—Joanna Macy[6]

We have stated that power is directed energy. What about personal power? How do we develop and maintain this power within a culture and educational system that teaches powerlessness as a way of fostering social cooperation? What happens when creative thinkers are seen as deviants to be ostracized from society while conformity is reinforced? Many parents train their children to be docile and well-behaved, but even obedience requires cooperation from our own will.

Social cooperation is certainly necessary; however, if it occurs through domination, it hardly deserves the term "cooperation" at all. It is then cooperation without desire, vitality, or the spark of fire characteristic of the third chakra. It becomes submission, which dampens and cripples our sense of power and will, and damages our self-esteem.

In order to develop and heal ourselves at the third chakra level, we must re-examine the concept of power that involves the domination of one part by another, commonly called "power over." Instead we can develop power as integration, "power within," the power of connecting with the forces of life. When we think about power, we can consider it an active verb rather than a noun, for indeed, power only exists in the doing, in the "powering" of changes or ideas. We can replace "power over" with "power to."

At this time in the world, I believe we are collectively passing through the latter stages of the third chakra. (See chapter 12, "An Evolutionary Perspective.") Our concepts of power and energy have become very complex. Through technology, the media, organized government, nuclear weapons, and mega-corporations, we are learning to control more with less. A few people make decisions for millions. A single plane can destroy an entire city. With little more than a phone call, most life on the planet could be annihilated. Issues of power, control, energy fuels, and political strength have become key themes in our current events. We have come a long way from iron spearheads to nuclear warheads, yet the disease of power used for control and domination has remained.

In order to pass through this chakra into the heart, we need to redefine our concept of power to become one that enhances, empowers, and strengthens. Our power structures must ensure, rather than threaten, continuance of our species, of our natural resources, and of our trust and ability to cooperate with each other. We need to see power that strengthens individuals and cultures simultaneously, rather than supporting one at the expense of the other. How can we change this?

Our dominant world view today is one that emphasizes separateness. Our sciences have looked at nature in reductionist terms—dissecting matter into smaller and smaller units. Western medicine treats the body as a collection of separate ailing units rather than seeing the mind/body as a whole. We look at people, countries, land, cultures, and races all as separate, isolated building blocks to be counted and carried, coordinated through control, rather than natural order.

"Power over" takes constant effort and vigilance. People are forced into submission, constantly intimidated and, thereafter, must be carefully guarded. Positions are never secure, but require greater and greater defenses. We overstep our bounds, depleting inner resources to steal wealth from some other place that we consider separate. In our diseased view, we see this as increasing our power—by increasing our dominion, increasing what we have "power over."

Through the lens of the Chakra System, power results from combining and integrating, rather than fighting and dominating. Each chakra level emerges, first of all, from the combination of the levels below it. It is then activated by the descending current of consciousness, which brings understanding to each level. Instead of finding our power through separation, power can come from unity and wholeness.

The true strength of any group or organism depends on its solidarity and its ability to combine and coordinate its inner forces. The strength of our planet will depend also on our ability to combine diversity and make something new out of the whole. Evolution, like the progression through the chakras, is a constant process of reorganization to more efficient levels—but always through an incorporation of what has come before. To focus on differences is to polarize, to separate, and estrange. To focus on unity is to strengthen.

When our world is ruled by strangers, we see only through machines; when our voice seems too small to be heard, estrangement is reinforced. It makes individuals easy to control, easily manipulated into serving some larger body that promises to return elements of our lost power to us piecemeal. Through participation in an alienating job, we receive a stipend of freedom known as a salary. The more thoroughly we participate, the greater the promise of reward; yet in reality, we often become further estranged.

Through estrangement, we have lost the concept of power *within*—the power of connection, union, fusion. Without this we stagnate, we lose our enthusiasm, our will, and our desires. We become automatons in an automatic world. Without our autonomy, we lose the desire to innovate, and remain stuck in the repetitive patterns of the lower chakras, unable to liberate, to find freedom. We need confidence to venture into the unknown. Without a strong third chakra, we cannot reach beyond into new levels, and instead remain stuck, clinging to security and sameness.

While bumper stickers may indeed advise us to "subvert the dominant paradigm," I believe we are, in fact, living in a *submissive paradigm*. This is a paradigm where there are far more people submitting than dominating. We are taught from a very young age to submit our will to another: first to parents, then to school teachers, clergy, bosses, military and government officials. Obviously, a certain amount of this is necessary for social cooperation. Yet many lose connection with their inner will in the process, and later find themselves powerless against alcohol, drugs, or destructive behaviors.

In a submissive paradigm, the power is placed outside ourselves. If we look for power outside, we look to others for direction, and find ourselves at their mercy, setting ourselves up for possible victimization. With an absence of power within, we may constantly seek stimulation, excitement, and activity, afraid to slow down, to feel the emptiness inside. We engage in activity as a way of getting acknowledged by others, a way of being seen, a way of having our ego strengthened. We may seek power for the sake of ego, rather than for the ability to better serve the larger whole. Power without purpose is mere whim, sometimes even dangerous.

Power is dependent on energy, just as survival is dependent on matter, and sexuality on movement. Power, from the Latin *podere*, "to be able," has the same meaning as Shakti, from the root of *shak*, "to be able." Shakti is our primordial energy field, ignited and given form by the spark of Shiva.

As electricity must be directed through wires in order for its power to be utilized, so must our life energy be directed by consciousness before we can make use of it with any true sense of power. Our cells metabolize and produce energy with little or no conscious direction from us. To have power, however, we need to be conscious. We must understand the relationships between things. We must be able to perceive and assimilate new information, to adjust our actions for maximum effect. We must be able to create and imagine events outside of present time and space. We must have knowledge, memory, and reasoning ability.

Power, then, is equally dependent on the upper chakras, though not at the expense of our lower ones. As we grow toward a greater understanding of consciousness and the spiritual world, we find that we will indeed evolve our concepts of power. This evolution will come from within each of us, from our core, our roots, and our guts, as well as our visions, our creativity, and our intelligence. Our future depends on it.

WILL

I assess the power of a will by how much resistance, pain, torture it endures and knows how to turn to its advantage.
—Friedrich Neitzche[7]

How do you make something happen? Do you sit still and make fervent wishes? Do you wait for circumstances to fall into place? Not likely, if you want to make any effective change. For that you need to exercise will.

Will is consciously controlled change. As the second chakra opens dualities, we are presented with choices. *Making those choices gives birth to the will.*

Will is the means by which we overcome lower chakra inertia, and the essential spark that ignites the flames of our power. Will is the combination of mind and action, the conscious direction of desire—the means through which we create our future. Personal power without will is impossible, making will a primary key to the development of the third chakra.

We all experience unpleasant events at various junctures of our lives. At the emotional level of the second chakra, we may feel like a victim of our circumstances. As a victim we feel powerless. Feeling this powerlessness and pain is an important step, as it puts us in touch with our needs. It becomes fuel for the will.

Getting to the third chakra, however, requires that we give up seeing ourselves as a victim, and realize that lasting change can only come from our own efforts. If we blame others, our only hope for improvement comes from hoping others will change—something we cannot control. When we take back responsibility, the changes come under the jurisdiction of our own will. Then we can truly heal from victimizing circumstances.

This is not to deny that victimization does exist and that many circumstances in our culture are hugely unjust. Nor is it touting the New Age belief that we are the sole creators of our own reality, created independently of all others.[8] Instead, will is the realization that we can regard each challenge as an opportunity to awaken to our highest potential. This does not deny what has come before, but incorporates it, using it as a springboard for the future. While we can't always control what happens to us, we can control what we do about it.

The task of the will is, first of all, to overcome inertia. As stated earlier, inertia occurs in rest or in movement. Simple lethargy or laziness can be an example of inertia at rest. Once we get up and get going, our muscles oxidize and our heart pumps, and we have more energy. Joggers, for instance, claim that they have far more energy on the days when they run despite the energy they expend. Energy begets energy, through the creation of momentum—and it is the will which begins this process. We also may find ourselves caught up in the momentum of something we would rather avoid. Here, we can use stillness to effect change, by refusing to be a part of this motion—and stopping it whenever it comes to us.

In the Kabbalistic Tree of Life, will is the conscious combination of force and form from the third level, which relates to *Hod* and *Netsach*. Netsach provides the radiant beauty, the energy, while Hod is the more intellectual state, the intelligence and form. These reflect the role of the upward and downward currents as they meet in the third chakra. Will is most effective when it is intelligent and strategic. This keeps us from wasting our energy by trying to do things through force alone. We are more efficient when we work smarter instead of harder.

At Manipura, force and form combine and evolve each other to higher and more efficient levels. Once the third chakra flame has been lit, the fire is less difficult to maintain. Once the light of understanding has dawned, the path to further understanding is illuminated. When Kundalini rises to this chakra, she makes herself apparent. Here she kindles the fire to destroy ignorance, karmic traps, and physical impurities. It is at this chakra that Kundalini begins to burn!

The first step in developing your will is to realize that you do have one, and that it is functioning quite well all the time. Look around you. All that you see in your personal midst, you have created with your will—the clothing you're wearing, the home you live in, the friends you keep. Feeling powerless is not due to lack of will, but failure to recognize and connect with our unconscious use of that will.

Failure to recognize that we have will is common. How many times in a day do you look at your tasks, exude a tired sigh, and say (or whine), "I *have to* do this." We tell ourselves we have to go to work, we have to do the dishes, we have to run this or that errand, or have to spend more time with our kids. It is disempowering to regard these circumstances as a dreary series of obligations, rather than choices we make actively. I don't *have to* do my dishes, but I *choose to* because I like a clean kitchen. I don't *have to* go to work, but I *choose to* because I like receiving a paycheck, or because I like to honor my agreements. This subtle change in attitude helps us befriend and realign with our will.

In talking about will, the distinction is often made between will and true will. If you do what someone tells you to do, when you really would rather not, you are still exercising your will, but deep inside, it is not your true will. You have essentially given your will over to another. To get it back, we must realize we have chosen to do this, and examine the reasons for that choice. Are we trying to please? Are we scared of the consequences? Are we out of touch with ourselves? How can we address these issues?

Only by answering these questions can we truly see what our will is serving. Is it in service of looking good? Being liked? Keeping the peace? Avoiding responsibility? Remaining invisible? Once we know what our will is serving, we must then ask what it might be betraying. Is looking good betraying your honest needs? Is keeping the peace perpetuating negative circumstances that might need to be confronted? Is pleasing others lowering your self esteem? To make these effects conscious is to empower ourselves to choose between them.

True will requires deep communication with the self, trust in your own volition, and the willingness to take risks and accept responsibility for those risks. If we dare to go against the grain by exercising our true will, then we risk criticism, ridicule, even abandonment. It's scary stuff, especially if our family environment was heavily invested in the *submissive paradigm.* It is through daring to use our will that a stronger sense of self is born, and through that strength the will is further developed. Like a muscle, we cannot strengthen our will without exercising it. And like all exercise, it serves us better when we do it wisely.

True will can be seen as an individual expression of a higher, divine will. It arises from our basic attunement with something larger. True will extends beyond the ego-self and embraces a higher purpose. It does not act for the sake of reward, but for the "rightness" of the action. As Aleister Crowley said, "True will, unassuaged of purpose, delivered from the lust of result, is every way perfect."[9] Therefore, if we are free from the ego's lust for results, the actions of our will take us to our destiny. While that destiny is not guaranteed to be pain-free, you can most certainly expect it to engage the third chakra, and ignite the very core of your being.

Detecting and using higher will is touchy business. There are many I know who use the concept of higher will as an escape from getting in touch with their own will, still seeing power as outside of themselves. "What does the universe want me to do in this situation? Why won't it give me a sign?" Every decision is preceded by numerous card readings, and endless seeking of advice from others. They may give their power over to others to decide for them, such as a psychic, teacher, therapist, or guru. Seeking guidance is often advisable, though we can sometimes avoid responsibility in this way. Perhaps a better question is: "What is my service to the world, and how can I best do this?" Power within is an openness to the flow of power around us, and our wills wrap themselves around our purpose gracefully when these powers are aligned.

Once we know our will, we return to a more practical level—how to effectively exercise it. First we must make sure we are grounded. Without grounding, we are not plugged in and we do not have the force of the liberating current running through us. We are more easily pushed around, often responding instead to another's will. This takes the form of an "intellectual will" and overrides the inner desires of the body. It's easily spotted by the preponderance of "shoulds" and "have-tos" in our internal dialogue. Self-discipline is important, but works better as a want than a should. Then our whole body/mind is in accord with it.

Like power, will is often associated with discipline, control, and manipulation, such as the will to go on a diet, get through school, or finish a project. While discipline is essential to accomplish most things, it is another aspect of control over separate parts if there is not an internal agreement within the body/mind. It takes discipline to sit here and edit this book, yet my will and desire are connected to my purpose. The parts I have to edit the most are the parts I wrote when I made myself do it, because it was my time of day to write rather than because the inspiration moved me. Those parts lacked power. Without agreement between will and desire, we lose our passion and our momentum, and thereby dissipate the power needed to carry out our will.

In order for our will to be engaged, we must also be in touch with our desires. How can we exert our will if we don't know what we want? While undue attachment to our desires may keep us trapped in lower chakras, suppression only blocks the force of the will. When a person feels deprived, unloved, or overworked, they are easier to manipulate. The will flourishes best when we are relaxed, happy, and in touch with ourselves.

However, will is not always in harmony with every desire. You may desire a piece of chocolate cake, but your greater will refuses it because you want to lose weight. You may not desire to take on a particular task and yet, quite peacefully, will yourself to do it anyway. We are still serving our desires, but we are choosing which desires are most important in the long run.

It is here that discipline becomes most important. The word discipline actually comes from disciple—the willingness to be a student of something. Here we are faced with the odd paradox of surrendering our will to a structure or form that brings about fulfillment of that will. In this act of discipline, there is a certain transcendence of feelings, in that we may not "feel like" doing our meditation on a particular day, or we may not "feel like" going to work. Yet, those feelings become irrelevant when our will is fixed to a larger purpose. In this way, the third chakra is both fueled by, and yet transcends, the feeling orientation of the second chakra.

Knowledge of the will, with its infinite and constant choices, comes from a deeper sense of purpose. This purpose is born out of our orientation to the world. It is born from who we are, what we love and loathe, what our talents apply to. Each of us has a purpose, and our ultimate will is to fulfill that purpose. This purpose can often sort out the difference between "will" and "whim," often hard to distinguish. Whim is momentary. Will has a larger purpose. We examine the long-range effects of our actions, and their part in our greater sense of purpose. We think in terms of far-reaching cause and effect. Our power, too, grows with our sense of purpose, for it gives us the direction that transforms mere energy into effective power.

If we are unclear about that purpose, then it's hard to know just what our will is in a given situation. The task of consciousness is an accurate assessment of who we are, for within that mystery lies the purpose our will must address. Once we know our will, its strength increases through use. Often using our power is merely a matter of understanding that we do indeed have the power to begin with. That understanding becomes solidified through use and experimentation, and results ultimately in gaining confidence.

All chakras have their positive and negative aspects, and the overuse of the personal will can keep us trapped at this level, especially if that will is not in harmony with the greater Cosmic Will of which it is a part. The intelligent and sensitive person must recognize when their will becomes detrimentally dominating and overly controlling. (And if they don't catch it, others will surely try to tell them!) Engaging this chakra requires developing the will, yet the passage beyond this chakra requires the ability to yield our will when appropriate. A person of true power should not have a need to dominate.

When personal will and divine will are one, then it is crucial that this will be followed. When personal will is out of tune with the greater will, it is equally critical that this difference be detected. From Crowley again: "A Man whose conscious Will is at odds with his True Will is wasting his strength. He cannot hope to influence his environment efficiently."[10] At this point the motives of our personal will must be re-examined. Failing to do this, we may find an undue number of obstacles in our way, making each step more difficult. Though many paths are difficult, the ones that are right for us have a coherency of flow that makes the difficulty easier to bear. It is the task of our intelligence to perceive the correct path. The task of the will is to follow that path.

SELF-ESTEEM

Let a man know his worth, and keep things under his feet.
—Ralph Waldo Emerson[11]

The third chakra attributes of power, will, vitality, and self-discipline are ultimately based on self-esteem. When our self-esteem is high, we are confident, assertive, proactive, disciplined, and basically excited about life. When self-esteem is low, we are filled with doubts and self-recrimination that act like check dams for the psychic momentum needed to get something done. If there are too many check dams, we lose our momentum entirely, and end up in a state of inertia. Once we find ourselves in that puddle of inertia, the self-doubt and recrimination only get worse, and the cycle can become paralyzing.

Then the demon of shame has entered the third chakra, and perhaps even taken over. Shame is the antithesis of self-esteem. It collapses the middle section of the body, depriving it of energy. It interrupts the fluidity coming up from the base, and overplays the constricting mental energy coming down from the top. Instead of moving outward, the energy turns against the self.

Self-esteem comes from a realistic sense of the self. Initially this comes from the body and the physical identity. This gives us our edges and boundaries. Next it comes from the second chakra and our emotional identity, which brings aliveness to our experience of self, and keeps us happy and in touch. Thirdly, self-esteem comes from trial and error as we reach out, take risks, succeed and fail, and in doing so, gain a realistic sense of our own abilities. Through self-discipline, we hone our skills. These form the foundation for self-esteem.

Our concept of self is further illuminated by interactions with others. If we are loved and accepted by others (fourth chakra) and feel we have something to give, we are more likely to love and accept ourselves. Through communication, we can get honest feedback about how others perceive us, and are able to communicate the interior of the self. And through the upper two chakras, we get the transpersonal elements that hold the self in a larger matrix.

Self-esteem forms a good foundation for opening the heart and maintaining successful relationships. If the lower chakras have done their job, then our partner doesn't need to make us secure, interpret our feelings, or bolster our ego. We can then move more completely into the delightful experience of love.

BREAKING POWERLESSNESS

Limitation is the first law of manifestation, therefore it is the first law of power.

—Dion Fortune[12]

Power, like any muscle in the body, must be developed consciously. In keeping with the well-known expression, "Knowledge is power," most powerlessness is the result of ignorance about how to behave effectively. It may be simply lack of awareness or attention. Increasing our awareness increases our power. Therefore, such things as meditation can help. As we raise energy up the spine, and as this energy pierces this third layer, feelings of power will naturally ensue. However, mere meditation is not enough.

The following are some simple concepts related to the development of the third chakra, followed by some physical exercises for opening this center.

Breaking Inertia

Do something different. If you are sluggish, get moving. If you are hyperactive, be still. Break boring repetitive patterns, and choose a challenge. Overcoming difficulties increases strength and confidence. Power is seldom developed by clinging to security. Give up being safe and your power chakra will awaken more quickly.

Avoid Invalidation

Criticism from those who do not understand your situation can sometimes be more detrimental than helpful, especially if you are a sensitive person who takes it to heart. Often when we are undertaking something new and uncertain, invalidation can be an instant power-crippler—stopping the sensitive person dead in their tracks. Remember, as Albert Einstein said, "New ideas meet their greatest opposition from those who misunderstand them."

Wiring and Resistors

Make sure that your energy travels in complete circuits—that what you put out has a way of coming back. Make sure that this energy is not unnecessarily caught up, interrupted, dissipated, or fragmented. Use the flow and momentum of the second chakra to fire up the will.

Effort and Resistance

Both effort and resistance are tiring and wear down our energy. They are both a sign that our power is not flowing harmoniously. When you find yourself straining with effort, stop. Think about what you are doing and imagine doing it without effort—smoothly, enjoyably. Ask yourself why you are so attached to this particular thing. Ask yourself why it's taking so much effort—what's missing that would make it flow smoothly?

If you are in constant resistance to some force, stop. Ask yourself why this force is manifesting in your life at this time. Resistance is often fear, the opposite of power. What is it you are afraid of? Imagine what would happen if you stopped resisting? How can your will protect you with less effort or resistance?

Breaking Attachments

Energy that is directed toward something that is not manifesting is energy that is "hung up," caught, or otherwise useless. If, after reasonable effort, something is not working, let it go. The energy you feel when the attachment no longer has control over you can be exhilarating. The more you release, the less friction there is on your energy. The lighter you become, the more you move toward spirit and away from matter. Be careful not to go too far, however, for the Earth plane is where the power manifests, and without some solidity the power may become too diffused.

Attention

Attention focuses energy. Pay it when it needs to be paid. Give it to yourself. Give and accept it from others. Notice where it goes. Where the attention goes, the rest of the energy will surely follow.

Grounding

We must be able to direct our attention to the here and now in order to manifest power. Grounding brings us into the present, into the power within our bodies, and consolidates and focuses our energy. Even though we are rising beyond this chakra, we never overcome the need for this simple practice.

Anger

Releasing blocked anger in a safe and effective way can sometimes help to unblock the third chakra. This is best done in conjunction with grounding and is an excellent way of using the energy within you to bring about change—at least in your state of mind, if not in your circumstances. Blocked power is very often blocked anger. Anger is a potent and cleansing force, but it is hard earned and should be spent wisely. It's not worth damaging loved ones for things we need to work out within ourselves.

Increasing Information

Knowledge is power and the more we learn, the more we can do and the fewer mistakes we theoretically make. Learning, under any circumstances, helps to increase one's power.

Love

Love is the unifying force that ties us all together, inspires us, and gives us strength to keep going. It is exhilarating, cleansing, energizing, healing, and feeds energy from the upper chakras into our third chakra. It gives us validation, contact and purpose, strengthens self-esteem, and inspires the will.

Laughter

Taking things too seriously can really make us lose touch with our power. If we can laugh at a situation, we have power over it. Whenever things seem at their worst, remember to laugh at yourself.

Take Care of Yourself

If you don't, no one else will. You know what you want and need better than anyone else. If you care for yourself, this decreases your need to get it from outside and need is often inversely proportional to power.

Empowerment Meditation

Think of a time when you felt powerless or victimized. Go back to that time and feel the fear, the hurt, the anger. Feel yourself at that stage of your life, as a young child, teenager, adult . . . . Let your body express the shape of your feelings at that time. How did you walk? How did you carry yourself? How did you speak?

Take a moment to step outside of this picture and examine it from a distance, as if you were an onlooker. See if you can be compassionate with yourself, accepting, noncritical. If you can, then next, see if you can laugh at yourself and become amused at the pathos, the pain, the seriousness.

Next, go back over the scene and replay it with a different outcome. Imagine yourself doing something that changes the situation: get mad, fight back, run away, laugh, stand firm—whatever you would see as an action of power. If you need to call in helpers, spirits, or friends, feel free to do so. Use whatever it takes to turn the situation around.

When you have resolved it, pat yourself on the back. Feel the sense of wholeness and satisfaction, and try to bring that through to your life right now.

Next, ask yourself if there is anyone you are currently blaming for the circumstances in your life. How much power are you investing in them? As an act of reclaiming your own power, write their name on a piece of paper and set fire to it, saying, "I hereby release you from responsibility for my life and its failures. I now take that responsibility myself." As you take back the energy, you are empowering yourself.

CHAKRA THREE EXERCISES

Breath of Fire

This is a rapid diaphragmatic breathing, designed to clean toxins from the body, raise internal fire, and stimulate the ascending current.

> Sit in an upright, comfortable posture with back straight and legs relaxed.

> Using the muscles of your abdomen, SNAP in your diaphragm, causing a quick exhale to escape through your nose. Keep the mouth closed.

> When you relax the abdomen, air will naturally enter your nose and chest, causing an inhale. You need not force this inhalation.

> Then SNAP the diaphragm once again, followed by relaxation, causing another exhale and inhale.

> When this process is comfortable, repeat quickly, causing several quick, sequential exhales. Do in sets of fifty or so, with a long, deep breath at the end of each set. Three sets of fifty or more make a good place to start. After a while you can pace yourself according to what feels right. Increase the number and the speed as the muscles become acclimated.

Jogging

Running is intense, high-energy physical exercise that gets the heart pumping, the lungs breathing, and the blood racing through the body. Of all the physical energizers, jogging is probably the best overall toner for overcoming inertia.

Stomach Crunches

As American and non-yogic as this may sound, ordinary sit-ups increase the muscle tone over the third chakra, and help tone the digestive organs.

Begin on your back, with knees bent and feet parallel. Lace your fingers behind your neck.

Tighten the stomach muscles until the head has lifted a few inches off the floor, exhaling. You need not sit all the way up. The muscles do their work in the first few inches of contraction.

Inhale as you lower your head, exhaling as you exert. Repeat as many times as you can, increasing the number over time.

The Woodchopper

The associated tone of the third chakra is a loud "ah" sound. This should accompany the motions in this exercise. This is also an excellent anger release.

Stand with feet planted firmly in the ground, with heels about two feet apart. Raise arms together, over the head, with hands joined. Arch your back slightly. (See Figure 4.3, page 178.)

Making the "ah" sound as you descend, swing the whole upper portion of the body downward, bringing your hands between your legs and through. (See Figure 4.3, page 178.) The motion should be smooth and rapid, and emit as much force and power as is possible.

Repeat five to ten times in a session and feel the energy break through into your upper body.

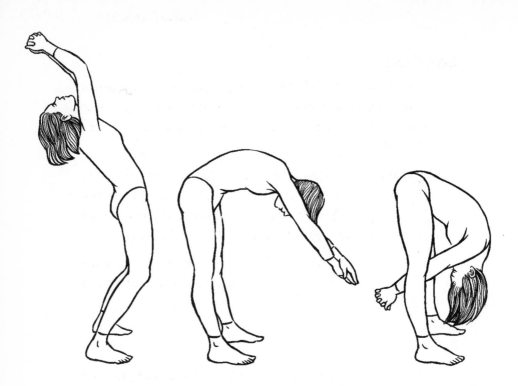

FIGURE 4.3
Woodchopper.

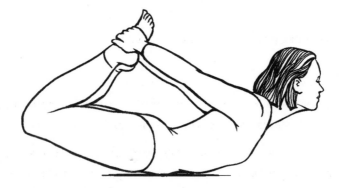

FIGURE 4.4
Bow Pose.

Bow Pose

Lie on your stomach, hands to the side, and relax. Take a deep breath and bend your knees and reach for your ankles. (If you can't reach, you can use a strap to bridge the difference.)

On an inhale, lift your head, press the sacrum down, and arch your back by lifting the chest and pulling on the ankles. Let your arms pull your shoulders back, and balance on your belly. (See Figure 4.4, page 178.) Breathe deeply.

Let your hands do the work of maintaining the arch while you relax the rest of your body as much as you can in this strange position.

Belly Push

From a seated position, push both feet out straight in front of you, with your palms placed on the ground by your hips.

Push your pelvis upward, approaching a slight arch from your feet to your head, pushing, especially through the solar plexus. (See Figure 4.5, page 180.)

Slowly relax and return to a seated position.

Pike Pose

Hard to maintain without practice, this little gem tightens tummy muscles and develops balance and self-control.

Resting on your back, bring your feet and legs up (knees as straight as possible) and your torso up, too, making a v-shape with your body. (See Figure 4.6, page 180.) Hold as long as possible, then relax.

For an easier version, try lifting one leg at a time, or placing your feet against a wall, so that you focus more on belly muscles than on the thigh muscles that may not be strong enough.

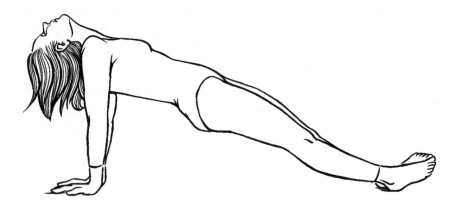

FIGURE 4.5
Belly Push.

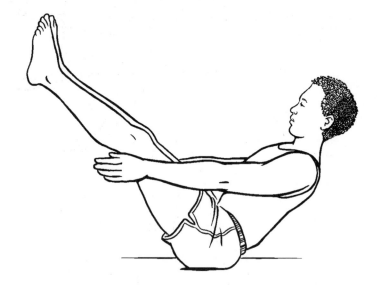

FIGURE 4.6
Pike Pose.

Making the Sun

The arms play an important part in the activation of power, for they make actual contact with the world. It is through the arms that we *do*, and doing is what the third chakra is all about. The strength of this exercise is that it involves visualization as well as physical movement. It works on moving energy from the heart and solar plexus out into the arms and hands.

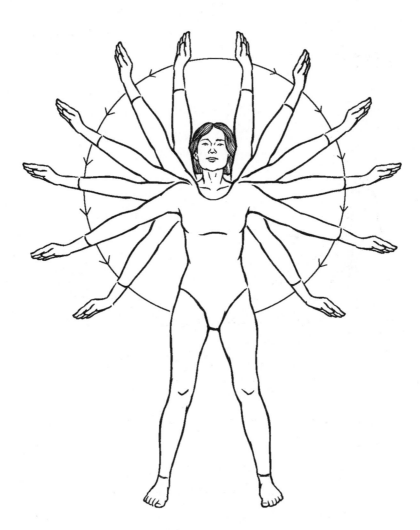

FIGURE 4.7
Making the Sun.

Stand upright, arms over your head, feet shoulder-width apart.

Take a deep breath, stretch your arms and fingers up as far as you can, and slowly bring them down to your sides, palms facing downward, arms reaching and stretching outward as long as possible at all times. (See Figure 4.7, page 181.)

About halfway down you should start to feel as if you were pushing against some invisible force. As you do this, imagine yourself as the center of the sun, your arms describing the circumference. As you feel the force you are pushing against, imagine it to be some block that you are working through. Feel your hands pushing it away. Imagine the tendrils of energy streaming out through your fingers, and when the circle is complete, take a moment to feel and imagine the solar glow around you.

Power Walk

Stand erect with arms bent at the elbows and hands in a fist at the chest.

Take a step and push one arm outward, as if you were pushing away obstacles. Then release the other arm.

Repeat.

Pretend you are clearing blocks out of your immediate vicinity as you do this, and ridiculous as you may feel, use words like "OUT" or "GO AWAY" to emphasize the action.

Laughing Circle

This is a children's game, done with a group of at least three, but better with four or more.

Everyone lie on the floor, each with their head on another's stomach. One person begins by saying an expulsive "ha" three times, followed by the next person and the next. As our heads bounce on the stomach below us, it's only a short time before the "ha's" become "ha-ha's" and uproarious laughter.

Basically, anything that gets the energy moving rapidly is good for the third chakra. The important thing is to overcome inertia. Once this is overcome, it becomes the domain of the will, where the combined force of desire and understanding channel the energy into action. It is an exhilarating step in the growth of our consciousness.

ENDNOTES

1. William Buck, *Mahabharata*, 49.

2. The crucial events in cell metabolism are the release of hydrogen atoms which are then transferred through compounds to oxygen, forming water. Energy is stored in the cells in the form of ATP (adenosine triphosphate) which requires a constant supply of oxygen to convert it from its lower phosphate form (ADP adenosine diphosphate) to the energy rich ATP. As our muscles do work we use the third phosphate, which must then be recycled to join again with oxygen to become ATP.

   It is interesting to note that hydrogen, relating to the third chakra (as in the sun) and oxygen, relating to the fourth chakra (as in the breath) are metabolized through action releasing water, an element of chakra two. This expresses on a chemical level the condensation process of descending through the chakras.

3. This can also relate to the first chakra needing extra weight for grounding. Normal grounding channels may be blocked, or a second chakra deficiency may exist as a way of warding off sexual feelings or advances.

4. While there seems to be no direct correlation here, it is interesting to note that the Nazi swastika represented some of the worst abuse of power we have known in human history.

5. *Sat-Chakra-Nirupana*, verse 21. Avalon, *Serpent Power*, 369.

6. Joanna Rogers Macy, *Despair and Personal Power in the Nuclear Age*, 31.

7. Friedrich Neitzsche, *The Will to Power*, Book 2, note 362 (1888; tr. 1967.)

8. We may create our own reality, but it is created within a field of six billion other people creating their reality as well. Our reality is not independent, but embedded within a larger structure which imposes certain limitations and challenges.

9. Aleister Crowley, *The Book of the Law*, verse 44, pages 23, 24.

10. Aleister Crowley, *Magick in Theory and Practice*, xv.

11. Ralph Waldo Emerson, Essays, "Self-Reliance," (First Series, 1841).

12. Dion Fortune, *The Cosmic Doctrine*, 112.

RECOMMENDED SUPPLEMENTAL READING FOR CHAKRA THREE

Assagioli, Roberto. *The Act of Will.* NY: Penguin Books, 1974.

Crowley, Aleister. *Magick in Theory and Practice.* NY: Dover Publications, 1976.

Denning, Melita and Osborne Phillips. *Psychic Self-Defense and Well-Being.* St. Paul, MN: Llewellyn Publications, 1980.

Macy, Joanna Rogers. *Despair and Personal Power in the Nuclear Age.* PA: New Society Publishers, 1983.

May, Rollo, Ph.D. *Love and Will.* NY: W.W. Norton, 1969.

Starhawk. *Truth of Dare: Encounters with Power, Authority, and Mystery.* San Francisco, CA: Harper & Row, 1987.

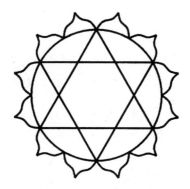

CHAKRA FOUR

Love

Air

Breath

Balance

Relationship

Affinity

Unity

Healing

Chapter 5

CHAKRA FOUR: LOVE

OPENING MEDITATION

FROM LOVE WERE WE MADE.
On passion's waves our spirit sparked
and down we came into our
mothers . . . mater . . . matter . . .
The pull of love calling us, deep into
the Earth,
As deep into the mother father
pushed.
Deep into the womb, we crawled—
the warm dark womb of earth
and water. The womb of love—

safe, dark, cradled, quiet.
  We grew.

In the dark there was but one sound—
the sound of life, the sound of love, the sound of the heart.
Beating . . . Beating . . . Beating . . . Beating . . . [1]

Hear it now in your own heart. Its rhythms pumping life and air and
    breath through every part of you, renewing you;
Bathing you in air, in space, in breath, in life.
Feel it now at the core of you, embrace it with your hands.
Feel it yearning, crying, loving, hoping, healing.
Feel it within you, old as you are, beating since the days from deep in the
    womb, feel how long it's been there,

Always beating. Never stopping.
Always beating. Never stopping.
Always beating. Never stopping.
Always beating. Never stopping.
Do you love that heart?

Breathe in deeply, drawing in the air . . . as softness, depth and wisdom.
As you breathe, spirit comes within your heart and touches you . . .
moving you . . . changing you.
Deeply, you accept as thirstily you drink.
Be thankful for this vessel that receives.

Faster now on waves of flame, we fling with joy up to the sky, above the
    Earth, above the water, beyond the fire, into the air.
We reach and spread our wings and fly, free to ride the winds. But soon
    get tossed about and cry:
Where is the heart? Where is the heart? Where is my home?

We listen for the beat and fly, deep unto its sound.
We reach for ground, slowing down.
We still ourselves to listen deeper, quiet is the sound.

Gently we reach, for the heart is tender. Softly we touch, for the heart
  is afraid.
We open our hands to the love inside, to unite, to touch, to heal.
Offer that love now. Ask for entry to your own heart.

Listen deep and hear inside, a silent sound.
Anahata, Anahata, Anahata, Anahata.
Listen deep and breathe into the sound, the breath, the winds of healing.
In . . . and out . . . in . . . and out . . . in . . . and out . . .
Inhaling that which is new, exhaling the old, each breath renewing.
Each breath a wind within you and around you, gentle zephyr, storm of
  life, winds of change.

For what does your heart cry? For what does it long? In what does it find
  peace? Release its hopes and dreams to fly upon the wings of change
  and then return on wings of love, fulfilled beyond your dreams.

You are not alone. Your cries are echoed in a thousand hearts the same.
If you listen, you can hear them: beating, beating, beating, beating.

Deep within each person find the heart.
Everywhere around you find the heart.
Deep within ourselves we find the heart.
Every time we touch, we touch the heart.

Within each one is love, awaiting sweet unfoldment.
Release that love upon the winds of breath, and reach beyond.
Touch the hearts inside the ones you love,
And listen to their breath that whistles in . . . and out . . . in . . . and out . . .

Like you, they laugh and cry and play,
Ceaseless rhythm through each day.
Feel the heart so like your own:
Hoping, healing, breathing, feeling.
Let there be no sound of striking,
Only that of love and liking.

Each unto the dance of love,
That joins the Earth to worlds above,
And joins ourselves unto each other,
Each one seen as sister, brother.
Within our hearts the seeds of peace
Lie, awaiting sweet release.
Upon the winds of change they fly
As deep within our hearts we cry:
Anahata, Anahata, Anahata, Anahata.
The sound of love.

CHAKRA FOUR
SYMBOLS AND CORRESPONDENCES

Sanskrit Name:	*Anahata*
Meaning:	Unstruck
Location:	Heart
Element:	Air
Outer State:	Gaseous
Function:	Love
Inner State:	Compassion, love
Glands:	Thymus
Other Body Parts:	Lungs, heart, pericardium, arms, hands
Malfunction:	Asthma, high blood pressure, heart disease, lung disease
Color:	Green
Seed Sound:	*Lam*
Vowel Sound:	Ay as in "play"
Petals:	Twelve

Tarot Suit:	Swords
Sephira:	Tiphareth
Celestial Bodies:	Venus
Metal:	Copper
Corresponding Verb:	I love
Sense:	Touch
Yoga Path:	Bhakti yoga
Herbs for Incense:	Lavender, jasmine, orris root, yarrow, marjoram, meadowsweet
Minerals:	Emerald, tourmaline, jade, rose quartz
Guna:	Rajas or sattvas
Animals:	Antelope, birds, dove
Lotus Symbols:	Twelve petals, within which is a six-pointed star. In the center is shiva lingam within a downward triangle (trikuna) within the seed symbol, yam. Depicted are Isvara, God of Unity, and Shakti Kakini. At the base of the star runs an antelope, symbol of freedom.
Hindu Deities:	Vishnu, Lakshmi (as Preservers), Krishna, Isvara, Kama, Vayu, Aditi, Urvasi
Other Pantheons:	Aphrodite, Freyja, Pan, Eros, Dian Cecht, Maat, Asclepius, Isis, Aeolus, Shu (also, Christ, though not technically a deity, would be the energy of the heart chakra)
Archangel:	Raphael
Chief Operating Quality:	Equilibrium

THE HEART OF THE SYSTEM

Love was born first, the gods cannot reach it, or the spirits, or men . . . . Far as heaven and earth extend, far as the waters go, high as the fire burns, you are greater, love! The wind cannot reach you, nor the fire, nor the sun, nor the moon: You are greater than them all, love!

—Atharva Veda 9.2.19

Now that we have ignited the fires of our will, taken control of our life, and burned through our stubbornest blocks, we can allow our fires to subside a bit. As they turn to warm embers, we turn toward our center, warmed, cleansed, and ready to embrace the next level of awareness.

From the active, fiery solar plexus, we are thrust into a new and different realm. From the realms of the body and manifestation, we move into the softer touch of spirit. From the focus on the self and its desires and actions, we embrace a larger pattern, and dance our small part within the greater web of relationships. We transcend our ego, and grow toward something greater, deeper, stronger. As we reach for the heavens, we expand.

We have now reached the central point of the Chakra System. Even in our language, the heart refers to the center of things, the essence, the kernal of truth, as in "to go to the heart of the matter." This is our spiritual center, our core, the place that unites forces from above and below, within and without. The task of chakra four is to integrate and balance the various aspects of our being. In so doing, it brings a radiant sense of wholeness to the entire organism, an acceptance of the exquisite interpenetration of both spirit and matter. Within this sense of wholeness lie the seeds of inner peace.

The heart chakra is the center of love. As spirit and matter are combined, Shiva and Shakti are united within the heart. In their eternal dance of creation, their love radiates throughout all existence, giving it the permanence that allows the universe to continue. In the form of Vishnu and Lakshmi, the Preservers, they rule over the middle part of our lives, bringing us steadiness and continuity. Their love can be thought of as the "binding" force that holds together all the building blocks of which life is made.

The love we experience at the level of the heart chakra is distinctly different from the more sexual and passionate love of the second chakra. Sexual love is object oriented—the passion is stimulated by the presence of a particular person. In the fourth chakra, love is not dependent on outside stimulation, but experienced within as a state of being. In this way it radiates outward, bringing love and compassion to whatever comes into our field. It is a divine presence of empathetic connection, rather than an extension of our need or desire. Hopefully, through the force of the will, our needs have been fulfilled or transcended. Love can emerge with the deep sense of peace that comes from lack of need, with a joyous acceptance of our place among all things, and the radiance that comes from inner harmony. Unlike the changing nature of the second chakra with its transitory passions, love from the heart is of an enduring quality, eternal and constant.

ANAHATA—THE STILL CENTER POINT

The symbol for the heart chakra is a circle of twelve lotus petals surrounding two intersecting triangles, forming a six-pointed star. (See Figure 5.1, page 194.) The triangles represent the descent of spirit into the body and the ascent of matter rising to meet spirit. This symbol (also known as the Star of David) represents the Sacred Marriage: the balanced interpenetration of masculine and feminine. This is the star of radiance that emanates from an open heart chakra. The six points can also be seen as relating to the six other chakras, as they are each integrated at this center.

In the body, this chakra relates to the cardiac plexus (see Figure 5.2, page 195.), and rules over the heart, lungs, and thymus gland. Just as each chakra can be seen as a disk of swirling energy, so, too, can the entire body/mind be seen as a chakra. If we follow a path from the crown chakra, spiraling through each center, we find that

God: Īsa   Goddess: Kākinī

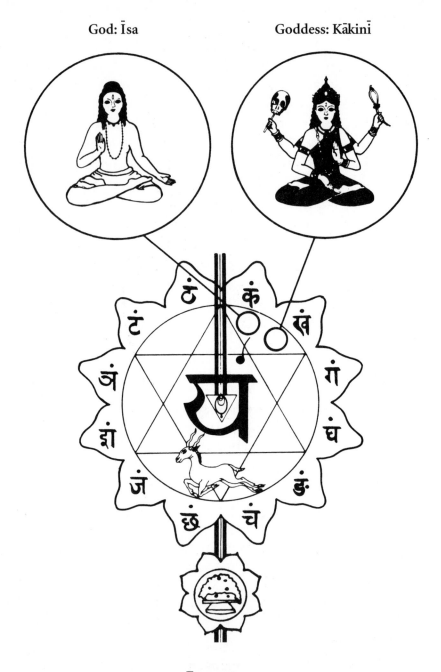

FIGURE 5.1
Anāhata chakra.
(Courtesy Timeless Books)

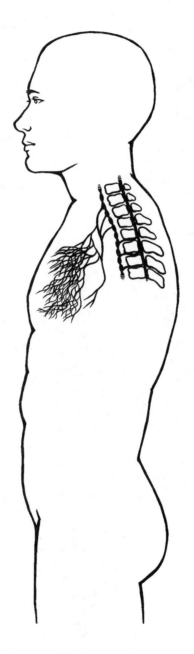

FIGURE 5.2
Chakra Four, the heart chakra.

the heart is the end point of the spiral—the center, the destination. (See Figure 5.3, page 197.) Here we find the eye of the storm, where calm prevails in the midst of fury. The heart is indeed a center of peace.

The Sanskrit name for this chakra is *Anahata*, meaning "sound that is made without any two things striking," as well as "unstruck," "unhurt," "fresh," and "clean." When the chakra is free of grief from old hurts, its opening is innocent, fresh, and radiant. The fight of the third chakra is replaced by acceptance in the fourth. If the third chakra has done its job, our circumstances are easier to accept.

The element of the fourth chakra is *air*, the least dense of our physical elements so far. As an element, air is commonly associated with knowledge and things that are expansive and spirited. Air represents freedom, as in the birds that fly. Air represents openness and freshness, as in the airing of a room. Air represents lightness, simplicity, and softness. When we fall in love, we feel like we are walking on air. Air implies spaciousness, which is achieved through letting go. When we cling too tightly to what we love, we suffocate our beloved, which is like depriving them of air. We talk about needing space when we want "room to breathe."

Air, the gaseous state of matter, differs from any element we have discussed because it tends to disperse itself evenly throughout any space it occupies (except gases that are notably lighter or heavier than our average atmosphere). Water sits at the bottom of the bowl. Earth stays rigid and fixed. Fire moves upward, but always clings to its fuel; yet air disperses. Incense burned on an altar gradually pervades the whole room. There is a sense of equilibrium, calm, and evenness. Likewise, the heart chakra reflects a kind of loving equanimity in regard to the complex interrelationships of all things.

Lastly, air represents *breath*, the vital process through which our cells are kept alive. The Hindus call it *prana* (from *pra*, "first," and *na*, "unit"). In yoga philosophy, prana is referred to as a vital energy in and of itself, a basic unit from which all life is made. This energy represents an interface between the physical world and the mental world. The

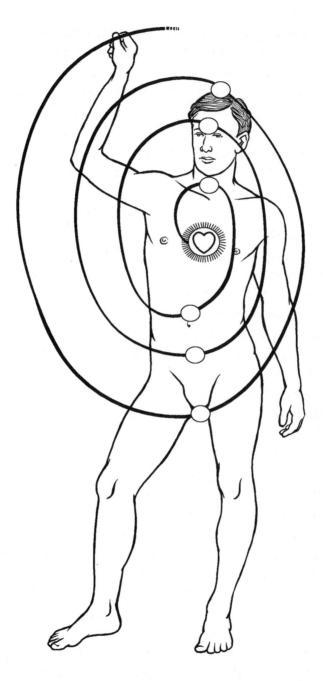

FIGURE 5.3
The heart as the end point of the spiral.

mind, if it wishes to influence the body, can do so through control of the breath. Likewise, control of the breath can quiet the mind. Prana is considered a vital link between the two—just as the heart chakra is the integrator between upper and lower chakras.

Opening the heart chakra requires a combination of technique and understanding. First, we learn to see the world in terms of relationships—what causes things to enter into and remain in combination with other things. This, of course, includes our personal relationships with others and with the world around us.

The heart requires an understanding and practice of balance—between mind and body, inner and outer realms, self and other, giving and receiving. Opening the heart requires a transcendence of ego, allowing us to surrender to forces larger than the self. Lastly, opening the heart chakra requires an understanding and control of the breath, for it is the tool of physical and mental transformation.

Each of these aspects of the heart will be discussed in the following pages. May they free your heart from its chains and bring you peace, for it says in the *Upanishads*:

> *When all the knots of the heart are unloosened, then even here in this human birth, the mortal becomes immortal. This is the whole teaching of the scriptures.*[2]

LOVE

Love is the attraction exercised on each unit of consciousness by the center of the universe in its course of taking shape.
—Teilhard de Chardin[3]

Love. Of all the words in the English language, this four-letter word probably has the most meaning, or at least the most elusive meaning. So basic to the soul of each one of us, love becomes the precious essence governing each of our lives. How do we find it? How do we maintain it? How do we share it? And beyond the power of words lies the question, "What is it?"

Love, like power, is something we all want and need. Few ever feel they have enough. Many live in fear of it. Nearly no one understands it. Yet we all search for it and gauge our lives by it when it is found. What is this mysterious force? Why does it have such power in our lives?

Love is a unifying force — it draws things together, and keeps them in relationship. From this unity, we can touch an underlying continuity that allows our separate parts to be held in relationship to something larger. From our parents we needed to learn that they would be there, day after day, in order to grow into security. A binding force allows something to hold together long enough to evolve its patterns to deeper and more cohesive states. Love allows change and freedom, but keeps coherence at the center.

In entering the fourth chakra, we transcend ego in order to loosen our self-defined boundaries and merge into the ecstasy of love. There is no greater way to invite love than to offer it first. Since it is something we all want and need, we gravitate towards those with whom we feel safe and appreciated. To offer that safety and acceptance to another invites the field of love to flourish. To offer loving energy, whether as verbal compliments, empathic acknowledgments, or physical nurturing, invites similar energy to be returned. Those who seek money or power are often merely seeking a way to receive love, usually in the form of admiration or acknowledgment. Going straight to the acknowledgement can bypass some of the less functional ways we behave in order to find love.

Love and approval are basic to our personal growth, as they promote self-acceptance—a necessary step to loving oneself. As young children we are conditioned and taught by approval, or lack thereof, from our parents. This feedback shapes our first ideas of who we are. "Oh, look what Sally made, isn't she creative?" This forms a positive feedback system. If I told you how nice you look today, you'd feel pleased. Most likely you'd want to find something nice to say to me as well. Then I would feel pleased. On it goes, each time making us feel more and more comfortable and appreciated by each other.

There are many things, however, which reduce the flow of loving energy from one person to another. Undue attachment to one person can reduce the flow of energy that could come from many others. Jealousy reduces the flow of love as it dictates that they must flow within narrow limits. Homophobia, ageism, and racism restrict love. "You cannot touch him—he's of the same sex!" "She's too old." "They are the wrong [color, size, or background]." Any of these demarcations destroy the understanding of oneness and interdependence that is integral to the heart chakra. If we see love as infinite, and approach it from abundance instead of scarcity, we see that in truth love is self-perpetuating.

Opening the heart chakra expands one's horizon for sharing loving energy. People of differing backgrounds are more likely to stimulate growth than those who are the same. The greater our understanding, the greater our capacity for love. The heart chakra perceives the world in its unity, not its separation.

Withholding usually decreases what we receive as well. It's a vicious cycle. "I don't think John likes me. He'd probably think I was silly if I said how much I admired him." Meanwhile, John is thinking about how cold and detached you are. Breaking this cycle removes some of the blocks between people on a heart chakra level. With third chakra empowerment literally under our belts, it is easier to make the first move.

Rejection is one of the most basic of human fears. This is not surprising when you consider how important it is that our core center remain healthy. Rejection threatens our basic internal balance and sense of self-acceptance. If the heart chakra is the integrator, then rejection may cause us to "dis-integrate." Our positive feedback system is short-circuited. We turn this "non-love" against ourselves and start to self-destruct. Instead of feeling connected, we are cut off, separate, and isolated. For some it is easier to live without love altogether than to risk opening, sharing, and failing.

This fear is integral to the understanding of the heart chakra. It works as a protective device, helping to balance the flow of input and output. It is the gatekeeper of the delicate heart chakra energy. Maintaining this gate, however, is a two-edged sword. The input and output of energy in a chakra increase together. The more tightly our gate closes, the more we restrict the passage of energy through all the chakras. This restriction not only inhibits energy passage to and from the outside world, but simultaneously restricts the flow between our upper and lower chakras, causing alienation between our minds and bodies. Eventually, the heart chakra becomes depleted, and we have walled ourselves into a world alone.

Learning to love takes energy on many levels. We need all of our chakras functioning in order to create and maintain it. We must be able to feel, we must be able to communicate, we must be able to have our own autonomy and power, and we need to be able to see and understand. Most important, we need to relax and let it happen. The heart chakra is yin, and sometimes the most profound love is that which can simply let things be the way they are.

Love is the expansion and equilibrium of air, the new dawn of the east, the gentleness of the dove, the spirit of peace. It is the field that envelops us. Through it we find our center, our core, our power, and our reason for living.

Love is not a matter of getting connected; it is a matter of seeing that we already are connected within an intricate web of relationships that extends throughout life. It is a realization of "no boundaries"—that we are all made of the same essence, riding through time on the same planet, faced with the same problems, the same hopes and fears. It is a connection at the core that makes irrelevant skin color, age, sex, looks, or money.

More than anything, love is the deep sense of spiritual connection, the sense of being touched, moved, and inspired to heights beyond our normal limits. It is a connection with a deep, fundamental truth that runs through all of life and connects us together. Love makes the mundane sacred—so that it is cared for and protected. When we lose our sense of connection with all life, we have lost the sacred, and we no longer care for and protect that which nourishes us.

We are that love. We are its life force, its expression, its manifestation, its vehicle. Through it we grow, we transcend, we triumph, and surrender to grow again even deeper. We are renewed, cut down, and renewed again. It is the force of the eternal, the stabilizer. Blessings be to the central wheel of life from which all others turn.

RELATIONSHIP AND BALANCE

The ideal situation for really understanding another is not so much how a person reacts to extreme stress, but rather how he or she suffers the vulnerability of falling in love.

—Aldo Carotenuto[4]

At the level of the fourth chakra, we step out of the minute cycles of the lower chakras and gain an overview of how they function together. Isvara, the deity within this lotus, is the God of Unity, representing the interdependence of the three fundamental tendencies (tamas, rajas, and sattvas). He represents the balance of these three qualities, sometimes thought of as illusion, for this state of balance is always in flux. To move from separation into unity first requires entering into relationship.

Let's review the building of our structure thus far, seeing the relationship among the lower chakras. Chakra one is about material objects that are separate, distinct, and solid. These objects range in size from subatomic particles (inasmuch as they can even be called objects) to planets and stars. At chakra two, we looked at how objects moved—the forces that acted on them. At chakra three, we looked at the reorganization that occurs from this movement as objects collide, change structure, combust, and release energy. We then saw how everything has these cycles within it, combining to form larger structures.

These cycles can only continue when they are in a certain kind of *relationship*. Poles do not attract when they are too far apart to be relevant. Not all fuel catches fire. There is a larger force that keeps these subroutines functioning—the force of chakra four—a force we call love. This force perpetuates the eternal dance of relationship, so that the smaller components can continue their subroutines and keep us functioning. Love for the body motivates us to take care of our physical needs. In a family, love keeps its members together, so they can conduct the business of life and raise their children. For a group, love of a common cause keeps its members relating, so they can accomplish their tasks. Love of learning makes us buy books or go to school. *It is love that keeps us in relationship.*

This mysterious force is full of paradox. It has gravitation as well as radiation. We *fall* in love, yet are *lifted* by the experience. Love binds together without limiting. It requires both closeness and distance. It is the essence of balance and equilibrium—dwelling at the core of each of us.

As our smaller patterns and cycles repeat, they are perceived and regulated by the mind, which, acting through the will, ensures their continuity. We see these aspects in terms of their relationships—we see the space between, rather than the things themselves. We view the world as an interlocking puzzle.

As between each of the chakras, the primary difference between the third and the fourth is one of awareness. Through the creation and repetition of pattern, the organism becomes self-aware. Our lower chakra activity has influenced and created consciousness. We have acted according to our instincts and emotions, learning from our mistakes. Our learning becomes ever more complex and is stored in the higher centers as concepts, memory, and logic, to descend downward again, where our consciousness can influence our actions.

Relationship is the interface between matter and information, and plays a part in all the levels that lie between. In fact, all information could be regarded as awareness of relationship. These patterns give us the concepts which form the basic structure of our thoughts, communication and perception. They are the foundation of who we are. The fourth chakra level of consciousness perceives the world as an intricate web of relationships, bound together by the force of love.

Once we perceive objects and their activities as relationships, we begin to perceive the perfection, balance, and eternal nature of these relationships. In viewing the planets, for example, we see an endless cycle of relationships, perfectly coordinated and balanced—the planets in orbit moving in balance with the pull of the sun, repeating their patterns eternally. We see each of the stars in its place in the heavens, though moving and pulsating; each blade of grass covers its own spot of turf, though it dies each year and is reborn.

As we perceive patterns in this way, we see that *all lasting patterns are a product of a dynamic equilibrium among its parts.* We then find each element of life woven into a greater pattern, each in its own place. We can then seek a point of balance between ourselves and our surroundings. This point becomes an integral part of the whole, giving it the coherence of a mandala, emanating from a central point. When we understand the perfection of the relationships around us, it beckons the heart to open.

In our interpersonal relationships, the same rule of balance applies. Relationships endure when an overall balance is maintained. They end when one or both partners feels the relationship has gotten out of balance and does not have the capacity to return. This can be due to an imbalance of taking and giving, an imbalance in basic life force, in spiritual evolution, money, sex, power, housework, childcare, communication, or any of the other elements that play out in the arena of relationship. It must be remembered that this balance is dynamic rather than static— it fluctuates over time. It is the overall totality that must contain a basic parity if the relationship is to survive.

Balance within ourselves gives us the best shot at maintaining balance in our relationships with others. Inner balance allows us to perceive and enter the equilibrium within the ordered pattern of the mandala, which then becomes a point of openness and stability. Neither the mind nor the body, nor any single chakra can do it alone. It must be done with the fullness of the heart as the center of being.

When the will has consciously tempered and fulfilled our needs, our mind can better enter into an understanding of relationship, and we find our "proper place." From this place, all our relationships, as well as their beginnings and endings, are in harmony with a greater pattern. Relationships with the greatest equilibrium and, therefore, the most grace, will necessarily be the most enduring. The ones that are more transitory are stepping stones in the swirling creation of a larger pattern.

This realization of perfection opens the heart to receive.

Each chakra receives its charge of energy by being in alignment with the sushumna, as the central column of energy. If we are not in balance with ourselves, our chakras fall out of alignment, much as the vertebrae in the spine can fall out of alignment. Unfortunately, there are no "chakra-practors" to put them back in place. This is something we must do ourselves.

The heart chakra, as the exact center of the personal mandala, suffers the greatest loss, and causes the greatest damage if it should fall too far out of its place. Imbalances within the heart (the central core) can throw the entire system off balance. Not only is balance between the upper and lower chakras and between the mind and body necessary, but also between inner and outer, between self and transcendence. In order to love there must be a certain transcendence of ego and loss of separateness that allows us to experience a greater unity. We give up some of our individuality for this union.

As this union is facilitated by moving along the liberating current, we experience the freeing, exhilarating effect of love—the union, the transcendence, a sacred and somewhat altered state of consciousness. Falling out of love is a return to a smaller place, the mundane self, alone and separated, fallen from the grace and idyllic high of this love state. We, therefore, become attached to maintaining the state of love.

The risk of the exhilarating lift of love is that we can easily lose our ground. In order to maintain love, we need a ground from which to nourish it and provide roots. We must retain a part of the individual self—a part of the substance from which passion and will emerge. If we transcend our separateness too much, we are no longer fully present. We have separated the flame from the fuel, and we come crashing down to Earth as it burns out. We have tipped our balance and we can no longer offer substance to the relationship at hand. When we lose ourselves, we lose our center, we lose our own heart, and displace our relationship to our loved ones. In the words of D. H. Lawrence, ". . . if one yields oneself up to the other entirely, there is a guttering mess. You have to balance love and individuality, and actually sacrifice a portion of each."[5]

Living in balance is living in a state of grace, of delicacy, of gentleness. Love is that which endures, and likewise, what is done with love will endure. That which is out of balance will not endure. Only by being balanced within ourselves can we hope to balance the world.

To maintain our balance we must be aware of all our parts. This is not something that occurs in an intellectual fashion, like taking inventory in a storeroom. Instead, it comes from a dynamic experience of our center—the heart itself—which organically organizes and balances if given the freedom to do so.

Lastly, the heart chakra needs to be balanced between input and output. Just as the breath equalizes its inhalations and exhalations, so, too, must our energy replenish itself in order to keep giving. When handled properly, there is an infinite supply of energy through any chakra. Love multiplies as it is given. Yet many people lose their alignment by giving too much, losing their ground, or giving when their energy is depleted. We are taught that selfishness is bad—that it is wrong to balance our accounts from time to time. Yet altering our own balance can alter the symmetry of the mandala around us. Constant overdrawing of the account can deplete the resources until we can't give at all. Then we can have a backlash that is not very loving at all.

In balance between all things, we need to get out of the polarities of "good" and "evil." We need not be puritanically good to stroke our delicate egos, nor need we be selfishly evil. True love flows from one center to another, allowing each the freedom to dance their own part in their own unique way. As Anahata is a yin chakra, one of its challenges is to allow "letting" to replace "doing" or "making." Only then can we truly perceive the pattern for what it is.

Love is not something that is attached to an object. Love is a state of being in harmony with oneself. Ken Dychtwald, after an extended fast where he meditated on the subject of love, came to describe it this way.

> *Love seems to be the appreciation that we are all little lumps in the same earthly soup which is a little lump in a larger cosmic soup. So, love is an awareness of this beautiful energetic relationship and a natural appreciation of this situation. It doesn't seem to be a matter of finding love . . . it's a matter of being aware of it. It's not a question of invention but rather of discovery.[6]*

Love is the natural relationship between healthy living things. We need only to believe that it is around us at all times and in all things to find it within ourselves.

AFFINITY

Affinity is a term used in chemistry to describe the tendency of one substance to enter into and remain in combination with another substance. This occurs because of an intrinsic fit within the atomic structure of the substance.

The result of affinity is bonding. When two substances with affinity for each other come together, they bond, forming a more permanent connection. Each has something the other is lacking. On a simplified level, it is the attraction of opposites seeking to balance themselves.

Human bonding can be so similar to chemical bonding that we often refer to it as "chemistry." We may not always understand why we feel drawn toward someone, but the feeling is there, nonetheless, and it is often irresistible.

Most often, the person has something in his or her energy field that we want and need. If we're lucky, we have something they need too, and a bonding can occur, good for the duration of the affinity feelings. As the heart chakra is the center of balance, it is fitting that love itself arises, initially, out of a natural tendency to merge and balance our energy with other living creatures.

Often this balance can be analyzed in terms of chakras. We've all felt the nonverbal ads: "White male, thirty-two, with dominant upper chakra awareness seeks grounded female; guaranteed to raise Kundalini;" or "Black female, highly creative, seeks second chakra partner for TLC." While these ads are not written in words in the newspaper, they are broadcasted at parties, and our psychic senses pick them up each time we meet someone.

This is not to say that we have an affinity only for those who are opposite to us. Many times, finding someone that shares our views can also give us that feeling of affinity—the peaceful sense of validation that comes from finding one who understands. The energy we project outward finds a matching energy reaching in. Again, our chakras, both open and closed, are searching for balance. It is not based on polarity as much as the organism seeking enhancement for its next stage of unfoldment. (See chapter 11, "Chakras and Relationships.")

The most important aspect of affinity, however, lies not in our chemical attraction to others, but in the development of affinity within the composite parts of the self. When we have this sense of affinity, we emanate a vibration that is loving, accepting, and joyful. This allows, and even encourages others to find their own sense of affinity.

So many people have minds that constantly war with their body: "You're too fat." "Work harder. Not until you finish this project can you rest." "What do you mean you're hungry? I just fed you an hour ago!" Many people take control of their bodies in a way that is harsh and unyielding.

The body, too, can war with the mind, like a spoiled child constantly demanding attention. "Feed me." "I'm too tired." Then, like a child, it needs to be "unspoiled," but in a way that is nurturing and supportive, making sure that the child gets the basic things it needs.

Self-acceptance is our first chance to practice unconditional love. It doesn't mean that we have to give up striving to be better, but that our self-love is not conditional on some future or imagined change. When this occurs within our heart, it then becomes easier to accept others, faults and all, with the unconditional love of the heart chakra. With acceptance and compassion for ourselves, it then becomes easier to make personal changes.

Affinity can also be seen as a vibrational quality. When we are "in affinity," the harmonious state we feel gives coherency to everything we say or do, like the tones of a scale in harmonic resonance. We radiate love because we have created a coherent center within ourselves, which in turn harmonizes the surrounding circumstances.

In the organ of the heart, each cell is beating continuously. If we were to dissect the heart, each cell would continue to beat by itself. As soon as we put these cells together with other heart cells (as on a microscope slide), the cells shift their rhythm so that they are pulsating together. They enter a state of rhythmic resonance (something we will discuss more fully in the fifth chakra). By tuning into our heartbeat, we tune ourselves into the resonance with the core rhythm of our organism and the rhythm of the world around us.

So how does one go about creating this sense of affinity? By taking a little quiet time to talk to yourself. All it really takes is checking in with yourself now and then. After you read these words, take time to close your eyes and take a deep breath, and say hello to your body. See if you get a hello in return. Begin a dialogue. Are there ways you could treat yourself better? Are there parts that need attention, parts that dominate unnecessarily? Do you treat yourself as well as you treat others? Is it time you threw a party to show your appreciation? Or do you need to just sit still and listen for awhile?

If there is strength in numbers, it is only when those numbers are united. We have many composite parts to ourselves. Our very strength lies in the unity and harmony within those parts. Only then are we able to effectively give to others. If those parts are all tuned into the center—the heart of the organism—they then are simultaneously tuned to each other and enter a natural state of affinity.

HEALING

Consciously or unconsciously every being is capable of healing himself or others. This instinct is inborn in insects, birds, and beasts, as well as in man. All these find their own medicine and heal themselves and each other in various ways.

—Sufi Inayat Khan[7]

To heal is to make whole. If the heart chakra is the integrator and unifier, then it follows that it is also the center of healing. Indeed, love is the ultimate healing force.

As we come up to the heart chakra, we encounter the arms. Upright, with arms outstretched, the body forms a kind of cross, the four points of which meet in the heart. (See Figure 5.4, page 211.) Just as the legs are connected to chakra one, the arms are an integral part of the middle chakras three, four, and five. The inside, yin channels of the arms contain three of the fourteen Chinese energy channels, called meridians. These particular meridians correspond to the heart, lungs, and pericardium (a loose sack covering the heart). (See Figure 5.5, page 212.) Obviously, these are all relevant to the heart chakra, and they carry energy from that center down to the arms and hands.

The channels of energy moving out from the heart toward the hands I call the healing channels, the means by which healing energy reaches out to others. There are also minor chakras in the hands. Hands are very sensitive extensions of the body/mind, having far more neural receptors than most parts of the body. The hands both create and receive and are sensory organs pulling in as much information as the eyes and ears. They are valuable tools in the perception and control of psychic energy. (To open the hand chakras, see the exercise on page 20.)

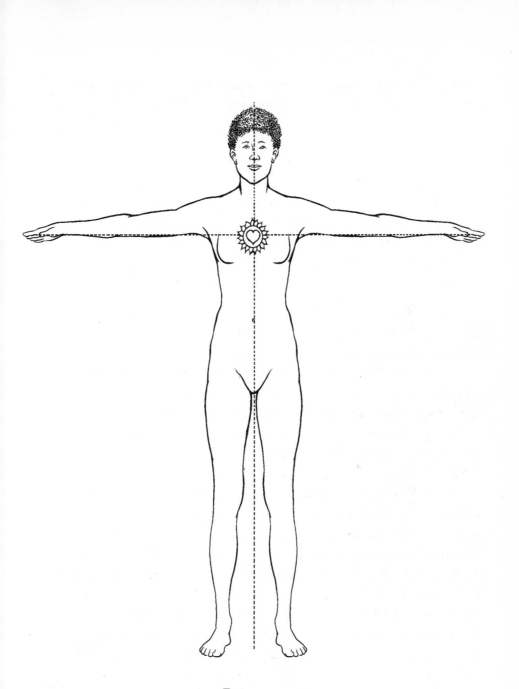

Figure 5.4
The cross of the heart chakra.

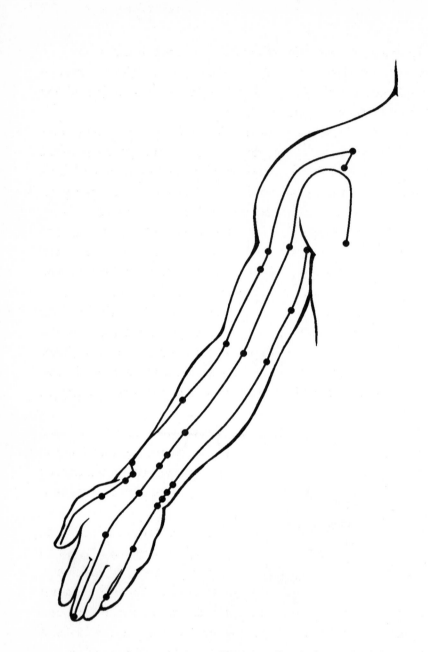

FIGURE 5.5
Meridians of the arm.

Healing is the restoration of balance to an organism or situation. It is believed that all disease, whether caused by germ, injury or stress, is the result of an "imbalance" that then fragments the organism and destroys its natural resonant affinity.

Opening the heart chakra and developing compassion, connection, and understanding for those around you naturally gives rise to the urge to heal. The realization that we are all one dictates that, like a Bodhisattva, we cannot advance alone while others are ailing. (A Bodhisattva is someone who is spiritually realized but avoids crossing into enlightenment until others can follow, instead staying behind to teach.) Like the Bodhisattva, we find we must take the time to heal others as we advance along our path. This brings into balance the lure of spirituality and the need to remain in the physical world.

Helping others also arises from a simple state of compassion—the center of the heart chakra. Through nonjudgmental compassion for others we cannot help but reach out in a healing manner. Our vision of the balance of all things underlines anything which is not in harmony with that balance. It is as natural as straightening a picture on the wall.

One need not be a professional healer, doctor, or possess supernatural power in order to have their healing channels open. The natural urge to help an elderly woman cross the street, comfort someone in tears, or rub a pair of tired shoulders is a potent expression of the heart chakra's healing energy.

Many people forget the lesson of balance in their healing efforts. You might call them meddlers. To properly heal someone, it is necessary that they come into balance with their own energy, which may not comply with the healer's concept of "correct." A true healer must tune into her subject, remaining grounded in her own energy, and allowing the subject to create his own sense of balance. The healer is merely a catalyst in the subject's own healing experience. When our heart chakras are open and balanced, our very presence radiates love and joy. This love is the essence of true healing.

BREATH—THE HEART OF LIFE

If your breathing is in any way restricted, to that degree, so is your life.

—Michael Grant White[8]

A normal human being inhales between 18,000 and 20,000 breaths per day,[9] totaling an average of 5,000 gallons of air. In weight alone, this is thirty-five times as much as we take in from food or drink. We can go weeks without food, days without water, hours without heat (in extreme cold) but only minutes without air. (How long can we go without thought?)

Breath, as related to the element air, is one of the primary keys to opening the heart chakra. Air is also the most quickly distributed element in the body. Unlike food, which takes hours or even days to digest, each inhalation of air immediately enters the bloodstream. Oxygen must be constantly supplied to each and every cell, or the cells quickly die. For this reason the body has a thorough and elaborate transportation system to distribute oxygen throughout the entire body. This is our circulatory system, mastered by the heart. Each breath nourishes and feeds this system.

The full importance of the breath cannot be expressed by these simple facts. Aside from maintaining basic life functions, the breath is one of our most powerful tools for transforming ourselves: for burning up toxins, releasing stored emotions, changing body structure and changing consciousness. Without breath we could not speak, for air is the force behind our voice. We could not metabolize our food without oxygen. Our brain could not think. Breathing is a grossly underestimated source of life-giving, healing, and purifying energy.

Unfortunately, the average person does not breathe very deeply. A normal pair of lungs can hold about two pints of air, while the average person breathes in about one pint or less per breath. You can confirm this for yourself by taking a normal breath and then seeing how much more air you can add to it. While you're doing this, notice how it feels to breathe deeply. Notice what parts of the chest feel tight, how it con-stricts the breath, and give those parts some gentle massage. Freeing up the chest and upper back through massage or emotional release helps to deepen the breath.

Most intellectual activity, since it requires so little physical exer-tion, leads to shallow breathing, which then becomes a habit. Frequent fear, anxiety, depression, smoking, or simply polluted air also lead to habitual breath deprivation. This habit, once formed, leads to slower metabolism, lower physical energy levels, and builds up toxins in the body, all of which contribute to a self-perpetuating cycle. As our metabolism is lowered we become lethargic, leading to greater reliance on conveniences such as driving when you could walk, ingesting stim-ulants for more energy, or smoking cigarettes to (paradoxically) stim-ulate the chest.[10] None of these things helps the breath.

The brain, too, relies critically on a constant source of oxygen. In the resting body, one-fourth of the oxygen consumed is used by the brain, even though it is only one-fiftieth of the body's mass. [11] Hold your breath and see how long you remain conscious.

The breath is also one of the few things in the body that comes under both voluntary and involuntary control. Involuntarily, the breath contracts when we are afraid—a carryover from survival instincts, when holding the breath helped us remain undetected by dangerous creatures. Similarly, we can combat fear by forcibly deepen-ing our breath, thus easing tension in our whole body.

By exercising the voluntary aspect and consciously trying to increase our breathing capacity, we gradually make deep breathing a habit. The breath can actually change the body structure, and once changed, the body hungers for this increased oxygen supply. It is an evolutionary and healing-oriented process.

The Hindus believe that breath is a gateway between the mind and body. Whole systems of yoga have been built on breathing techniques, called *pranayama*, which are designed to expand consciousness and purify the body. When the thoughts are quiet, the breath is calm as well, and a soothing and healing rhythm runs throughout the whole body. The mind also can be calmed through control of the breath. The flow of breath, as it constantly enters and leaves the body, is a dynamically moving energy field that continually fills your body shape, and returns, formless again, to the outside world.

Pranayama techniques are designed to nourish the psychic and spiritual pathways in the body, such as the major nadis and acupuncture meridians. These channels are charged by this process, and raise the subtle vibrations within the entire organism. Yogis make a distinction between the gross physical ingestion of air *(sthula prana)* and the subtle movement of energy that results from the breath *(sukshma prana)*. It is important in doing breathwork to pay attention to the subtler movements that occur. We can then direct that energy toward specific areas or chakras through visualization or use of postures.

Breathing Exercises

Pranayama breathing exercises are many and varied. If you are really interested in working with this powerful tool, there are several books on yoga that list more exercises than there is room for here. A few basic exercises follow:

Deep breathing, or the complete breath

This is as simple as it sounds. Sit down in any comfortable position and watch the path of your breath, making both inhalation and exhalation as full as possible. Breathe deep into your belly, then into your chest and finally into your shoulders and throat. Exhale, reversing the order, and repeat several times.

Breath of fire

This is a rapid, diaphragmatic breathing using fast, short breaths created by snapping in the muscles of your abdomen in rapid succession, described more fully in the third chakra on page 176.

Alternate nostril breathing

This is a slow, methodical breath which works on the central nervous system and leads to increased relaxation and deeper sleep. Close off your right nostril with your right hand and breathe deeply through your left nostril. When the breath is full, close off your left nostril and exhale through your right side. When the breath is again empty, inhale again through your right side, switching when full and exhaling on the left. The pattern is to inhale, switch, exhale, inhale, switch, exhale. Continue this 20 times or more on each side. Practicing this exercise brings profound changes in consciousness.

Bandhas

"Bandha" means lock, and the bandhas of pranayama are methods of holding the breath and locking it into certain parts of the body. There are three basic bandhas: the chin lock, the abdominal lock, and the anal lock that work on retention of the breath in the three major areas of the body.

The chin lock, or *jalandhara-bandha*, sends energy into the head, and stimulates the thyroid gland and throat chakra. Simply inhale fully, contract the throat, and lower your head toward your chest, keeping the back straight. Hold the breath as long as comfortable, but don't push it, for it can make you feel quite faint if done improperly.

The abdominal lock, or *uddiyana-bandha* is done in a standing position. It helps to massage internal digestive organs, and purify the body. Inhale fully and exhale deeply. While the body is empty of air, hold your breath empty, and pull in the stomach and abdomen as far as you can, being careful not to inhale. Hold as long as comfortable, and inhale by slowly relaxing the abdominal muscles.

The *mulabandha* or anal lock tones the root chakra. It is

practiced by tightening the perineum and anal sphincter after inhalation while the breath is held. This stimulates sleeping Kundalini.

CHAKRA FOUR EXERCISES

Chest Opener

Put your arms behind your back, clasp your hands together and rotate your arms so that your elbows lock. This should press your shoulders back and your chest out. Take a deep breath. Throw your head back and use your arms as momentum to rotate your torso, loosening the tight muscles you may have there. Continue your deep breathing. (See Figure 5.6, page 219.)

For added stretching and opening of the pectoral muscles around the chest, grab a belt, towel, or tie and hold it overhead with your arms forming a triangle. Keeping your elbows straight, stretch your arms back behind you, still holding the belt to provide a good stretch. If you cannot keep your elbows straight, move the hands farther apart on the belt. If you cannot feel a good stretch, move the hands closer together.

The Cobra

This is a yogic exercise, wonderful to do upon first waking up in the morning. It works on the upper thoracic vertebrae, and helps alleviate the rounded back that comes from a collapsed chest.

Lie flat on your stomach with arms bent and palms placed face down by your shoulders. Without using your arms as support, slowly lift your head, shoulders, and back as far as you can go comfortably. Then relax. Lift again, going as far

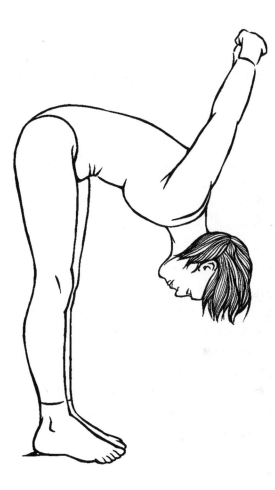

FIGURE 5.6
Chest Opener.

as you can, and then using your arms, push yourself up just a little farther. Do not straighten the elbows completely, but work to open the chest, keeping the shoulders down and relaxed, the head held high. Stretch the stomach and chest, take a deep breath and relax. Repeat as often as you like. (See Figure 5.7, page 221.)

The Fish

This is another yoga asana, designed to expand the chest cavity. Begin by lying flat on your back and stretch the legs along the floor. Place your hands just under your hips, palms down. Pressing down against the elbows, lift the chest upward, arching the neck back and touching the head (if possible) to the floor. Breathe deeply. Hold as long as is comfortable and then relax. Breathe deeply again. (See Figure 5.8, page 221.)

(If this is too difficult, you can place a bolster behind your shoulder blades and arch over it to loosen the upper spine.)

The Windmill

We have all done this exercise as little children. Stand with arms stretched outward to each side and twist the torso back and forth. This sends energy from the body down into the arms and hands, and loosens the tight muscles of the chest and abdomen.

Arm Circles

This stimulates the muscles of the upper arms and upper back (the wings). Stretch the arms out straight to each side and rotate in small circles in one direction, gradually moving to larger and larger circles. Then switch directions and repeat. You can also (in keeping with the element of air) pretend you are flapping your arms like wings and flying, taking deep, deep breaths as you do. (See Figure 5.9, page 223.)

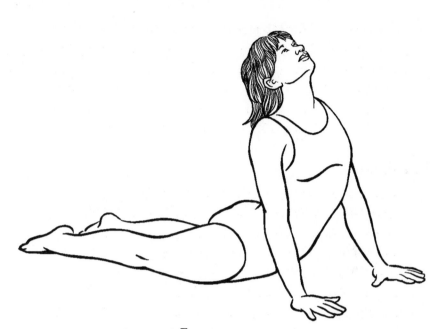

FIGURE 5.7
The Cobra.

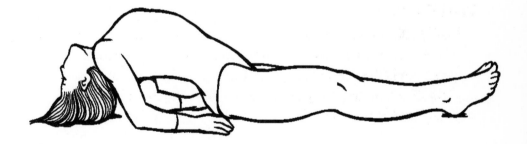

FIGURE 5.8
The Fish.

Opening the Hand Chakras

Since the heart chakra energy is so often expressed through the hands, the exercise on page 20 is also relevant to the heart chakra.

MEDITATIONS

Kalpataru—The Wishing Tree

(A note of caution for this exercise: Be careful what you ask for—you may get it.)

Just below the heart chakra is a tiny lotus of eight petals, the Anandakanda Lotus, within which is the "celestial wishing tree" from the Heaven of Indra, the *Kalpataru*. This magic tree, in front of which is a jeweled altar, is said to hold the deepest wishes of the heart—not what we think we want, but the deeper longing of the soul within. It is believed that when we truly wish upon this tree, and release those wishes, the Kalpataru bestows even more than is desired, leading to freedom *(moksa)*.

Lie down comfortably. Take a few moments to ground yourself, get centered, relax your muscles. Make sure you are in an environment that feels safe and comfortable.

Breathe deeply, in . . . and out . . . in . . . and out . . . in . . . and out . . . Become aware of your heartbeat. Listen to its rhythm. Imagine each pulsation of your heart pumping blood all through your body, through the intricate network of arteries and veins. Imagine each of these pathways above your heart as branches of a tree, below your heart, as roots to the tree, teeming with life. Follow the path of oxygen as it is pumped out through the heart, out through your chest, your shoulders, down your arms, into your hands, and back again. Follow it again down your belly, your legs, knees and feet, and back up again through your body, and home, to the core. Every drop of blood that passes through the heart returns to be refreshed again with breath, air, and life.

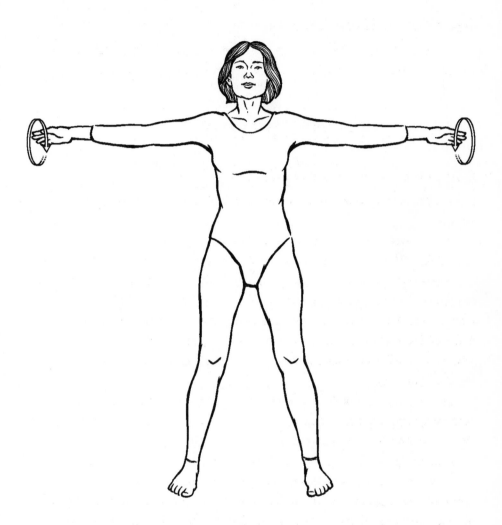

FIGURE 5.9
Arm Circles.

Your heart is a sacred tree. Its branches are threads of a web of life extending all through your body, and then out into the world. The trunk of the tree is you—your core, your being, your central self. From this core dig roots, the foundation of the tree. Their pathways find the food and water that support and give us substance. From this core spring branches, their leaves but wishes of the heart. They collect the sun and wind that make you grow. They flower and fruit and fall upon the ground to grow again. All that is expressed eventually returns.

In front of this tree, lies a jeweled altar. Make an offering to this altar, either something you are willing to give up, like a bad habit, or something you are willing to give of yourself, like creativity, loyalty, or healing. Make this offering as a symbol of exchange for granting your wish.

Next, breathe into your heart and feel its pain and joy. Feel the deep longings of the soul within. Do not define this longing specifically, but feel its essence. Let the feelings increase, breathing into them. Feel them through your whole body, pulsing outward, returning, pulsing outward again. Allow this longing to fill the branches of the tree.

When the tree is saturated with the deepest wishes of your heart, imagine that a single bird comes into the tree. The bird flies to the center of the tree, cocks its head to one side, cocks its head to the other, and listens deeply to the longing and wishes that have been expressed. Have a moment of communion with this bird that lives inside your heart. As you do, hold the bird close into your heart and let your heart (not your mind) speak its wishes to the bird. Let it come from the yearning; if specific images come to mind, fine, but don't search for them. When you feel complete, kiss the bird good-bye and gently release it to fly away. Set it free to do your work. Let it go and forget about it. The bird will carry your wishes to the powers that be, so that they may be fulfilled in the best way possible for all concerned.

Appreciation Ritual

Make a circle with a group of friends you feel close to, who are all close to each other; or sit opposite a lover or friend with whom you have a deep connection.

Cast a circle if you are magically oriented, or take some time to ensure that your time and space will be protected from distraction. Take time to ground and center, breathe deeply and relax.

Look around the circle. Look into the eyes of each one there, one at a time. Think about that person's value in your life—the experiences you have had together, the trials, the joys. Think about those experiences from their point of view: what their struggles were, their fears, their joys. Take as much time as is necessary and then close your eyes and go inside.

Beginning in the east of the circle, take the person sitting there and put them in the middle. Let everyone else in the circle chant their name three or four times, softly. After the chanting, beginning with the person to the left of where the subject was standing, go around clockwise, and let each person take a few moments to tell the one in the middle what they appreciate about them. "I really liked the time you helped me get my car started." "I appreciate the way you always listen." "I like the way you make me laugh." Do not allow any comments, criticism, or suggestions. Do allow hugs and gifts if they feel appropriate.

When you've been all the way around the circle with appreciation, the person in the middle calls the name of the next person, and returns to the circle as the group chants that name, and the whole process is repeated until each member of the group has had a turn in the middle. Ground and close the circle with a chant, a sharing of food and drink, music, if possible, and of course, a group hug.

Empathy Exercise

This exercise is often a good one for couples who are having problems with each other over a specific issue. To do this, imagine you are the person you are having trouble with. Tell the story from his or her point of view, beginning, middle, and end. Put yourself in the other person's place as you do. Ask if you got it right, or if you left out anything important. Then switch roles and have the other person tell your story from your point of view.

Compassion Meditation

This meditation can be done alone (with imagination), with a group, or best of all, in a crowded place like a bus station, restaurant, or park bench.

Pick a spot to sit comfortably and relax. Close your eyes, center yourself, and begin breathing deeply, down into your belly, down into your feet, down into the Earth. Tune into your heartbeat and feel its rhythm pulsing all through your body. Breathe into it, feeling your heart, accepting yourself unconditionally, filling yourself with love, and exhale.

Open your eyes and look around you. Look at each person you can focus on clearly, one at a time, looking at their eyes, listening to their voice, watching their actions. (If alone, imagine someone you know or see often.) Using the breath to keep things circulating through your body, look at each person without judgment, criticism, aversion or desire. Just look at them and allow yourself to focus on their heart. Look at how the body has shaped itself around that heart—imagine its hopes and dreams, its buried sorrows and fears. Allow a sense of compassion to build up within your heart for that person. Breathe into it, let yourself feel it, but don't hang on to it. Breathe it out again with each exhalation.

Without words or movement, imagine a beam of energy running from your heart to theirs. Send them love, and then release it. Do not hang on to the connection or make yourself responsible in any way. Let the bond go, and then move on to someone else.

When you've had enough, close your eyes and return to your own center. Feel your own heart in the same way you looked at the others. Give yourself the same sense of compassion and love. Breathe into it, sending it deeper. Release.

ENDNOTES

1. Helpful to have drum beat as heart rhythm.

2. Katha Upanishad, *The Upanishads,* (NY: Dover Publications, 1962). 11.6.15 from Max Muller.

3. Pierre Teilhard de Chardin, *Let Me Explain*, 66.

4. Aldo Carotenuto, *Eros and Pathos: Shades of Love and Suffering,* (Toronto: Inner City Books, 1989), 54.

5. D.H. Lawrence, "The Stream of Desire," in *Challenge of the Heart,* John Welwood, 48.

6. Ken Dychtwald, *Body-Mind,* 149.

7. Sufi Inayat Khan, *The Development of Spiritual Healing*, 89.

8. Michael Grant White, "The Breathing Coach" is known to me personally as an expert extraordinaire on the breath. This quote was taken from his website at www.breathing.com

9. Swami Rama, Rudolph Ballentine, M.D., Alan Hymes, M.D., *Science of Breath, a Practical Guide,* 59.

10. I find that smoking gives one a false impression of energy in the heart chakra, and often comes out of a need to mask an emptiness that otherwise resides there. Of course, it does not solve the problem, but merely enables one to cope with maintaining the emptiness.

11. Isaac Asimov, *The Human Brain: Its Capacities and Functions.*

RECOMMENDED READING FOR CHAKRA FOUR

Farhi, Donna. *The Breathing Book: Vitality and Good Health through Essential Breath Work.* NY: Henry Holt, 1996.

Hendricks, Gay. *Conscious Breathing: Breathwork for Health, Stress Release, and Personal Mastery.* NY: Bantam, 1995.

Hendricks, Gay, Ph.D. and Kathlyn Hendricks, Ph.D. *Conscious Loving: The Journey to Co-commitment.* NY: Bantam, 1990.

Stone, Hal, Ph.D. and Sidra Winkelman, Ph.D. *Embracing Each Other: Relationship as Teacher, Healer, and Guide.* Mill Valley, CA: Nataraj Publishing, 1989.

Welwood, John. *Challenge of the Heart.* Boston, MA: Shambhala, 1985.

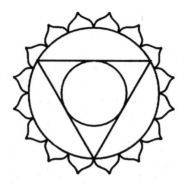

CHAKRA FIVE

Ether

Sound

Vibration

Communication

Mantras

Telepathy

Creativity

Chapter 6

CHAKRA FIVE: SOUND

OPENING MEDITATION

*Before the beginning, all was
darkness and all was void
The face of the cosmos was deep and
unmanifest,
Indeed, not a face at all but endless
nothing.
No light, no sound, no movement, no
life, no time.
All was null and the universe was not
yet created*

Nor even conceived.
For there was no form in which to conceive or be conceived

In its emptiness the darkness fell upon itself
And became aware that it was nothing.
Alone and dark, unborn, unmanifest, silent.
Can you imagine this silence, the silence of nothing?
Can you quiet yourself enough to hear it?
Can you listen to the silence within you?

Breathe deeply, but slowly so the breath is silent in your lungs.
Feel your throat expand with the air coming in.
Listen for the nothing, listen for the quiet,
Listen deep within yourself for the place of stillness.
Slowly breathe into this void, a deep and peaceful breath.
In its infinite quiet, darkness fell upon itself
And in its emptiness, knew itself to be alone
And alone it desired another
In this desire, a ripple moved across the void
to fold and fold again upon itself
Until it was no longer empty and the void was full with birth.

In the beginning the great, unmanifest
became vibration in its own recognition of being.
And that vibration was a sound from which all other sounds were born.
It came from Brahma in his first emanation.
It came from Sarasvati, in her eternal answers.
In their union, the sound arose and spread through all the void and filled
it.
And the sound became one, and the sound became many, and the sound
became the wheel that turned and turned the worlds unto the dance
of life, forever singing, always moving.

If you listen, you can hear it now. It is in your breath, it is in your heart, it
*   is in the wind, the waters, the trees and the sky. It is in your own*
*   mind, in the rhythm of each and every thought.*
From one sound does it all emerge and to one sound shall it return.
And the sound is
AUM . . . Aaa-ooo-uuu-mmmmmmmmm . . . Aum . . .

Chant it now inside you quietly. Let it build within your breath.
Let the sacred sound escape you, moving on the wings of air.
Rhythm building, deep vibration, rising up from deep within.
Chant the sound of all creation, sound that makes the chakras spin.
Louder now the voice arises, joins with other sounds and chants.
Deeper now the rhythms weaving all into a sacred dance.
Rhythms pounding, voices growing, echoing the dance of life.
Sounds to words and words to music, riding on the wheels of life.
Guiding us along our journey, moving spirit deep within.
Chant the voice that is within you. This is where we must begin.
Up from silence, breath and body, calling now into the void.
Hear its answer in the darkness, fear and pain have been destroyed.
Brahma is the first vibration, Sarasvati is the flow.
Sound unites us in our vision, harmonizing all we know.
Soon the silence comes again, with echoes of primordial sound,
Purifying all vibration, echo of the truth profound.

CHAKRA FIVE
SYMBOLS AND CORRESPONDENCES

Sanskrit Name:	Visuddha
Meaning:	Purification
Location:	Throat
Element:	Sound
Function:	Communication, creativity
Inner State:	Synthesis of ideas into symbols
Outer Manifestation:	Vibration
Glands:	Thyroid, parathyroid
Other Body Parts:	Neck, shoulders, arms, hands
Malfunction:	Sore throat, stiff neck, colds, thyroid problems, hearing problems
Color:	Bright blue
Sense:	Hearing
Seed Sound:	Ham
Vowel Sound:	Eee
Petals:	Sixteen, all the Sanskrit vowels
Sephira:	Geburah, Chesed
Planet:	Mercury
Metal:	Mercury
Foods:	Fruits
Corresponding Verb:	I speak
Yoga Path:	Mantra yoga
Herbs for Incense:	Frankincense, benzoin, mace
Minerals:	Turquoise, aquamarine, celestite
Animals:	Elephant, bull, lion

Guna:	Rajas
Lotus Symbols:	Downward triangle, within which is a white circle, thought to represent the full moon. In the circle is a white elephant, over which is the Bija symbol, *ham.* The deities in the lotus are Sadasiva, a three-eyed, five-faced, ten-armed form of Shiva, seated on a white bull, clothed in a tiger skin with garland of snakes. The Goddess is Gauri, shining one, consort of Shiva, thought by some to be a corn goddess. Gauri is also the name of a class of goddesses which includes Uma, Parvati, Rambha, Totala, and Tripura.
Hindu Deities:	Ganga (river goddess, related to purification), Sarasvati
Other Pantheons:	Hermes, the Muses, Apollo, Brigit, Seshat, Nabu
Chief Operating Quality:	Resonance

GATEWAY TO CONSCIOUSNESS

Sound . . . rhythm . . . vibration . . . words. Powerful rulers of our lives, we take these things for granted. Using them, responding to them, creating them anew each day, we are the subjects of rhythm upon rhythm, endlessly interweaving the fabric of experience. From the first cries of a newborn child to the harmonies of a symphony, we are immersed in an infinite web of communication.

Communication is the connecting principle that makes life possible. From the DNA encoded messages of living cells to the spoken or written word, from the nerve impulses connecting mind and body to the broadcast waves connecting continent to continent, communication is the coordinating principle of all life. It is the means whereby consciousness extends itself from one place to another.

Within the body, communication is crucial. Without electrical communication between brain waves and muscle tissue, we couldn't move. Without chemical communication of hormones to cells there would be no growth, no cues for cyclic changes, no defenses against disease. If it were not for the ability of DNA to communicate genetic information, life could not exist.

Our civilization is equally dependent on communication as the connecting fabric through which we coordinate the complex tasks of cooperative culture, much as the body's cells work together to form one organism. Our communication networks are a cultural nervous system, connecting us all.

Chakra five is the center related to communication through sound, vibration, self-expression, and creativity. It is the realm of consciousness that controls, creates, transmits, and receives communication, both within ourselves and between each other. It is the center of dynamic creativity, of synthesizing old ideas into something new. Its attributes include listening, speaking, writing, chanting, telepathy, and any of the arts—especially those related to sound and language.

Communication is the process of transmitting and receiving information through symbols. As written or spoken words, as musical patterns, omens, or electrical impulses to the brain, the fifth chakra is the center that translates these symbols into information. Communication, due to its symbolic nature, is an essential key to accessing the inner planes. With symbols, we have the means to represent the world in a more efficient way—one that gives us infinite storage capacity in the brain. We can discuss things before we do them; we can absorb and store information in a concise form; we can synthesize thoughts into concrete images and store the images again as thoughts—all through the symbolic representation of perceived patterns.

As we climb to this fifth level, we are taking yet another step away from the physical. Communication is our first level of physical transcendence in that it enables us to transcend the ordinary limitations of the body. By telephoning New York, we can avoid going there physically. The call takes only minutes, costs little, yet the limitations of time and space have been transcended as nonchalantly as if we were crossing the street. We can record voices on tape, read diaries of the deceased, and decipher ancient patterns in the DNA of fossils, all through an interpretation of symbols.

As stated earlier, the lower chakras are highly individual. Our bodies, for example, are clearly separate, with our edges defined by our skin. As we climb up the chakra column, our boundaries become less defined. When we reach pure consciousness, the ideal of the seventh chakra, it becomes impossible to draw a border around this consciousness and say, "This is mine, and that is yours." Information and ideas are like the breath we breathe—an invisible field surrounding us, from which we take what we need. There are no separations in this field. Each step upward decreases boundaries and separation and takes us closer to unity. *We arrive at this unity through the ability of consciousness to make connections.*

Communication is an act of connection. It is one of the uniting principles of the upper chakras. If I give a talk to a group of people on the subject of healing, I am uniting their consciousness, if only momentarily, around certain ideas. Due to the communication that has occurred, there is now a subset of information shared by all the people in the audience as they leave the hall. If I give the lecture several times, this subset of shared consciousness grows even larger. Previously diverging minds have information in common after communication has occurred.

Communication is a way of extending ourselves beyond our ordinary limitations. Through communication, information contained in your brain that is not in my brain becomes accessible to me. You may have never been to China, for example, but through the communication of books, movies, pictures, and conversations, you're still able to have some knowledge of China's customs and landscapes. As communication unites, it also expands, allowing our world to become larger. This expansion mirrors the pattern of the ascending current of consciousness.

In the descending direction of the chakras we are moving toward limitation and manifestation. We are taking patterns of thought and making them specific through the process of *naming*. Naming focuses consciousness by drawing limits around something, saying it is this and not that. To name a thing is to clarify it, to set its boundaries, to specify. Naming gives structure and meaning to our thoughts.

Communication shapes our reality and creates the future. If I say to you, "Bring me a glass of water," I am creating a future for myself which contains a glass of water in my hand. If I say, "Please leave me alone," I am creating a future without you. From presidential speeches and corporate board meetings to marital fights or children's bedtime stories, communication is creating the world at each and every moment.

It is clear that communication can direct consciousness in both directions of the chakra spectrum. Communicaton can be seen as a *symbolic system that mediates between the abstract and manifested idea.* It formulates our thoughts into controlled physical vibrations, which in turn can create manifestations on the physical plane. With words, consciousness has a tool through which it can order or organize the universe around it, including itself! Therefore, this chakra occupies a crucial place in the gateway between mind and body. It is not a central place of balance like the heart; rather it mirrors the transformative properties of fire—a medium in the transition from one dimension to another.

In this chapter we will explore communication from the theoretical to the practical. We will examine the principles of vibration, sound, mantras, language, telepathy, creativity, and media as petals in the lotus of the fifth chakra.

VISUDDHA—THE PURIFIER

O Devi! O Sarasvati!
Reside Thou ever in my speech.
Reside Thou ever on my tongue tip.
O Divine Mother, giver of faultless poetry.
—Swami Sivananda Radha[1]

The chakra of communication, commonly called the throat chakra, is located in the region of the neck and shoulders. Its color is blue—a bright, cerulean blue, as opposed to the indigo blue of chakra six. It is a lotus with sixteen petals, which contains all the vowels of the Sanskrit language. In Sanskrit, vowels are typically thought to represent spirit, while consonants represent the harder stuff of matter.

This lotus is called *Visuddha,* which means "purification." This implies two things about this center: 1) To successfully reach and open the fifth chakra, the body must attain a certain level of purification. The subtler aspects of the upper chakras require greater sensitivity, and purification of the body opens us to these subtleties. 2) Sound, as a vibration and a force inherent in all things, has a purifying nature. Sound can and does affect the cellular structure of matter. It also has the ability to harmonize otherwise dissonant frequencies both within and around us. We'll examine these principles more closely a little further on.

Within the chakra we again see Airavata, the many tusked white elephant. He is within a circle inside a triangle pointing downward, symbolizing the manifestation of speech. The deities are the God Sadasiva (a version of Shiva, also known as Pancanana, the five-fold one) and the Goddess Gauri (an epithet meaning fair one, yellow, or brilliant one). Gauri is also the name of a class of Goddesses which includes *Uma, Parvati, Rambha, Totala,* and *Tripura.*[2] Each of the deities in this chakra is shown with five faces. (See Figure 6.1, page 240.)

The associated element of the fifth chakra is *ether,* otherwise known as *Akasha* or spirit. It is in the fifth chakra that we refine our

God: Sadāśiva Goddess: Gaurī (Eternal)

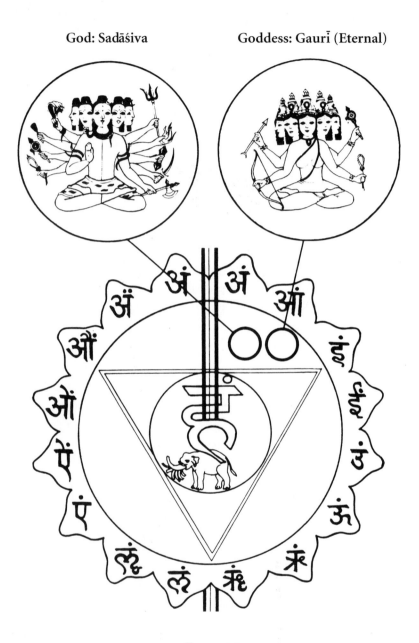

FIGURE 6.1
Viśuddha Chakra.
(from *Kundalini Yoga for the West*)

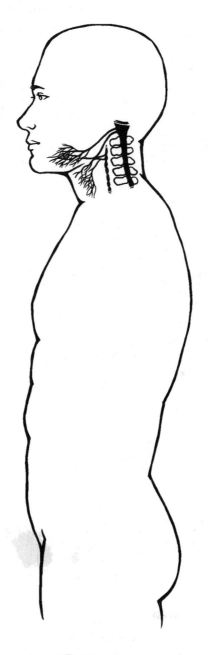

FIGURE 6.2
Chakra Five.

awareness enough to perceive the subtle field of vibrations known as the etheric plane. This plane is the vibrating field of subtle matter that functions as both a cause and a result of our thoughts, emotions, and physical states.

Few people, especially in light of modern parapsychological research, can deny that there exists some sort of plane through which phenomena, impossible to explain by the laws of ordinary reality, can and do occur quite regularly. Examples of remote viewing, telepathic communication, and distance healing are only a few of the types of phenomena that occur by supernormal means. Kirlian photography is a technology that can visually record the otherwise invisible field surrounding living things, showing how this field reveals states of health or disease. Richard Gerber, M.D., in his groundbreaking book, *Vibrational Medicine*, describes how "in reality, it is the organizing principle of the etheric body which maintains and sustains the growth of the physical body."[3] Diseases tend to show up first in the etheric body, before they manifest in the tissues. Likewise, healing can be brought about by techniques that primarily treat the subtle body, such as acupuncture, homeopathy, and psychic healing.

The element ether represents a world of vibrations—the emanations of living things that we experience as the aura, as sound, and as the subtle plane of whispered impressions on the mind into which our more solid realities are enfolded.

While most metaphysical systems postulate four elements (earth, water, fire, and air), ether, or spirit, is the generally universal element added when a system encompasses five elements. In some cases, it is called "space," being the non-physical element beyond earth, air, fire, and water. In these systems, the four elements describe the physical world and the spirit is left for the unexplainable non-physical realm.

The fifth chakra is the last of the seven chakras to have any element associated with it according to classical associations, so the spirit realm is shared by the top three chakras. In my interpretation of the system, I have correlated *sound* to be the element associated with this chakra, as sound is the gross representation of an invisible field of vibrations, and operates in a similar way to subtle vibrations. As Arthur Avalon states in *Serpent Power*: "Sound . . . is that by which the existence of the ether is known."[4] I have then assigned *light* and *thought* to the sixth and seventh chakras respectively as progressively subtler vibrational phenomenon.

THE SUBTLE WORLD OF VIBRATION

All things . . . are aggregations of atoms that dance and by their movements produce sounds. When the rhythm of the dance changes, the sound it produces also changes . . . Each atom perpetually sings its song, and the sound, at every moment, creates dense and subtle forms.

—Fritjof Capra[5]

Ether can be equated with the all-encompassing and unifying field of subtle vibrations found throughout the universe. Any vibration, be it a sound wave or a dancing particle, is in contact with other vibrations, and all vibrations can and do affect each other. To enter the fifth chakra is to tune our consciousness into the subtle vibrational field that is all around us.

Let's take something we're all familiar with: the automobile. We know that our cars are powered by an engine with numerous parts. We have solid matter in the form of pistons and valves, liquid gas and oil, spark plugs firing, and compressed air (the first four elements). Intricately timed movement allows all these parts to work together in precise relationships. When we open the hood, however, we see only vibration. Because we can't see the small parts inside the motor, we see it only from a kind of macro-perspective. A running engine looks like a vibrating block of metal, emitting a whirring sound. We can tell if our car is running well by listening to the sound it makes. When the sound is different than what we know it should be, that tells us something is wrong.

In the same way, we experience the overall vibrations of a person or situation, even though we may not know the minute details. We can tell if something is off. The sum total of vibrations *includes* all the levels within it. In the fifth chakra, as we refine our consciousness, we begin to perceive these subtle vibrational messages. The etheric field is a kind of blueprint for the vibrational patterns of our tissues, organs, emotions, activities, experiences, memories, and thoughts.

Even the most solid aspects of matter are constantly vibrating at high speeds. In fact, it is only by this constant movement that we perceive the emptiness of matter as a solid field. The movement of atomic particles, bound to a very small space, becomes more like vibration or oscillation, vibrating at the rate of about 10^{15} Hz.[6] (Hz = cycles per second) Vibration, even at our most fundamental units, exists throughout all forms of matter, energy, and consciousness.

Vibration is a manifestation of rhythm. Dion Fortune, in *The Cosmic Doctrine*, describes vibration as "the impact of the rhythm of one plane upon the substance of another."[7] As we climb up the chakra column, each plane is said to vibrate at a higher, faster, and more efficient level than the chakra below it. Light is a faster vibration than sound (by about forty octaves), and thought is a subtler vibration than light. Our consciousness vibrates upon the substance of our bodies, energy affecting movement and movement affecting matter.

In the 1800s, a scientist by the name of Ernst Chladni did some experiments demonstrating how vibration affects matter. Chladni put sand on a fixed steel plate and then rubbed a rosined violin bow along the edge of the plate. He found that the vibration that was "played" onto the disk "danced" the sand into beautiful mandala-like patterns. As the frequency of the vibration varied so did the pattern. (See Figure 6.3, page 245.) A plate of sand over a stereo speaker will also produce similar patterns if the tones are from a simple frequency.

This is a clear-cut example of the way sound affects matter—an example of the rhythm of one plane impacting the substance of another. It is not, however, a haphazard pattern that is created by these

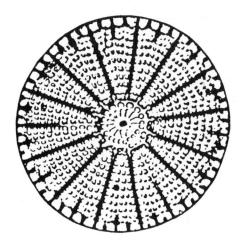

The bacterium Arachnoidiscus (x600).

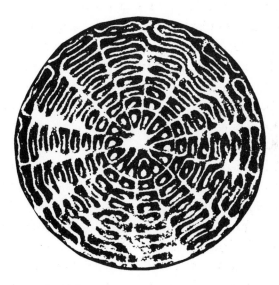

A Chladni figure formed by vibrating a
sand-covered disc to specific frequencies.

FIGURE 6.3

tones, but a mandala-like design, arranged geometrically around a center point—just like a pattern of a chakra. One can't help asking what effect sound has on the minute cellular and atomic structures or on the less visible etheric field.

Subsequent experiments have shown that sound waves, projected into various mediums, such as water, powders, pastes, or oil, produce patterns with remarkable similarity to forms found in nature, such as spiral galaxies, cellular division in an embryo, or the iris and pupil of the human eye. Study of this phenomenon is called *Cymatics* and was largely developed by a swiss scientist named Hans Jenny.[8]

The Hindus believe that vibration, working through various levels of density from *Brahma*, the creator, to *Vaikhari*, audible sound, is the basic emanation from which matter was created. In fact, in Hindu scripture it is said, "OM—this whole world is that syllable! . . . For this, Brahma is the whole."[9] While Hinduism may differ greatly from Christianity in many aspects, one cannot deny the similarity to the statement in I John, "In the beginning was the Word, and the Word was with God and the Word was God."[10] Both describe how sound, as an emanation of the divine, creates the manifested world.

All vibrations are characterized by rhythm, a repeated, regular pattern of movement through time and space. These rhythmical patterns are deeply ingrained functions of our consciousness. The turning of the seasons, the diurnal rhythms of day and night, the cycles of the moon, women's menstruation, the movement of breath, and the constant beating of our hearts are a few examples. No living thing escapes these rhythms. Rhythm, like change, is a fundamental aspect of all life and consciousness.

Operating from the fifth chakra, a person becomes aware of things on a vibrational level. We may respond to the tone of a voice more than the actual words spoken. The effect of the more "abstract" plane upon our consciousness is subtler than that of the grosser actions, yet is no less profound. Unfortunately, most of us are not consciously aware of our actions and reactions on this plane.

Even our perceptions, through any of the senses, are a function of perceiving rhythm. Hearing sound waves and seeing light waves are only two. The very mechanism through which nerve fibers feed information to our brain is through rhythmic pulsations of energy. From the first contractions of our mother's womb at birth to our last dying gasps we are rhythmic, dancing creatures, dancing in what Ram Dass calls "the only dance there is."

George Leonard, in his wonderful book, *The Silent Pulse*, defines rhythm as "the play of patterned frequencies against the matrix of time."[11] He states that the primary role of rhythm is to integrate various parts of a system. We are like a symphony orchestra. The various aspects of the system are the strings, the horns, the woodwinds, and the percussion, yet only through the uniting power of rhythm can we make music. The rhythm is the heartbeat of the system!

What many of us lack in our lives is this resonant rhythm, the integrating aspect that connects us from the very core of our being to the heartbeat of the universe. Consequently, we are at odds with the world and with ourselves. We lack coordination, cohesiveness, and grace.

Furthermore, rhythms, like chakra patterns, tend to perpetuate themselves. The person who starts each day from a calm, centered state of mind will find his interactions more calm and centered. On the other hand, the person who drives to work every morning during rush hour and works a high-pressure, fast-paced job is involved with different kinds of vibrations each day. This rhythm affects one down to the cellular level of his or her being, and necessarily affects one's thoughts, actions, and emotions. After working all day, then driving home in rush hour traffic, one can't help manifesting this rhythm in his or her home life, eating patterns and interactions with others. Spouse and children are subject to the bombardment of these rhythms and may be stimulated or irritated by it, either consciously or unconsciously. They may (and probably will) react on the same vibrational level, adding further aggravation. If the heartbeat is a conductor of our internal rhythms, no wonder so many executives suffer from heart failure!

We all affect each other, as well as everything around us, by the vibrations we carry within our minds and bodies. We don't pay much attention to them—for the level is subtle, difficult to pinpoint or describe—but they affect us profoundly, nonetheless. Few people use conscious effort to temper these vibrations. There are many relatively simple techniques and principles that make this possible for anyone. Their use can be a great help to the development of our own consciousness, as well as the enhancement of the evolutionary well-being of everyone around us.

RESONANCE

At the heart of each of us, whatever our imperfections, there exists a silent pulse of perfect rhythm, a complex of wave forms and resonances, which is absolutely individual and unique and yet which connects us to everything in the universe. The act of getting in touch with this pulse can transform our personal experience and in some way alter the world around us.[12]

—George Leonard

All sounds can be described as wave-forms, vibrating at a particular frequency. *Rhythm entrainment*, also known as *sympathetic vibration*, or simply *resonance*, is where two wave-forms of similar frequency "lock into phase" with each other, meaning that the waves oscillate together at exactly the same rate. The resulting wave is a combination of the two original waves: it has the same frequency but increased amplitude (See Figure 6.4, page 249). Amplitude is the distance a wave travels from crest to trough. In sound waves increased amplitude means increased energy and volume, as in amplified music. In other words, power and depth are increased when the wave-forms are in resonance.

We can understand this by paying a visit to a shop that sells grandfather clocks. Suppose we walk in and none of the clocks have been wound. The shopkeeper, assuring us that the clocks do indeed work, goes around and winds each clock, setting the pendulums in motion. At first, these one-second tick-tock swings of the pendulum are not coordinated with each other, but may be off by a half or quarter second. As time passes, we notice that there are fewer ticks and tocks. Soon all the pendulums are swinging back and forth in unison. Their rhythms have become entrained.

Two oscillating vibrations, *if they are near enough to each other in frequency,* will eventually entrain. Musical choirs, for example, will hold their last note until the voices reach resonance. If you have a trained ear, you can perceive these pulsations as subtle beats. It's what

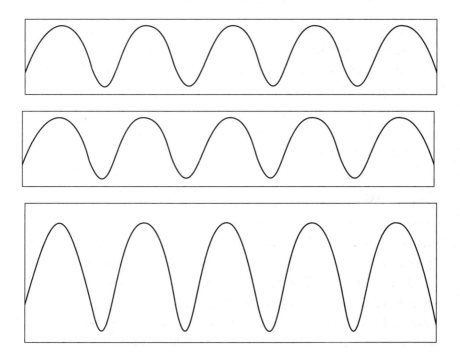

FIGURE 6.4
Constructive interference of sound waves.

gives that clean, clear ring that echoes through the auditorium when the note is cut off. The sound waves have locked into phase with each other, creating a resonance that is pleasant to experience.

This principle of rhythm entrainment also occurs with just one wave triggering a vibration in a resting source. If, for example, we both have violins tuned to concert pitch, I can set the D string on your violin vibrating merely by playing my own D string nearby. This is how tuning forks are used in remote control television units. When we push the button, it strikes a tone that is remotely activated in the TV set several feet away.

While similar waves will lock into phase with each other, creating resonance, waves of differing frequency may instead create dissonance. A pure tone of a flute, for example, is a coherent sine wave, which will tune to other flutes. The noise of a bus is many complex sound waves that are dissonant.

People who live in the same household become rhythm entrained to each other's subtle vibrations. It has been long known that women who live together long enough will tend to menstruate at the same time of the month. Couples married for a long time often come to look alike, and their speech exhibits similar rhythms. As a culture, we become rhythm entrained to our neighbors, friends and peers. We are influenced by our environment, not only in visual, psychological, and physiological factors (e.g. billboards, social pressure, air pollution) but on a deep, subconscious level of inner vibrations.

The Transcendental Meditation Society, more commonly known as TM, has a meditational philosophy based on this principle. They believe that the brain-wave rhythms created by mantra meditation can positively influence the world of non-meditators. The more meditators there are, the more likely this rhythm entrainment is to occur. They have even put this assumption to a test in Atlanta, Georgia, where every night at a certain hour, meditators agreed to meditate. It was shown that there was a remarkable reduction in crime during that hour.[13]

All speech has rhythm. This means that conversation is also subject to the principles of rhythm entrainment, with some fascinating implications, as demonstrated by the work of Dr. William S. Condon, of Boston University School of Medicine, described below.

In order to more accurately see the subtler aspects of communication, Dr. Condon filmed numerous conversations, and then analyzed the films at very slow speeds (1/48 second). By breaking simple words into fundamental units of sound (such as the word "sound" being s— ah—oo—nnn—d), each lasting a fraction of a second, he found that the body movements of both the listener and the speaker *were in precise synchrony with the voice* at all times that communication was occurring. These movements might be a raising of the eyebrows, a tilt of the head, or a flexing of a finger. With each new set of sounds, a new set of movements would occur. What's most amazing about this is that the listener's movements were *entrained* to the speaker, rather than occurring as a delayed response. Dr. Condon makes this comment:

> *Listeners were observed to move in precise shared synchrony with the speaker's speech. This appears to be a form of entrainment since there is no discernible lag even at 1/48 second . . . It also appears to be a universal characteristic of human communication, and perhaps characterizes much of animal behavior in general. Communication is thus like a dance, with everyone engaged in intricate and shared movements across many dimensions, yet all strangely oblivious that they are doing so. Even total strangers will display this synchronization . . . .* [14]

He further describes how the content of the message only seems to come across once entrainment occurs. Before that point, there is often misunderstanding. During the sixties, George Leonard and Dr. Price Cobbs, a black psychiatrist, conducted weekend interracial encounter groups, where black and white participants had marked variations in their speech rhythms. Participants were encouraged to pour out their resentments, fears, and anger. The beginnings of the marathon would be discouraging and painful, but at a certain point in the weekend they would find the rhythms approaching fever pitch, with everyone talking and shouting and stamping their feet, reaching a fevered crescendo. They descibe:

Near the end of the section, some of the shouts and curses began turning to laughter. Then a strange thing happens: the entire group suddenly stops, then begins again, then stops, then begins and more quietly—all in perfect rhythm. After this the encounter resumes with a new tone of tenderness and ease. It's as if the pendulums of understanding are swinging together, the heart cells beating as one.[15]

It was not until the group entered resonance that communication really began to occur. Perhaps communication is really a rhythmic dance rather than a stimulus-response phenomenon, as we usually think of it. For we see that the listener is not *reacting* to the speaker but is instead *resonating* with the speaker when communication is truly occurring.

Further studies by Dr. Condon examined the behavior of disturbed and autistic children in regard to this auditory rhythm entrainment. The children showed a time-lag response between the listener and the speaker, and acted as if they were responding to an echo of the original sounds. Their micromovements put them out of harmony with the world around them, hence the feeling of alienation and confusion that characterizes their condition. George Leonard, in his analysis of this data, concludes that "Our ability to have a world depends on our ability to entrain with it."[16]

This is a very important concept for understanding the fifth chakra. If we are unable to entrain with the vibratory frequencies around us, we cannot experience our connection with the world. If we cannot entrain, we cannot communicate. Without communication we are isolated, separate, and cut off from the nourishing energy so vital to health. Just as the Hindus believe that sound creates all matter, communication—be it oral, chemical, mental, or electrical—creates and maintains life. Without it we die, both spiritually and physically.

Perhaps our concept of verbal interchange as comprising the most significant aspects of communication is merely another manifestation of the great Maya, which veils the nature of its underlying reality. Perhaps communication is nothing but rhythmic interchange. Yet, language is the tip of the iceberg of communication, and our prime indication of just what and where that iceberg is.

If simple vibration can move matter into coherent, harmonic patterns, resonant vibrations can only deepen that effect. When we truly resonate with something, it affects us deeply. We can play our own part in the evolution of our environment by being aware of this principle of sympathetic vibration. Our own vibrations may trigger a new thought or vibration in a resting source, awakening consciousness in another. We can choose to contribute "good" vibrations or "bad": those in harmony with the vibrations around us, or those out of phase, in disharmony.

Chakras also exhibit vibrational patterns, spanning from the slower, grosser vibrations of solid matter in the first chakra to the highest and fastest vibrations of pure consciousness. An active chakra in one person can, through its vibrations, trigger the opening of an inactive chakra in another.

In San Francisco there is a place called "Exploratorium" which is filled with scientific exhibits that teach by involving the observer. There is one exhibit there, created by Tom Tompkin, called "Resonant Rings," that illustrates sympathetic vibration. The exhibit is a beautiful example of how chakras vibrate in the body.[17]

Fastened to a rubber plate over a speaker chamber are several circular bands of metal, each describing a circle varying in size from approximately two inches to six inches. (See Figure 6.5, page 254.) The observer can then turn a knob that emits sound through the speaker and vibrates the plate at a particular frequency. Adjusting the knob adjusts the frequency.

At low frequencies only the large circles vibrate with a slow, undulating motion, emitting a low-pitched sound. At higher frequencies

Rubber plate over speaker chamber

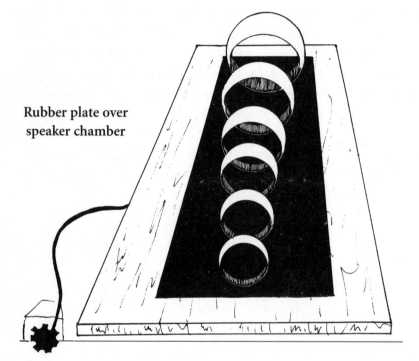

FIGURE 6.5
Resonant Rings.

only the smaller circles vibrate with a smooth, high-pitched whir. Intermediate frequencies vibrate the middle circles. You can control which circles vibrate by adjusting the knob to different pitches.

Our bodies are the "plate" that vibrates the chakras. The general vibrational pattern of our life—our actions, thoughts, emotions, eating patterns, and environment—sets off the vibrations of our chakras. We can activate different chakras by changing the vibrational rhythm of our lives. That which is slow allows the first chakra to open. Higher frequencies stimulate the third chakra. Beyond that it must be remembered that we deal with subtler vibrations—moving the physical body faster won't open up the higher chakras, but meditation may allow the brain to process "higher" vibrations. As we get out of the limitations of time and space, our vibrations are less hindered. On a vibration level, enlightenment could be thought of as the omnipresence of a waveform with infinite frequency and infinite amplitude.

MANTRAS

The essence of all beings is earth, the essence of earth is water, the essence of water is plants, the essence of plants is man, the essence of man is speech, the essence of speech is the Holy Knowledge (Veda) the essence of Veda is Sama-Veda (word, tone, sound), the essence of Sama-Veda is OM.
—Chandogya Upanishad

The Chladni disk and the principles of rhythm entrainment show us that sound waves can and do affect matter. It is not surprising that they would affect consciousness as well.

This is the basic idea behind sacred sounds used in meditation and chanting, called *mantras*. The word comes from "man," meaning mind, and "tra," which means protection or instrument. Thus, a mantra is a tool for protecting our minds from the traps of non-productive cycles of thought and action. Mantras serve as focusing devices for making the mind one-pointed and calm. The vibration of the mantra has been likened to the vibration of someone shaking your shoulders to wake you up from sleep.[18] A mantra is designed to awaken the mind from its habitual sleep of ignorance.

Just as a particular vibration on the Chladni disk created a mandala out of a pile of sand, so can the chanting of a simple mantra, such as OM, change our random pile of thoughts and emotions into a cohesive and graceful pattern. It is not necessary to intellectualize the meaning or symbology of a mantra for the sound to have this effect upon us. The rhythm of the sound will work on a subconscious level and permeate our inner rhythms. In fact, it is part of the mantra's magic that one not think about the meaning, for then we transcend the fragmented aspects of the conscious mind and perceive an underlying wholeness.

If, however, meaning is ascribed to a particular sound, as in the use of an affirmation that we repeat to ourselves every day, such as: "I am love" the rhythm of the repetition helps to infuse that meaning into our consciousness.

Spoken aloud for a few minutes in the morning, an effective mantra can reverberate silently in the mind all day long, carrying with it the imprints of its vibration, image, and meaning. With each reverberation, it is believed that the mantra is working its magic on the fabric of both mind and body, creating greater order and harmony. Actions may take on a new rhythm, dancing to the drumbeat of the mantra. If a fast mantra is chosen, it can be used to generate energy and overcome inertia. If a slow, peaceful mantra is used, it can help bring a state of relaxation and calm throughout the day.

Seed Sounds of the Chakras

Hindu metaphysics states that everything in the universe is made of sound. Within each thing there is a symbolic representation of the energy patterns that compose it, known as a seed sound, or *bija* mantra. These mantras are designed to set the chanting person into resonance with the object of the seed sound. Through knowledge of bija mantras, one gains control over the essence of that thing, and can therefore create, destroy, or otherwise alter it. Hazrat Inayat Khan has said, "He who knows the secret of the sounds knows the mystery of the whole universe."[19]

Each chakra has its own associated seed sound which is said to contain the essence, and therefore the secrets, of that chakra. As each chakra has its own associated element, we find that the seed sounds are believed to give access to the qualities of that element. The seed sounds or bija mantras for each chakra are as follows:

Chakra One	Earth, Muladhara	LAM
Chakra Two	Water, Swadhisthana	VAM
Chakra Three	Fire, Manipura	RAM
Chakra Four	Air, Anahata	YAM (or SAM)
Chakra Five	Ether, Visuddha	HAM
Chakra Six	Ajna (light)	OM
Chakra Seven	Sahasrara (thought)	(no mantra)

The M in each of these sounds is said to represent the maternal and material aspect of the universe. The A sound in turn represents the Father, the nonmaterial. L (lam, earth) is a heavy, closing sound, while H in HAM (ether) is a light, airy, ethereal sound, and R (ram, fire) is an energetic, fiery sound. In addition to the seed sounds, each chakra has a particular number of petals, each of which is named by a letter of the Sanskrit alphabet. Typically, consonants have come to reflect the hard, material aspects of the world, while vowels represent the spiritual or etheric aspects. Chakra five, then, is the carrier of the vowel sounds, as only vowels appear on its petals. Control of these letters is said to be in the hands of the Goddess *Kali*, whose name means "time." Kali is the destructive aspect of the Hindu goddesses, who destroys the world by removing the letters from the petals of the chakras, hence removing sound or speech.[20] Without the sound that is the essence of all things, nothing can exist.

We are not helpless victims of disharmonious vibrations, and we can send out vibrations of our own. The uttering of mantras is a way of taking control of our rhythms and guiding the development of our minds and bodies at the fundamental etheric level.

The following table lists a few commonly used mantras and their purposes. This list is minute in comparison to the possibilities that exist for effective mantras. The importance of a mantra lies in its rhythm and overall vibration. Mantras are experienced within—you can perceive which ones are effective for you as you try them out. It does, however, take some time for a mantra to become fully effective. Take one on for a week or a month to fully assess the real benefit.

OM or AUM: The great primordial sound, the original sound from which the universe was created, the sound of all sounds together.

(For Christians, the mantra AMEN is similar to AUM.)

OM AH HUM: Three syllables of great power used for the following purposes: to purify an atmosphere prior to embarking upon a ritual or meditation; or to transmute material offerings to their spiritual counterparts.

OM MANI PADME HUM: "The jewel of the lotus resides within." MANI PADME represents the jewel in the lotus, the essential wisdom lying at the heart of Buddhist doctrine, the divine essence, while HUM represents the limitless reality embodied within the limits of the individual being. HUM unites the individual with the universal.

GATE GATE PARAGATE PARASAM GATE BODHI SWAHA: Tibetan Smaller Heart Sutra.

I AM THAT I AM: An English version also designed to unite the individual with the universal.

OM NAMA SHIVAYA: "In the name of Shiva." One of the many mantras uttering god names. Any god or goddess name may be used to create a mantra.

***ISIS, ASTARTE, DIANA, HECATE, DEMETER, KALI—
INANNA:*** A popular Pagan chant of Goddess names, from Charlie
Murphy's record "The Burning Times." Subsequent verses can be
added to this, for the God: NEPTUNE, OSIRIS, MERLIN, MANANON,
HELIOS, SHIVA—HORNED ONE. (The dash indicates a slight
pause.)

***THE EARTH, THE WATER, THE FIRE, AND THE AIR—
RETURN, RETURN, RETURN, RETURN:*** Along the same lines as
the Goddess mantra above, this is also a ritual chant for acknowledging the elements.

There are thousands of chants and mantras from different cultures
and religions around the world. Some have similarities of tone and
rhythm while others do not. The deepest value of a mantra has to do
with how much we invest in it—how much we use the sound in our
meditations, in our work, in our thoughts throughout the day. If many
people use a common mantra, then the sound collects resonance on
the subtle planes and becomes more potent. Each time we use a mantra we become more entrained with it.

While there are mantras that have been used for centuries to create
particular effects, there is nothing wrong with making up your own
mantras. Affirmations, put into the form of a mantra, have a more
powerful effect, for in any language, words are a form of the object's
internal structure. Thus, the affirmation, "I will be strong" carries
within it the particular aspects of strength we are seeking. However,
the affirmation, "I am strong!" creates even more strength by only a
slight change of words. Mantras must be chosen carefully to create the
effects we want. Mantras have long been a secret esoteric tradition in
most mystical schools. Their power is subtle and is usually not even
detected by the insensitive or uninitiated. Their power is felt through
experience only. Their use employs only the simple "idiot-proof " technique of repetition, and their benefits can be felt by any sincere seeker.

They are a basic, fundamental key allowing human beings to unlock some of the mysteries of our own inner harmony.

Vowel Sounds and the Chakras

The seed sounds for each chakra listed previously only differ in their consonants, so the sustained sound of the vowel of each seed sound is the same (except chakra six). What I have found to be far more effective for resonating the chakras is working with various vowel sounds. While research has shown differences from one system to another, the following list represents the most common correlation of different systems. You can best validate this by chanting the sounds yourself, and experiencing which chakras seem to vibrate with which sounds. Feel free to experiment. Your own chakras may resonate to slightly different tones.

These sounds are equally effective, if not more so, when used as a silent mantra or as a meditation device. Pick the chakra or chakras you want to work on most and use the vowel sounds to help awaken them.

Muladhara:	O as in Om
Svadhisthana:	U as in Cool
Manipura:	A as in Father
Anahata:	E as in Play
isuddha:	I as in Seed
Ajna:	mm
Sahasrara:	nng as in sing, or just silence

TELEPATHY

The key to the mastery is always silence, at all levels, because
in the silence we discern the vibrations and to discern them is
to be able to capture them.

—Sri Aurobindo[21]

Telepathy is the art of communicating across time and space without using any of the "normal" five senses. There are relatively few people adept at this form of communication, yet it is something we all respond to on a subliminal level. With a well-developed fifth chakra this type of communication becomes accessible.

As we learn to refine our chakras, calm our minds, and quiet our thoughts, the fabric of our consciousness becomes smoother and smoother. Our vibrations become steadier and our perceptions more direct. In this state it is far easier to become aware of the subtler ripples of vibrations in our energy field. The quieter levels of telepathic communication become apparent when the grosser vibrations of our lives are no longer creating interference.

Let us make an analogy of telepathic communication by amplifying our phenomenon. If you're at a noisy party where everyone is talking at once, music is playing loudly, and people are dancing, you'll have to raise your voice considerably to have any kind of conversation. If, for some strange reason, your partner is only whispering, you won't hear her at all. In order to hear her whispering, you'd have to be in a silent room, where there were few or no interference patterns to your communication.

Telepathy could be defined as *the art of hearing the whispers of another's mind.* In order to do this, we must be quiet within our own minds. Most of us, by nature, have a party going on inside our own heads. We're always conversing with ourselves or running tapes through our heads. When added to the usual din around us, this dulls the receptivity of the fifth chakra. We're accustomed to using technological devices to send our messages beyond the limits of our voices. We're not accustomed to listening for the subtle stirs in the ether that can bring us communication across time and space.

And why should we be? Isn't gross, physical communication more accurate, more specific, and less subject to loss or error? If you send a telepathic message, how can you be sure it's received? Or received accurately?

Consciousness is not really a verbal process. In order to communicate, we must translate our consciousness into a symbolic structure. In order to receive the communication, we must translate symbols back into consciousness. While this may seem instantaneous, we are downgrading consciousness from its purer form. As any linguist knows, the essence of a communication is often distorted in translation.

Seen in this light, telepathic communication can be more precise and immediate than verbal communication, which can often contain lies and omissions.

While few people are really adept at this form of communication, there are even fewer people who have never experienced it at all. Two people saying the same thing at the same time, finding a busy signal because your friend is simultaneously calling you, or getting the psychic hit that a family member is in danger are a few examples of the common ways telepathy can occur.

If we accept the ether as a connective field of gross and subtle vibrations, then communication occurs through a perceptible alteration in that field. Telepathic communication is merely a subtler alteration, perceptible only when the grosser vibrations are quieted. Telepathy may result when two or more minds are rhythm-entrained such that a variation in the pattern of one rhythm results in a similar variation in the other. Entrained rhythms increase the amplitude of the wave. A wave of higher amplitude has more potency, more chance of being heard.

Whatever the explanation, examples of telepathic communication indicate a kind of mental connectivity floating through the ether that permits an exchange of information on a non-physical plane. As thoughts become more and more dense, they begin to manifest—they are recognized by one mind, then two, and become denser and denser until they are real. The old adage that "thoughts are things" becomes believable.

Whether we are initiators or receivers, there is little doubt that there exists some medium through which we can tap into a realm where the vibrations of minds converge. Through the refinement of our chakras and attention to the vibrational world that surrounds and creates us, we can gain access to this unifying level of consciousness. As we approach the upper chakras, we approach a universality of mind transcending the physical limitations of time and space that keep us separate. We need not create it. We need only to quiet our minds and listen. It is already there, and we are already playing a part in it. We can choose to make that part conscious.

CREATIVITY

Communication is a creative process. The more adept we are at this art, the more creative the process becomes. A young child, when first learning to speak, merely mimics his parents' words. Soon, however, the child understands that certain words bring particular results and he begins to experiment. As his vocabulary grows, the child has more and more elements with which he can become creative. He begins to use words, sounds, and gestures to create his reality— as he will for the rest of his life.

While many people have associated creativity with the second chakra, (since that's where we create babies) I believe creativity is ultimately a form of *expression*, related to chakra five. Creating life in the womb is not a conscious process. We do not decide to make fingers or toes, blue eyes or brown. While the emotional states of the second chakra may fuel creative impulses, it takes will (chakra three)[22] and abstract consciousness (upper chakras in general) to create.

The arts have always existed on the turning edge of culture. Be they visual, auditory, kinesthetic, dramatic, or even literary, the arts, precisely by their nonregimented, nonconformist character are able to reach into the vast uncharted realm of the future and illustrate ideas and concepts in a way that affects consciousness on an immediate and whole brain level.

In the words of Marshall McLuhan, master analyst of media:

I am curious to know what would happen if art were suddenly seen for what it is, namely, exact information of how to rearrange one's psyche in order to anticipate the next blow from our own extended faculties . . . . The artist is always engaged in writing a detailed history of the future because he is the only person aware of the nature of the present.[23]

Art forms are generally more abstract than any other forms of communication. Leaving room for the imagination, they invite participation of the most innovative components of our consciousness. Saying less, perhaps we can hear more. As we approach the more abstract planes of consciousness, it is only fitting that we turn to our more abstract means of communication in order to embrace these planes.

The process of creation is a process of inner discovery. In creating a work of art, we open ourselves to the very mysteries of the universe. We become channels for spiritual information, learning a language more universal than human tongues.

The process of creativity is a delicate one. Regimented lives do not lend themselves to it, and are instead threatened by it. Creativity releases our inner power much as language "releases the unknown from limbo, making it so the whole brain can know it."[24]

Presently there is a new birth of therapies utilizing the creative process. Using visual art, psychodrama, movement, dance, and the calming effect of music, one can access the deeper and generally healthier regions of the mind and body while releasing the inner frustrations that fragment our wholeness.

Survival and health in the twenty-first century will require innovation and flexibility. Creativity is the key to unlocking these qualities. We must honor it in ourselves and in each other. We must honor the means which make it possible and protect ourselves from those phenomena which threaten to shut down this basic life force. Our very future depends upon it.

MEDIA

Television, radio, newspapers, and other public forms of communication can be seen as the cultural expression of the fifth chakra, acting as a connecting nervous system for us all. If communication is the passage of knowledge and understanding, the mass content of our collective consciousness is, for better or worse, heavily influenced by the media and those who control it. Whether we are forced to hear about a politician's private sex life, made to look at countless murders on television, or hear honest data about the environment, the media directs the public attention to archetypal themes that *they deem* to be of concern to public consciousness. Media directs our attention, and where the attention goes, the rest of the energy generally follows. If media feels violence is more appropriate for our children to watch than lovemaking, they are setting cultural values for us all.

Media is also the most potent means we have of cultural transformation. Media can be a potent feedback system, allowing us to see ourselves as we are—in our beauty and our ignorance. It was the pictures on the news of the Vietnam war that allowed people to get it touch with its atrocities, *while it was still going on*, and create the anti-war protests. Media lets us know the state of the planet's ecology, the condition of people in other places, and helps wire up the global brain.

Media can also show us ways of being different. A movie can make a hypothetical reality seem so real that our imagination is filled with new possibilites. Media can express creativity, communicating from the depths of the collective unconscious. Media can show us the fronts of cultural transformation by bringing the hidden innovators to light and letting their voices be heard.

It is important to demand integrity of those who control the media. If it is the cultural nervous system most influential to the ways we live our collective reality, then it is imperative that we keep our media from being polluted with mindless garbage, sensational gossip, propaganda, and lies. Otherwise we risk being collectively manipulated by those who, in actuality, have more power than most of our elected representatives. If the fifth chakra name *Vissudha* means purification, then our collective fifth chakras must be purified with the resonance of truth that can enlighten us all.

CHAKRA FIVE EXERCISES

Playing Charades

Spend an hour with someone in total silence, yet engaged in active communication. Pick challenging things to communicate about. Notice what methods you use to communicate, such as gestures, hand symbols, physical manipulation, eye movements. Notice how much easier it gets toward the end of the hour. Notice what points are especially difficult. This exercise can actually help build communication between two or more parties.

Vow of Silence

Listening is an essential and too-often-overlooked component of communication. Yogis often take vows of silence for extended periods of time to purify their vibrations of audible sound and better tune into subtle sounds. By avoiding verbal communication, one can open up other avenues of communication, namely communication with higher consciousness. Begin with a few hours, then try a whole day or longer.

Voice Recording

Make a recording of your voice during ordinary conversation. See how much you talk and how much you listen, whether you interrupt, or falter in your speech. Notice your tone of voice. If you didn't know this person, what would you intuit about them from the voice?

Neck Rolls

The neck is the narrowest part of the torso. Much of the time it acts as a filter between the abundant flow of energy between the mind and the body. This causes it to be extremely subject to tension and stiffness. Loosening the neck is an essential beginning for any work on the fifth chakra.

> Lift your head up away from your shoulders, and then slowly roll your head in a circular motion, stretching your neck. Stop at any point that feels tense or uncomfortable, and massage with your fingers. Pause in the tight places until it relaxes some, Then move on. Go both clockwise and counterclockwise. (See Figure 6.6, page 268.)

Head Lift

This stimulates the thyroid gland and helps strengthen the neck.

> Lie flat on your back and relax. Slowly lift your head, leaving your shoulders on the floor, so that you are looking at your toes. (See Figure 6.7, page 268.) Hold this position until you feel the energy move into your neck.

Shoulder Stand

To make this pose easier on the neck, it is helpful to first fold a blanket or towel (about 2-3 inches thick) so that when you lie flat, your head touches the floor, but your upper thoracic vertebrae lie on the blanket.

> Lie flat on your back, arms at your sides, and relax. Bend your knees and lift your legs toward the chest, rounding the back.

> As your hips rise, allow your arms to bend at the elbows, so that the heel of your hand can support your waist.

> Slowly straighten the legs above you, using your arms for support. Hold for as long as is comfortable. (See Figure 6.8, page 269.)

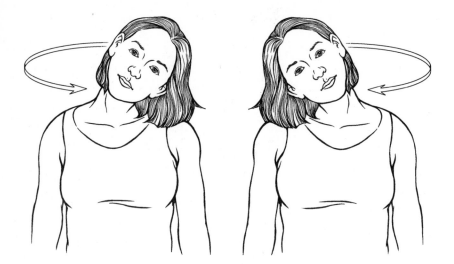

FIGURE 6.6
Neck Rolls.

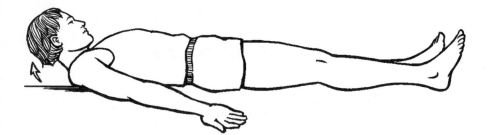

FIGURE 6.7
Head Lift.

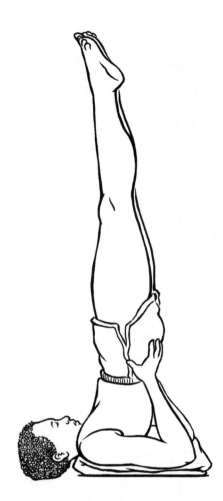

FIGURE 6.8
Shoulder Stand.

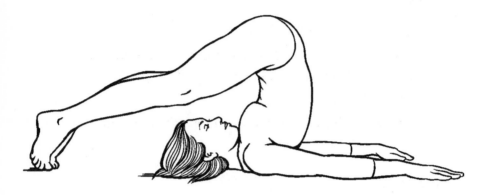

Figure 6.9
Plough.

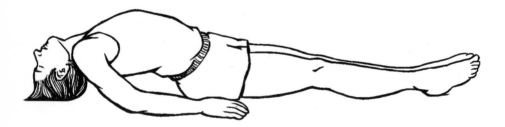

Figure 6.10
Fish Pose.

The Plough

If the shoulder stand was successful, you might want to try the plough.

Return to the shoulder stand.

Lower your legs behind your head, touching your feet to the ground, keeping your knees as straight as possible. (See Figure 6.9, page 270.)

For less flexible bodies, you can have a chair behind your head and lay your thighs on it.

Fish Pose

This often follows the shoulder stand or plough as it gives the neck and back a complementary stretch. This also helps open the chest cavity and stimulates the thyroid.

Lie flat on your back. With hands on hips, prop your upper body up on your elbows, lifting your chest toward the ceiling and arching your neck backward until your head touches the floor. (See Figure 6.10, page 270.)

ENDNOTES

1. Swami Sivananda Radha, *Kundalini Yoga for the West,* 231.

2. Stutley, Margaret and James, *Harper's Dictionary of Hinduism,* 96.

3. Richard Gerber, *Vibrational Medicine,* 302.

4. Arthur Avalon, from his discussion on the *bhutas,* or elements, *The Serpent Power,* 71. Further on he quotes the Hatha-yoga-pradipika, "Whatever is heard in the the form of sound is Sakti . . . So long as there is the notion of Ether, so long is sound heard." Ch. IV, vv 101, 102, quoted in *The Serpent Power,* 99.

5. Fritjof Capra, *The Tao of Physics,* (NY: Bantam Books, 1975), 229.

6. Itzhak Bentov, *Stalking the Wild Pendulum,* 68.

7. Dion Fortune, *The Cosmic Doctrine,* 57.

8. For a visual feast of this phenomenon, see the video *Cymatics: The Healing Nature of Sound*, put out by MACROmedia, P.O. Box 279, Epping, NH, 03042.

9. Patrick Olivelle, *The Early Upanishads: Annotated Text and Translation,* From the Mandukya Upanishad, (NY: Oxford University Press, 1998), 475.

10. I John, King James Bible.

11. George Leonard, *The Silent Pulse,* 10.

12. Ibid., xii.

13. Arthur Aron, in a paper available through Center for Scientific Research, Maharishi International University, Fairfield, Iowa.

14. William S. Condon, "Multiple Response to Sound in Dysfunctional Children." Journal of Autism and Schizophrenia 5:1 (1975), 43.

15. George Leonard, *The Silent Pulse,* 23.

16. Ibid, 18.

17. Tom Tompkin, Exploratorium, Palace of Fine Arts, San Francisco, CA, 1986.

18. Arthur Avalon, *The Serpent Power,* 97.

19. Hazrat Inayat Khan, *The Sufi Message, Vol. 2,* (London: Barrie and Rockcliff, 2nd ed. 1972.)

20. Arthur Avalon, *The Serpent Power,* 100.

21. As quoted by Satprem in *Sri Aurobindo, or the Adventure of Consciousness,* 71.

22. Some people, such as Edgar Cayce and Carolyn Myss, place will in the fifth chakra. I believe that will occurs much sooner, or we don't even get to the fifth chakra. Furthermore, it leaves communication entirely out of the chakra system. We may express our will in this chakra, but inner power and will are initially a silent process.

23. Marshall McLuhan, *Understanding Media,* 70–71.

24. Marilyn Ferguson, *The Aquarian Conspiracy,* 80.

RECOMMENDED SUPPLEMENTAL READING FOR CHAKRA FIVE

Gardner, Kay. *Sounding the Inner Landscape: Music as Medicine*. Stonington, ME: Caduceus Publications, 1990.

Gardner-Gordon, Joy. *The Healing Voice*. Freedom, CA: The Crossing Press, 1993.

Gerber, Richard, M.D. *Vibrational Medicine*. Santa Fe, NM: Bear & Co., 1988.

Hamel, Peter Michael. *Through Music to the Self*. Boulder, CO: Shambhala, 1979.

Leonard, George. *The Silent Pulse*. NY: E.P. Dutton, 1978.

CHAKRA SIX

Light

Color

Seeing

Intuition

Visualization

Imagination

Clairvoyance

Vision

Chapter 7

CHAKRA SIX: LIGHT

OPENING MEDITATION

IT IS DARK. EYES CLOSED, WE LIE AS if asleep, dreamless, ignorant of all around us. Floating in a sea of emptiness, we are cradled in darkness— unseeing, unknowing, at peace. We breathe slowly, in and out, in and out, stretching and relaxing our bodies as we settle into the warm, peaceful darkness inside. We are home. We are safe. We are deep within ourselves, feeling, hearing, being—but not yet seeing.

Become this darkness—all-knowing, yet unknowing, empty and free. Let the dark wash over you, soothe you, as you empty your mind into the infinity of the void, the womb of darkness—the birthplace of our dreams to come.

Somewhere, in the darkness, we hear a sound—a distant note, a voice, a scuffle of movement. We feel the flutter of a breeze upon our face, feel a warmth upon our shoulders, feel the pull to rise and flow and follow but we know not where. Our bodies cannot see and dare not move. They are dark and still.

They call to us for direction, wisdom, guidance. They call to intelligence, they call to memory, they call for clarification of the pattern. They call to light.

And afraid to leave the darkness and safety of our ignorance, we hear this call.

We hear this call and our own mind, hungry for answers, quests outward. We long to see, to know, to behold at once the wonders that surround us. To fill our minds with recognition, the certain steps of knowing, the safety and the peace that light, too, can bring.

We open our mind. We open our eyes. We look about.

Images pour forth in myriad kaleidoscopic forms, tumbling inward, pattern upon pattern, endlessly interweaving.

Colors, shapes, and forms reflecting space around us, reflecting back into us, recording life in patterns that our minds can clearly see.

The mind opens and receives.

But there is too much and the light is blinding.

We call to the dark to shade us, to temper, to bind the patterns into meaning.

And the dark comes softly, hand in hand and shadow to the light, defining, shading, intertwining, ordering.

The light comes more gently now, rainbow colors, healing, soothing, illuminating, coming at will. Active yellow, healing green, soothing blue, potent violet. All that is alive glows with light. Shape and essence in form revealed for us to see and know.

What do we wish to see? What do we call forth to our inner vision?
What does the light bring?

Beauty of a thousand suns, beauty of a single Moon,
patterns of the life we're leading, all the truth we are perceiving.
Gently now on wings of light, our petals flutter through the night,
Reaching out to worlds beyond, events forthcoming, days long gone.
Holographic matrix net escapes the boundaries by time set.
All the truth can be contained by patterns in the mind retained
Red and yellow, green and blue, interlace in varied hue.
Shape and form, insight revealed, nothing can remain concealed
From inner vision reaching out, seeing truth, removing doubt.
Inside we open, watch and wait, while wisdom's visions spin our fate.
Illumination shows the way, our inner light turns night to day. And
though the dark shall yet return, we fear it not for we have learned
the way the dark and light combine, letting patterns be defined
Dark to light and night to day
Within our minds, we light the way.

CHAKRA SIX
SYMBOLS AND CORRESPONDENCES

Sanskrit Name:	Ajna
Meaning:	To perceive, to command
Location:	Center of the head slightly above eye level
Element:	Light
Essential Form:	Image
Function:	Seeing, intuition
Gland:	Pineal
Other Body Parts:	Eyes

Malfunction:	Blindness, headaches, nightmares, eyestrain, blurred vision
Color:	Indigo
Seed Sound:	Om
Vowel Sound:	(not really a vowel in this case) mmmm
Petals:	Two
Sephira:	Binah, Chokmah
Planets:	Jupiter, Neptune
Metal:	Silver
Foods:	Entheogens
Corresponding Verb:	I see
Yoga Path:	Yantra yoga
Herbs for Incense:	Mugwort, star anise, acacia, saffron
Minerals:	Lapis lazuli, quartz, star sapphire
Animals:	Owl
Guna:	Sattva
Lotus Symbols:	Two white petals around a circle, within which is a golden triangle pointing downward (tri-kuna) containing the lingam, and the seed sound om; in the pericarp, the Shakti, Hakini, with six red faces and six arms, seated on a white lotus; above her, a crescent moon, the Bindu dot of manifestation, Shiva in the form of lightning flashes.
Hindu Deities:	Shakti Hakini, Paramasiva (form of Shiva), Krishna
Other Pantheons:	Themis, Hecate, Tara, Isis, Iris, Morpheus, Belenos, Apollo

THE WINGED PERCEIVER

Imagination is more important than knowledge.
—Albert Einstein

From the dawning of ages, darkness and light have intertwined to bring us one of the greatest gifts of consciousness—the ability to see. To witness the wonders of the universe, whether light years away in the twinkling dome of stars, or blossoming in the flowers of our backyard, the gift of sight allows us to behold the beauty of creation. Seeing gives us the ability to instantaneously take in enormous amounts of information about our surroundings. Shape and form distilled into light waves create an internal map of the world around us. From our dreams, images spring from the unconscious and connect us to the soul. With intuition, we see our way through situations, gleaning wisdom to guide us in difficult moments.

It is this gift of seeing—both inner and outer—that is the essence and function of chakra six. Through seeing, we have both a means of internalizing the outer world, and a symbolic language for externalizing the inner world. Through our perception of spatial relationships, we have building blocks for both memory of the past and imagination of the future. Thus, this chakra transcends time.

The "brow chakra," as it is often called, is located in the center of the head behind the forehead—either at eye level or slightly above, varying from person to person. It is associated with the third eye, an etheric organ of psychic perception floating between our two physical eyes. The third eye can be seen as the psychic organ of the sixth chakra, just as our physical eyes are tools of perception for the brain. The chakra itself includes the inner screen and vast storehouse of images that comprise our visual thinking process. The third eye sees beyond the physical world, bringing us added insight, just as reading between the lines of written material brings us deeper understanding.

The Sanskrit name of this chakra is *ajna*, which originally meant "to perceive" and later "to command." This speaks to the twofold nature of this chakra—to take in images through perception, but also to form inner images from which we command our reality, commonly known as creative visualization. To hold an image in our mind increases the possibility that it will materialize. This image becomes like a stained glass window through which the light of consciousness shines on its way to manifestation. If there is no interference, the form on the manifested plane is just what we visualized, just like the projected image of the stained glass window if there is no furniture in the way. One reason our visualizations don't always manifest is because so often we do encounter interference along the descent to manifestation. That interference could be someone else's circumstances, fears from the unconscious, or simply lack of clarity in our visualization.

While our petals have been steadily increasing in number as we climb up the Sushumna, we suddenly have only two petals at the ajna chakra.[1] (See Figure 7.1, page 283.) There are many possible interpretations of their meaning: the two worlds of reality—manifest and unmanifest; the intertwining nadis, Ida and Pingala, which meet at this point; and the two physical eyes that surround the third eye. The petals also resemble wings, and symbolize the ability of this chakra to transcend time and space, allowing the inner spirit to "fly" to distant times and places. It is interesting to note that if you compare the caduceus to the chakras and nadis, the two wings occur where the sixth chakra would be. One further interpretation is that the two petals, surrounding a circle, resemble the whites of the eye itself, as it surrounds the iris.

The corresponding element to this chakra is *light*. Through the sensory interpretation of light we obtain information about the world around us. How much we are able to see depends upon how open or developed this chakra is, including, to some degree, the acuity of our normal eyesight. The gamut of visual and psychic ability can run from those who are extremely observant of the physical world to those who are gifted in psychic perception, who can see auras, chakras, details of the astral plane, precognition (the "seeing" of future events) and remote viewing (seeing things in other places).

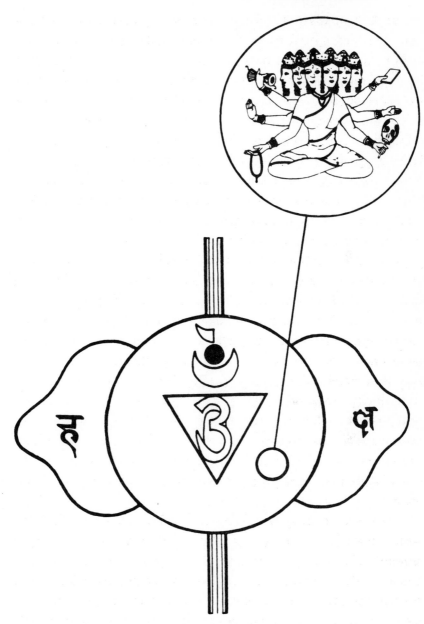

Goddess: Hākinī

FIGURE 7.1
Ājñā Chakra.
(from *Kundalini Yoga for the West*)

Unlike the five lower chakras, which are situated in the body, the brow chakra is located in the head. Therefore, its nature is more mental than any of the previous chakras. Our visual perceptions must become translated into other forms, such as language, actions, or emotions, before they can be tangibly shared. As we become more mental, we leave behind the limitations of time and space and enter a transpersonal dimension.

As each chakra corresponds to a gland, chakra six is related to the *pineal gland*, a tiny (10 x 6 mm) cone-shaped gland located in the geometric center of the head at approximately eye level. (See Figure 7.2, page 285.) It is possible that this gland was, at one time, located nearer to the top of the head. In some species of reptiles it still is, forming a kind of light-sensitive perceptual organ, resembling another eye.[2]

The pineal gland, sometimes called the "seat of the soul," acts as a light meter for the body, translating variations in light to hormonal messages relayed to the body through the autonomic nervous system. Over 100 body functions have daily rhythms which are influenced by exposure to light.[3] The pineal reaches the height of its development at age seven, and has been thought to influence the maturation of the sex glands.[4] Embryologically, the pineal gland is derived from a third eye that begins to develop early in the embryo and later degenerates.[5] The pineal has some tranquilizing effect on the nervous system and removal of the pineal can predispose an animal to seizures.

Melatonin, a hormone relevant to pigment cells, has been isolated from the pineal. It is suggested that the production of melatonin is triggered by exposure of the eyes to light, even in small amounts.[6] Melatonin, now widely researched as a sleeping aid, is believed to strengthen our immune system, reduce stress, and retard aging.[7] Melatonin production decreases as we age, and low melatonin levels are commonly found in depression, and consequently, higher than normal levels in manic states.[8]

Because the pineal gland is located just above the pituitary, some people correlate the pineal to chakra seven and the pituitary to chakra

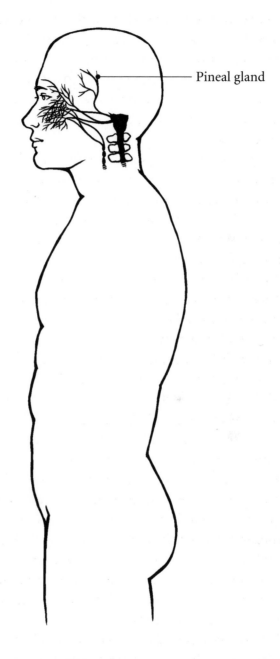

Pineal gland

FIGURE 7.2
Chakra Six.

six. I strongly feel that since the pituitary is the master gland that controls the other glands, this relates to the master chakra of the crown. Since the pineal is a light sensitive organ, it seems clear that the pineal is related to chakra six.

Is the immaturity of our culture at this sixth chakra level relevant to the atrophy of the pineal gland? Does this gland have a mystic function that presently lies dormant, waiting for some sort of spiritual or cultural awakening? Studies have shown that light has a definite effect on the health and behavior of plants and mammals.[9] Could it be that the pineal gland plays some secret role in the link between light and the chemistry of the body?

At this point there is not enough evidence to say. Melatonin, as a sleeping aid, increases dreaming, showing that it has some relevance to inner vision. Melatonin is chemically similar to native plants known to induce visions and can cycle into a compound called 10-methoxyharmalan, which is potentially hallucinogenic. Some psychotropic drugs, such as LSD, increase melatonin synthesis.[10] There may indeed be chemical properties associated with the pineal in advanced humans that trigger the phenomenon of inner vision. Now that melatonin has become so widely used as a sleeping tonic, it will be interesting to see over time what effect this may have on our pineal glands or our psychic sensitivity.

LIGHT

If therefore thine eye be single, thy whole body shall be filled with light.

—Matthew 6:22

At the fifth chakra level of awareness, we experienced vibration as an underlying manifestation of form. At chakra six we encounter a higher, faster vibration than that of sound, though of a fundamentally different character. Here we embrace the part of the electromagnetic spectrum that we perceive as visible light. Ultraviolet radiation, radio waves, x-rays, and microwaves are just a few of the many wave forms within this spectrum that are not visible to the eye. Light is the form directly perceivable by consciousness. Whereas sound is expressed through a wavelike oscillation of air molecules, light is a far finer vibrational energy, produced by radiative emission from atomic and molecular systems as they undergo energy-level transitions. In a very real sense, light is the voice of atoms and molecules, whereas sound is the voice of larger structures.[11]

Visible light consists of wave packets called photons, which exhibit either wave-like or particle-like properties, depending on the method of observation. Because light is wavelike, some of the principles we discussed with sound waves apply equally well to light, such as wave-forms that can be coherent. Variations in frequency give us the different colors, just as frequency in sound gave us different pitches. Since light is also particle-like, we can think of it as discreet packets or photons, each containing information that allows us to see.

Light travels the fastest of any of the elements discussed so far. Extreme wind, which may reach over 200 miles per hour, and even sound, at 720 miles per hour, are left far behind by light at 186,000 miles per second—the fastest known speed of any material phenomenon.[12] Again, we step further out of the physical limitations of time and space with each new dimension, and the extreme speed of light distorts and transcends our very sense of time. Indeed, if one were to travel at the speed of light, time would cease to pass. This too becomes important at the sixth level, for as Vissudha transcended distance, the Ajna chakra transcends time. In this way, we may see a star in the sky, thousands of light years away, which may even have gone nova and disappeared — but the light of that phenomenon has not yet reached our eyes.

Light is electromagnetic energy. Though the photons are without mass, light can induce an electric current upon striking metal, a phenomenon known as the photoelectric effect. Photons, striking the metal, displace electrons in the metal, which induces a current. The interesting thing about this effect is that the lower frequencies of light—such as red light, for example—do not have enough energy to induce a current, regardless of their intensity. At higher frequencies, such as blue or violet, a current is produced, which then will vary with the intensity of the light.

This implies that in the nearly nonphysical dimension of light, quantity of light is far less important than quality, and quality is dependent upon frequency, which we experience as color. For this reason, any study of light must include an excursion into color.

COLOR

Color, like features, follow the changes of the emotions.
—Pablo Picasso[13]

Color is the form through which we perceive light. Vivid in experience, rich in depth, color is the very fabric of our seeing. Color is produced by different frequencies in the wavelengths of light. The "hotter" colors—such as reds, oranges, and yellows—are of a lower frequency than the "cooler" colors of green, blue and violet, and therefore the photons have less energy. (Hot and cool are our own subjective assessments, and say little about the actual energy of the light.)

Light is produced by the excitation and de-excitation of electrons within the atom. Electrons lose or gain energy by "leaping" from one energy level to another. Each leap is called a quantum jump, a discrete step and amount of energy much like the steps on a stairway. When an electron jumps to a higher level, it must absorb a certain amount of energy. When it falls back again toward the nucleus, that energy is released as a photon of light. An electron falling through two levels releases more energy than an electron falling through only one level. Therefore, the photon emits light at a higher frequency, giving us the blues and violets of the upper chakras.

Color carries very definite psychological effects. Red, which physiologically stimulates the heart and nervous system, is also associated with aggressive and initiatory energies—anger, blood, beginnings of things. Blues, by contrast, are associated with peace and tranquillity, and have exactly that effect on most people. Even wavelengths beyond the visible spectrum have an effect on our health and state of mind. Fluorescent lights, for example, which do not contain the invisible ultraviolet rays, have been shown to have a negative influence on health, both in plants and animals.[14] By contrast, full sunlight, containing the complete spectrum, have in some instances helped heal arthritis, cancer, and other diseases.[15]

If we consider that a large percentage of our information comes to us in visual form, and that visual information is perceived as patterns of color, the subtle changes in frequency exhibited by light must have an enormous affect upon our minds and bodies.

If sound waves affect the physical arrangement of subtle energy, it would follow that color, being such a high octave of material manifestation, could influence matter in much the same way. For this reason, color has been used in healing, with remarkable success. Recent studies have shown some colors of light can be 500% more effective in stimulating certain bodily enzymes.[16] This art was known by healers in the early part of the century, (before such things were scoffed upon by the medical profession) as witnessed by the following quote from a practicing physician versed in the art of color therapy :

> *For about six years I have given close attention to the action of colors in restoring the body functions, and I am perfectly honest in saying that, after nearly thirty-seven years of active hospital and private practice in medicine and surgery, I can produce quicker and more accurate results with colors than with any or all other methods combined—and with less strain on the patient. In many cases, the functions have been restored after the classical remedies have failed . . . . Sprains, bruises, and traumata of all sorts respond to color as to no other treatment. Septic conditions*

yield, regardless of the specific organism. Cardiac lesions, asthma,
hay fever, pneumonia, inflammatory conditions of the eyes, corneal
ulcers, glaucoma, and cataracts are relieved by the treatment.[17]

Various theories on the healing effects of color have been written and documented in the last century or so. Using methods such as bathing a person in sunlight passing through a stained glass of a particular color, or drinking water that collected sunlight in a colored glass, has had a remarkable healing effect in many cases. Treatments of blue light, for instance, have been known to provide permanent relief in cases of sciatica and inflammation. In one case the patient had had unrelenting symptoms for eleven years and was relieved within a week of color treatments, with no relapse.[18] In other cases, yellow light has been used to bring mental clarity, red to combat physical exhaustion, and golden-orange has helped diabetics.[19] If diseases begin at the subtle level, should they not be treated at a subtle level as well, using such things as color—especially in conjunction with positive visualization?

The colors of the chakras follow a logical progression through the spectrum, correlating the lowest frequency of light, which is red, to the lowest chakra, matching the rest of the chakras to the spectrum accordingly. This seems to be both the most sensible and the most universal system of coordination to the chakras, but it is *by no means the only system*, and should not be confused with the colors that the chakras appear to be when viewed clairvoyantly, or the colors described in Tantric texts. Some clairvoyant studies, however, such as those conducted by Valerie Hunt, completely corroborate the "rainbow" system as witnessed by the following quote:

Chakras frequently carried the colors stated in the metaphysical
literature, i.e. kundalini–red; hypogastric–orange, spleen–yellow,
heart–green; throat–blue, third eye–violet, crown–white. Activity
in certain chakras seemed to trigger increased activity in another.
The heart chakra was consistently the most active. [20]

In addition, Jacob Lieberman, Ph.D., found in his research that when people were unreceptive to a particular color, it correlated nearly 100 percent of the time to stress, disease, or injury in the part of the body related to the chakra of that color.[21]

According to the rainbow spectrum, the colors for the chakras (according to modern systems) are as follows:

Chakra One:	Red
Chakra Two:	Orange
Chakra Three:	Yellow
Chakra Four:	Green
Chakra Five:	Blue
Chakra Six:	Indigo
Chakra Seven:	Violet

Various Tantric texts describe the chakras differently, saying the first chakra is yellow, the second white, the third red, the fourth smoky, the fifth blue, with the sixth gold and the seventh lustrous beyond color. Perhaps as we evolve, our chakra vibrations are changing frequency, and the colors are now becoming more aligned to the pure colors of the spectrum.

When viewing chakras clairvoyantly, it is equally unlikely that one would see a set of chakras exactly reflecting the above rainbow description, for these are optimum colors occurring in chakras that are fully developed and clear. (In Valerie Hunt's study, subjects were observed throughout weeks of intense rolfing therapy—the clearer colors occurred only toward the end of therapy.)[22] From my own experience, it is far more common to see many colors in each chakra, twisting in and out of the chakra and forming patterns and images that relate to that person's life.

You can also use the associated colors as meditational or mnemonic devices to gain access to your chakras or to find out more about them. First, we can take a small reading of our own chakras through examination of the colors we tend to surround ourselves with—as in our clothing and home decor. Do you always pick the purples and blues or do you consistently go for the vibrant reds and oranges? Are you fond of dark or light colors? Is it a mere coincidence that some monks, who practice celibacy, wear saffron (pale orange) robes, a color related to the second chakra?

Secondly, we can choose colors that complement the chakras we feel are the weakest. For a long time I was aware of an absence of yellow in my auric field which was also confirmed by many friends and psychics who looked at me. Simultaneously, I had metabolic problems, and many issues related to the third chakra, such as low energy and feelings of powerlessness. I found that wearing a yellow gemstone (topaz) and yellow clothing helped my attitude considerably, to the point where other people remarked about an improvement. On a subtle level, this brought balance into my personal energy system.

Colors can also be used in visualization for self-healing. In the above case, especially on darker days, I would sit and visualize my aura as a bright yellow; or alternately, visualize golden rays of energy coming to me from the sun. What I projected outward from myself gradually became manifest around me. When Selene Vega and I teach our chakra workshops, we encourage students to wear colored clothing to match the chakra we are studying each day. In this way, we immerse ourselves in the vibrational spectrum of that particular chakra. Colors, like the sounds associated with each chakra, are another form of expression of the seven planes associated with this system.

THE HOLOGRAPHIC THEORY

In the Heaven of Indra, there is said to be a network of pearls so arranged that if you look at one you see all others reflected in it. In the same way, each object in the world is not merely itself but involves every other object, and in fact, IS every other object.

—Hindu Sutra [23]

How do light and visual process connect to what we experience in perception? Why do so many mystics claim to see patterns of light when they meditate, eyes closed? Why do dream images seem so real? And what constitutes memory?

The most plausible theory put forth to answer these questions comes from a neuroscientist named Karl Pribram, and is based on a model of the mind as a hologram. A hologram is a three-dimensional image formed by two intersecting laser beams. This is analogous to dropping two pebbles into a pond at different locations, and quickly freezing the water. The intersections of ripples would be permanently recorded onto the ice, just as the interference of the light beams are recorded onto the holographic plate.

In the creation of a hologram, a beam of light produced by a laser is reflected from an object, and recorded on a light-sensitive plate. The plate also receives another beam of the same frequency, called the *reference beam*, which goes directly from the source to the plate. Looking at the plate itself, we would see only a meaningless pattern of dark and light swirls. This is the coded information of the intersection of the two beams, much as the grooves on a record are the coded representation of a sound track.

When the plate is later "reenacted" by a reference beam that contains the same frequency as the original laser, the image of the holographed object eerily jumps out at you in three dimensions. You can move to the side of the hologram and see the side of the object as if it were really there, yet since it is only light you can pass your hand right through it.

There are many remarkable things about holograms. The first is that the information is stored "omnipresently" on the plate. In other words, if the plate were to break into pieces, any piece of the plate would be capable of reproducing the whole picture, though with increasingly less detail as the pieces diminish in size. The second remarkable thing about holograms is that they are nonspatial. Many holograms can be superimposed upon one another in one "space," or on one plate by using laser's of different frequencies. Karl Pribram's theory states that the brain itself functions like a hologram through constant interpretation of interference patterns between brain waves. This is fundamentally different from previous brain models, where each bit of information is stored in a particular place. This theory has shaken the foundations of physics and physiology, creating a paradigm shift in the study of consciousness. Its ramifications are far reaching in the understanding of the mind as well as the world around us. This model seems particularly relevant to the understanding of the ajna chakra. Let's look at how this theory developed:

Pribram first began by doing brain research on rats and monkeys in 1946. Working with Karl Lashley, he dissected numerous brains, looking for the mysterious basic unit of memory, called the engram. Thinking, as many did at that time, that memories were stored in various nerve cells in the brain, they expected that certain memories would be wiped out by removing brain tissue.

Not so. Instead, they found that memory seemed to be stored omnipresently throughout the brain, much as the plate stores holographic information. When tissue was removed, memories became fuzzier but didn't disappear. This explained why memories survived massive brain damage, why the brain can store an entire lifetime of memory, and why memories were often triggered by certain associations, or "reference beams."

When we view an object, light is transformed into neural frequency patterns in the brain. The brain is filled with some thirteen billion neurons. The number of possible connections between these neurons numbers in the trillions. Where scientists have previously looked at the neurons themselves as significant to brain activity, they are now looking at the *junctions between the neurons*. While the actual cells exhibit a kind of on-off reflex action, the junctions at the nerve endings exhibit wavelike qualities when viewed as a whole. In Pribram's own words: "If you look at a whole series of these (nerve endings) together, they constitute a wavefront. One comes this way, another that way, and they interact. And all of a sudden you've got your interference pattern!"[24]

As impulses travel through the brain, the wavelike qualities create what we experience as perception and memory. These perceptions are stored as encoded wavefront frequencies in the brain and can be activated by an appropriate stimulus, triggering the original wave forms. This could explain why a familiar face brings up recognition, even though that face may look different from the last time you saw it. It may explain why mention of roses brings to mind a particular smell, and why snakes may generate fear even when there is no particular threat.

Our perception of the world around us seems to be a reconstruction of a neural hologram within the brain. This applies to language, thought, and all the senses as well as to the perception of visual information. In the words of Pribram: "Mind isn't located in a place. What we have is a holograph-like machinery that turns out images, which we perceive as existing somewhere outside the machinery."[25]

Because this model hints at each of our brains containing access to all information, even that of other time dimensions, it can explain many things beyond the normal functions of memory and perception such as remote viewing, clairvoyance, mystic visions, and precognition.

Contemporary to Pribram's holographic brain theory, theoretical physicist David Bohm has described a model which suggests that the universe itself may be a kind of hologram.[26] His term for this is holoflux, as hologram is static and not fitting for a universe so filled with movement and change.

According to Bohm, the universe is "enfolded" or spread as a whole throughout a kind of cosmic medium, much as we would enfold egg whites into a cake batter. This enfoldment allows for an infinite number of interference capabilities, giving us the forms and energies that we experience with our holographic minds. In this context, then, the brain itself is part of a larger hologram, and would therefore contain information about the whole. Just as we perceive the world in a holographic fashion, so may the world itself be a larger hologram in which we are just small pieces. But as pieces, we each reflect the whole.

If this is true—if there is an inner and outer world, both of which mirror the entire creation in any of its parts—then we, as parts, contain the information of the whole, as does everything around us. Not only does a grain of sand describe the universe in which it occurs, but each of our minds also contains the encoded information of a greater intelligence, just waiting for the right reference beam to trigger the image. Perhaps this is why gurus can trigger shaktipat, and sympathetic vibration can trigger altered states of consciousness.

If both inner and outer worlds appear to function holographically, then the question must be asked: Is there any difference between them? Are we, ourselves, also holograms? As we slowly dissolve our self-created ego boundaries and embrace more universal states of being, are we merging our consciousness with a greater hologram? If each piece of the hologram contains information about the whole, though less clearly, is that why we gain clarity each time a new piece of information fits into the puzzle? As we grow and expand our understanding, do we not see things more and more as one interpenetrating web of energies, one picture?

At this time these questions have no definitive answers. Few could argue that what is considered "external" does influence our perceptions, thoughts, and memories, becoming "internal." Few could argue that there is a structure inside of us which encompasses energies above and beyond the external world. Doesn't this internal structure, in turn, influence the external world? Can the construction of our mental holograms be projected outward to take form on the material planes? Karl Pribram seems to think so, and in a most down-to-earth fashion:

> Not only do we construct our perceptions of the world, but we also go out and construct those perceptions IN the world. We make tables and bicycles and musical instruments because we can think of them.[27]

It is this principle that best illustrates the abilities of the ajna chakra—to perceive and to command—and the psychic reception and projection of imagery with the outside world.

SEEING

All that we see are our visualizations. We see not with the eye, but with the soul.[28]

It has been estimated that in the sighted person ninety percent of our information comes through our eyes—more than through any other organ or sensory means. It follows then that a large portion of our memory and thought processes are also coded with visual information. This of course varies from person to person, as some people are more visually oriented than others. While the visual experience of the world may often be limited or misleading, there is no doubt that it is a fundamentally important level of consciousness.

Visual information can be defined as a pattern which communicates spatial relationships, reaching us without the necessity of physical contact (as in touch). These relationships describe form, as in size and shape, color, intensity, location, movement, and behavior.

The physical eyes see by focusing reflected rays of light onto the retina. The focusing is done by the cornea, which takes a larger pattern of light and reduces it, inverted, onto the retina. The retina is made up of rods and cones which are stimulated by varying intensities of light. When light hits these cells, a chemical reaction takes place, triggering nerve impulses. These impulses are then conducted along the optic chiasm to the cerebral cortex of the brain, in the form of electrical impulses. No actual light enters the brain.

It is not really our eyes that see, but our minds. The eyes are merely focal lenses for transcribing information from the outer world to the inner. The brain does not actually receive photons of light, but rather encoded electrical impulses. It is up to the mind/brain to interpret the electrical impulses traveling along the optic nerves into meaningful patterns. This is a learned ability. In persons blind from birth whose sight is later restored by surgery, it is found that their first perceptions are only of light and they must struggle to learn to make meaningful images of this perception.[29]

We also must remember that it is not matter that we perceive, but light. When we look at the world around us, we think that we see objects, but what we are really seeing is the light reflected by these objects—we see what they are not, we see the spaces between them, the spaces around them, but we cannot see into the actual objects. If we see red, then the object absorbs all frequencies *except* red light. We confirm its presence by touch—but our hand moves through the empty space. It too cannot feel the object, but only the edge of the object. What it feels is the textured boundaries of the empty space. From this perspective, matter can be seen as a kind of no man's land— a world we cannot enter except perhaps in very thin slices—penetrable by light under a microscope, or through glass and crystals. We experience our world through a dimension of empty space.

CLAIRVOYANCE

In order to see, you have to stop being in the middle of the picture.

—Sri Aurobindo[30]

The most significant aspect of consciousness at the level of the sixth chakra is the development of psychic abilities. While psychic perception is not always visual, as in clairaudience (from chakra five), or clairsentience (chakra two), the timelessness of clairvoyant information allows it to encompass a greater scope than any psychic abilities discussed thus far.

The term clairvoyance means clear seeing. This is seeing that is not muddled by the opaque world of material objects normally defining our limited sense of space and time. The words *clear* and *seeing* quite accurately describe the processes involved: to be clairvoyant, we need to look in the spaces that are clear—to look at the *fields* of energy, not at the objects themselves; to look at relationships, not things; to see the world as a whole, and to reach with our minds directly and clearly for the information we want. The more clarity we have within ourselves, the better we're able to see the subtle properties of the world around us.

To *see* implies a far deeper perception than to look—as exemplified by Don Juan in the Carlos Castaneda series. When Castaneda looked at a person, he only perceived a body, facial expressions, clothing. When he learned to *see*, he perceived a luminous egg surrounding the body—the web of interpenetrating energies we call the aura. When Don Juan looked at his brother dying, he was deeply grieved, but when he instead changed his mode to seeing, he understood the greater process involved and could learn from it.

Looking is the action of seeing, but seeing is the internalizing of the image into understanding. Take, for example, the common expression, "I see." It generally means that someone has been able to take a small part of information and fit it into a scheme of the whole. Just as each bit of a hologram clarifies the whole picture, each new thing we look at becomes immediately incorporated into our sense of wholeness, bringing more clarity to our internal picture.

How do we do this? According to Pribram's model of the hologram, our mind/brain acts as a kind of stage upon which our visual images play. When the proper cue is given (the holographic reference beam), the images appear on the stage. But where and what are the actors?

The actors are the slides, stored holographically, as colors, shapes, sounds, and tactile patterns. There is no carousel in the brain keeping complete and separate images, but instead portions of the brain may produce qualities such as red, warm, fast, or quiet. These qualities combine in unique ways to create the images we see.

We can think of the third eye as a mental screen upon which we cast our slides for viewing. If you close your eyes and remember your first car, you may be able to see the color, the texture of the upholstery, perhaps a small dent on one side. In your mind's eye you can walk around the car, seeing the front and the back as you choose, just like the three-dimensional effect of a hologram. The actual car need not currently exist. The image exists apart from it. By focusing our attention, the image is retrieved.

In your mind's eye, you can see what you choose to look at. If I ask you the color of your lover's hair, you can mentally retrieve that "slide," look at it, and tell me what it is. Our memories are holographic.

Can you create an equally vivid picture of a car you would like to have? Can you picture the color, the make, the vanity plate on the back? Can you visualize yourself driving it, going down a country road, the feel of the steering wheel in your hand?

That car may never be yours to own, so your visualization is called *imagination*, even though it may seem just as real as your memory. If, however, you won a sweepstakes, and a car such as the one you just visualized came to you, then your visualization could be considered *precognitive*—a form of clairvoyance. The difference lies in the result, *but the process is the same.* Through development of visualization and imagination, we simultaneously develop the means for clairvoyance.

The process of clairvoyance is one of specified visualization. It is a matter of systematically being able to call up relevant information on demand, regardless of whether it had been previously known. Our minds are using a self-made reference beam in the form of a question, to retrieve previously unknown data from the holographic memory bank. For instance, you may ask yourself to look at the area around someone's heart chakra with a specific question that needs answering, such as something about their health or relationship. That question becomes the reference beam that "lights up" that particular piece of information in the holographic pattern.

We have stated that we transcend time in the sixth chakra. We need not limit accessible information to what has been learned in the past— we can also retrieve information from the future. The only difference is that we are actively creating the reference beam that will bring forth the image, rather than waiting for some point in future time where circumstance will call it forth. To quote novelist Marion Zimmer Bradley, "I don't decide where my stories are going. I just peek into the future and write down what happened."[31]

Few people believe they can see something outside ordinary knowing, something they haven't literally seen or been told. There is no permission to have that information and no current explanation for it, so most people don't even bother to look for it. In order to see something, one needs to know where and how to look. We look for things in places where they are likely to be. We need not have put them there ourselves—*we need only understand the basic order in which those things occur.* The decimal system at the library is a prime example. So is finding the appropriate item in an unfamiliar grocery store. You survey the store, noting its general layout, you know what category the item belongs in, you superimpose the two mental images and head to that section to look more closely. Voila! Your mental cross-referencing clicks in place as the sight of the item fits into your precreated mental niche.

Accessing mental information is really no different. If you tried to remember who told you a particular joke at a party, you would review the people at the party, the people you had personal conversations with, all the time keeping the joke in your mind, waiting for the right piece of data to fall into place. When you hit the correct memory, the image would "light up" in your mind—as if illuminated by a clarity that the other images did not have. In this process we look through thousands of bits of data, sorting and deciphering, until we "see" the pieces that fit.

Once we know *where* to look for data, we need to know *how* to look. How many times have you looked for something you knew was in a particular place and still been unable to find it? How many times have you looked right at something and failed to see it? How many times have you accessed your memory and failed to bring forth the information you knew was there?

Accessing memory is a process of finding the right code (the right reference beam) to bring the holographic image back to life. Just as a computer contains data that is accessible only with the right command, so do our mental images require the proper mental image to unlock them.

The development of clairvoyance depends on the development of the visual screen and the creation of an ordering system with which to access information for the screen. If we don't label our slides, we won't know what it is we're looking at. The development of visualization is the ability to retrieve, create, and project images onto the mental screen. Once this is done, *seeing depends largely on asking the right questions.*

We are not limited to slides we have "holographed" ourselves. If the holographic model has any validity, then we have access to an infinity of images, each created by an infinity of brain wave patterns. We need only call it up by finding the correct "reference beam."

Many people begin with Tarot cards, palmistry, or astrology to use as a structure that can provide the reference beam. The card brings up a variety of images, the person you are reading brings up another variety of images. What points seem most important? What points seem to "light up"? Where do the waves of information cross and become strongest?

To look at something clairvoyantly, we not only need a reference point with which to retrieve the data, but also a blank screen to view the information. This comes with practice, patience, and a quiet and open mind. Emptying the mind of images, through meditation, paradoxically allows one to better see what images there are. Learning to focus the mind, creating a one-pointedness, allows one to look deeper, and therefore see more. In clairvoyance there are no substitutes for a clear and quiet mind.

Because these nuances are so subtle, it is common to ignore or invalidate them. Just as we cannot hear the whispers of telepathy in a noisy world, we can't see the subtle movements of the etheric realms if we expect them to be outlined in neon. Following is a typical exchange involving a new student of clairvoyance:

AJ: Have you ever seen an aura?

Student: I don't think so. I don't see auras.

AJ: Have you ever looked?

Student: I've tried. But I don't see colors around the body.

AJ: What do you see when you look for an aura?

Student: I just see the body. Around the edge I see the things in the room behind the body.

AJ: You are looking through space, not at it. Close your eyes and feel the aura. Then tell me what color it feels like.

Student: It feels dark. No color. There's a little bit of gold color over the heart, I guess. But I don't know if I'm really seeing it. I kinda think I maybe see a little red in the legs, especially on the right. But I don't know.

AJ: I thought you couldn't see auras.

Student: But I don't, really. Only with my eyes closed—I mean, it's just my imagination isn't it?

AJ: I don't know. Why don't you check it out first? Ask the person how they are feeling—if the colors fit. Reach out and test it.

Third Person: Well, I was running in the sunshine today, which I love doing, but I tripped on a root and fell. I kinda banged my knee a little and it's still sore. I guess that's relevant.

(enter validation!)

Student: Wow! I really did see something! Yeah, the red was around your knee. (then timidly) Did you bump your head, too?

Third Person: Yes, as a matter of fact. But not as hard.

AJ: How did you know that?

Student: Well, I didn't really see it, but the head looked kinda sore. But there were no colors—just a feeling.

AJ: It looked sore but you didn't see it. O.K. Now look at that other person there.

Student: (eyes half-closed) Well, I see green around the head, blue in the throat—nothing much in the stomach, but a lot of light in the hands.

AJ: And you still say you can't see auras?

Whether a parapsychologist would consider this kind of seeing to be a "hit" or a fraud is beside the point because this exchange is not with a developed clairvoyant, but with a beginning student just learning to see. The process begins with learning to notice what you already see. This is heightened by validation of subtleties. The best way to obtain legitimate validation is to ask! The more we test our perceptions, the more we learn about our abilities and the more we can trust our strong points and develop our weak ones. In a world so bombarded with physical visual stimuli, and so ignorant of the internal images, validation is crucial.

In searching for validation, it is also important to realize that it's O.K. to be wrong—at least while learning. Being wrong doesn't mean that it is impossible, or that you have no psychic ability. Instead use that feedback to refine the seeing: look over what you thought you saw; search for the grain of truth; see if you can find some correlation in your mind's eye to the objective information you've been given. So often when people "guess" wrongly their reaction is, "Darn! That answer was my first impression but I discarded it!" Unless you are purely shooting in the dark, there is usually some grain of truth to all honest perceptions.

Clairvoyance, then, is a matter of seeing the inner relationships of things—the fitting of the part into the whole. It is done by searching for the cross-point, or interference pattern between our question (the reference beam) and the piece of information that best fits the space we have created for it. The potency of the image that clicks into place sets it apart from the infinite number of other possible answers. Through meditation, visualization, and training, we can develop our abilities to perceive the subtle difference between the information we request and the countless other possibilities.

CHAKRA SIX EXERCISES

Yogic Eye Exercise

This is an exercise for strengthening and centering the physical eyes; also good for eyestrain, vision improvement, and general fatigue from doing a lot of paperwork or heavy reading.

Begin in a seated meditation position, spine straight. Close your eyes and bathe them in the darkness. Bring your awareness to the point between your eyes, in the center of the head. Feel the darkness there, and let yourself bask in its quiet calm.

When you feel centered, open your eyes and gaze straight ahead. Slowly look upward, stretching your eyes skyward, without moving your head. Then trace a straight line downward, gazing as low as your vision can reach, still without moving your head. Repeat upward, and then downward again, then return your eyes to center, and close them, returning to the darkness.

Open your eyes again and center them. Then repeat the above movements, going instead from corner to corner, first from upper right to lower left, two times, then from upper left to lower right, also two times. Return again to darkness.

Repeat again, moving from far right to far left, returning to darkness after two times. The final time, after centering your eyes, make half circles, first on the top, then on the bottom, and finish by rolling your eyes "around the clock," making a complete rotation, stretching your eyes as far as they can go, both clockwise and counterclockwise.

Close your eyes again. Rub your palms together briskly, until you feel your hands become warm. When the heat feels sufficient, place your warmed palms over your eyelids and let your eyes bask in the warmth and darkness. (See Figure 7.3, page 307.) As the heat dissipates, slowly stroke your eyelids, massaging your forehead and face. From here you can either go into a deeper meditation or return to the outside world.

Color Meditation

This is a simple visualization for healing and cleansing the chakras, and developing the ability of the inner eye to create and perceive color.

Begin in a meditation position, preferably seated. Ground and center your energy.

When you are sufficiently grounded, imagine a bright disk of white light, floating directly above your head, from which you can draw each color.

Let the first color be red, pulling it down through your crown chakra, down through your whole spinal column and filling up the first chakra with a vibrant red color. Hold that color in your first chakra for a few moments. Notice how your body feels with this color. Does it like it? Does it feel energized or uncomfortable?

Next, return to the area above the crown chakra and pull orange light out of the white disk. Run it down through your body, noticing what effect this color has on you. Bring it down to your second chakra, and fill your belly with a vibrant, orange color.

Return to the crown and find a golden yellow light to pull through the body down to the third chakra. Imagine a warm golden glow coming out of your body at the solar plexus, with rays streaming through each part of your body, filling and warming it. As the third chakra has to do with energy distribution throughout the body, these rays are important for spreading the sense of inner fire.

Now we come to the heart, and the color green. Feel this color wash over you, bringing with it a sense of love and affinity for the world around you. See it as a warm emerald glow around your heart.

Next, we reach into our white disk for the color blue, pulling it down into the throat chakra. Allow it to soothe your throat as well as relax your arms and shoulders. Feel the blue rays extend all around your throat, communicating with all that is around you.

Next, we come to the third eye itself, usually seen as a deep indigo blue. Feel the coolness of this color as it bathes your

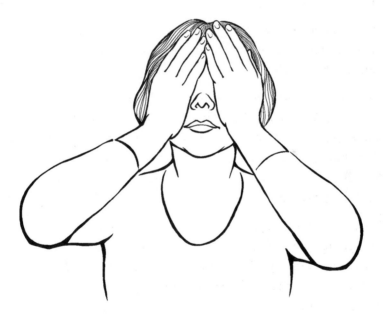

Figure 7.3
Palming the Eyes.

third eye. Allow it to wash any foreign images away, cleansing and soothing your inner screen.

And lastly, the crown chakra is seen as a bright vibrant violet color. Feel this violet light streaming into your crown chakra, energizing and balancing each of the chakras.

Check all of the chakras to see if they are retaining their colors. Take a glimpse of your whole body and see if you can "see" it as a continuous rainbow. As you check over your body, notice which colors are the strongest or brightest. Notice how the different colors felt—which ones were more nourishing or energizing. The colors that felt the most welcome probably represent energies that you need most at this time. The colors that felt the least welcome represent areas that you typcially avoid or where there may be difficulty. Pale or washed-out colors represent weak areas; strong colors, places of strength and solidity. Play internally with the colors until they feel balanced to you. This helps to balance the aura as well.

Photo Blink

This exercise is a simple way to get a sense of someone's aura if you normally don't see auras. It also helps to improve visual observation.

Place the person you want to look at directly opposite you, about six to ten feet away. Close your eyes and clear your mental screen. Wait until you feel grounded and centered, with no particular thoughts or images running through your mind.

Very quickly open and close your eyes once—the opposite of a blink—so that you get only a quick glimpse of the person in front of you, making a sort of frozen "photographic" image imprinted in your mind. Hold that image and examine it. What characteristics do you notice? Do you see an afterimage or a glow around the body? Do certain colors or body positions stand out? As the image fades, quickly open and close your eyes again to strengthen it. See how much detail you can decipher in this "afterimage." Which parts fade first, and which characteristics linger? All these things tell you about the strengths and weaknesses of that person's aura.

Meditation

The most useful exercise for strengthening the third eye is simple meditation, focusing the attention on the center of the head or the point between the eyebrows. Visualizations of colors or shapes can be added, or you can simply focus on clearing the mind screen until it is clean and blank.

> Once the screen is blank, visualizations can be willed in answer to questions you may have. If you want to know about someone's health, for example, visualize a picture of their body shape, and allow black or white to show areas of health and disease. Be creative in finding a visual metaphor for your question. The limits of this system are only the limits of your imagination, and the more we open this center, the more we expand our imagination!
>
> Another way to perceive how we feel about a certain decision is to phrase the question so that it can be answered with a simple yes or no. Then make a visualization to represent each answer—put yes on one side of your screen, no on the other. Then imagine a gauge with a needle pointing straight up, and on the count of three, let the needle point to the answer most appropriate. Don't control the needle—let it go where it will. You may be surprised!

Note: The ability to visualize successfully depends on constant use, like a muscle. Get in the habit of imagining a face before you answer the telephone; retrace all your steps of getting to work in the morning as if you were watching from the outside; reconstruct memories of your childhood bedroom, playmates, or first sweetheart. Visualize a task completed before you begin it and find out if it makes the doing easier; visualize larger numbers in your check register; visualize meeting someone new.

Visualization is active dreaming. The more we do it, the more vivid and capable our mind's creations. The opportunities for practice are endless. Once it becomes a habit, it develops naturally.

ENDNOTES

1. Leadbeater postulates 96 petals for the brow chakra, which is two times the sum of all the lower petals or 2 x (4 + 6 +10+ 12+16) = 96. C. W. Leadbeater, *The Chakras,* 14.

2. *Encyclopedia Americana,* s.v., "pineal gland."

3. Jacob Lieberman, *Light, Medicine of the Future,* (Sante Fe, NM : Bear & Co., 1991), 32.

4. Ibid. It keeps sexual characteristics from maturing too soon.

5. Arthur C., Guyton, *Textbook of Medical Physiology*, 884.

6. Jacob Lieberman, *Light, Medicine of the Future,* (Sante Fe, NM: Bear & Co., 1991), 32.

7. Alan E Lewis, and Dallas Clouatre, Ph.D. *Melatonin and Biological Clock,*   7–8.

8. Ibid., 16.

9. John N. Ott, *Health and Light.*

10. Alan E. Lewis and Dallas Clouatre, Ph.D. *Melatonin and the Biological Clock,* 23.

11. Stephanie Sonnleitner, Ph.D., personal conversation.

12. There are hypothetical subatomic particles called tachyons which are believed to travel faster than light speed, but are unable to slow down to the speed of light.

13. Pablo Picasso, Conversations avec Picasso, in *Cahiers d'Art,* vol. 10, no 10 Paris, 1935. Translated in *Picasso, Fifty Years of his Art* by Alfred H. Barr, Jr., 1946.

14. John N. Ott, "Color and Light: Their Effects on Plants, Animals, and People," Journal of Biosocial Research 7, part 1, 1985.

15. John N. Ott, *Health and Light,* 70 ff.

16. K. Martinek and I.V. Berezin, "Artificial Light—Sensitive Enzymatic Systems as Chemical Amplifiers of Weak Light Signals," Photochemistry and Biology 29 (March 1979), 637–650. (as quoted by Jacob Lieberman, *Light, Medicine of the Future,* 9).

17. Kate W. Baldwin, M.D., F.A.C.S., "The Atlantic Medical Journal," April, 1927, as quoted in *The Ancient Art of Color Therapy,* by Linda Clark, 18–19.

18. Edward W. Babbitt, *The Principles of Light and Color,* 40.

19. Linda Clark, *The Ancient Art of Color Therapy,* 112.

20. Valerie Hunt, Ph.D., " A Study of Structural Integration from Neuromuscular, Energy Field, and Emotional Approaches." now published in *Wheels of Light: A Study of the Chakras,* Rosalyn Bruyere, (Sierra Madre, CA: Bon Productions, 1989), 197 ff.

21. Jacob Lieberman, O.D., Ph.D., *Light, Medicine of the Future,* (Santa Fe, NM: Bear & Co., 1991), 189.

22. Valerie Hunt, op. cit., 197 ff.

23. As quoted in *The Holographic Paradigm and Other Paradoxes,* Ken Wilbur, ed., 25.

24. Karl Pribram, "Interview: Omni Magazine, October, 1982, 170.

25. Ibid., 172.

26. "The Enfolding-Unfolding Universe: A Conversation with David Bohm" conducted by Renee Weber in *The Holographic Paradigm and Other Paradoxes,* Ken Wilbur, ed., 44–104.

27. Ibid., 139. This is also similar to Rupert Sheldrake's theory of morphogenetic fields.

28. Mike Samuels, *Seeing with the Mind's Eye,* xviii.

29. Ibid., 57–59.

30. Satprem, *Sri Aurobindo, or the Adventures of Consciousness.*

31. Marion Zimmer Bradley, personal conversation.

RECOMMENDED READING FOR CHAKRA SIX

Clark, Linda. *The Ancient Art of Color Therapy.* NY: Pocket Books, 1975.

Friedlander, John and Gloria Hemsher. *Basic Psychic Development.* York Beach, ME: Samuel Weiser, Inc., 1998.

Gawain, Shakti. *Creative Visualization.* CA: Whatever Publishing, 1978.

Lieberman, Jacob, O.D., Ph.D. *Light, Medicine of the Future.* Santa Fe, NM: Bear & Co., 1991.

Samuels and Samuels. *Seeing With the Mind's Eye.* NY: Random House, 1976.

Wallace, Amy and Bill Henkin. *The Psychic Healing Book.* Wingbow Press, 1981.

Wilber, Ken, ed. *The Holographic Paradigm and Other Paradoxes.* Boston, MA: Shambhala, 1982.

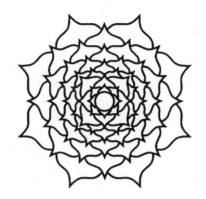

CHAKRA SEVEN

Consciousness

Thought

Information

Knowing

Understanding

Transcendence

Immanence

Meditation

Chapter 8

CHAKRA SEVEN: THOUGHT

OPENING MEDITATION

You have gone on a journey.
You have touched, you have tasted, you
*   have seen, and you have heard.*
You have loved and lost and loved
*   again.*
You have learned. You have grown.
*   You have arrived at your destina-*
*   tion intact.*

And now, at the end of the journey, you are almost home.
There is but one step left—the biggest and the smallest of them all.
It is the biggest for it takes us the farthest.
It is the smallest because we are already there.
There is one more door to open—and it contains the key to all that lies
beyond
You hold that key, but you cannot see it. It is not a thing, it is not a way.
It is a mystery.
Allow yourself to review the places you have gone . . .
Remembering the touch of flesh to Earth, the flow of movement and
power, the song of love in your heart, the memories imprinted in your
mind . . .
Who is it that remembers?
Who has traveled on this journey?
Is it your body? Then what has guided you? What is it that has grown?
Through what have you traveled?
Who now would hold that key that can't be seen, the key that cannot
lock?
The answer to this is the key itself.
All wisdom is within you. Nothing is beyond you. The kingdom is before
you, within you, around you. It is in your mind, which is but one
mind in a sea of many; connected, contained, intelligent, divine.
It is the seat of the gods, the pattern of creation, the immensity of the infi-
nite, the endless unfolding petals of the lotus, fully blooming and con-
nected all the way to Earth.
We find it in our thoughts.
Beyond form, beyond sound, beyond light, beyond space, beyond time,
Our thoughts flow.
Below, behind, above, around and through our thoughts flow.
Within, without, before and after, our thoughts flow.
Droplets in an endless sea, the song of mind is infinite.
We have come full circle and the pattern is complete.
We are the thoughts that make the pattern,
And we are the pattern that makes the thoughts.

From whence do our thoughts arise?
Where do they go when they rest?
And who is it that perceives them?
Deep within ourselves we find a place to open up our mind.
Through starry heavens ever climbing, matter's solid threads unbinding.
Out beyond far Heaven's veil, the Father rules the starlit trail.
In patterns bright, perceived by sight, our thoughts turn over day
    through night, Through our thinking, ever linking, winding, weav-
    ing, wisdom's webs,
Ancient patterns, flows and ebbs.
Auspicious Shiva, Lord of Sleep, your meditations bring us deep
To ancient wisdom found within, a sacred place where we begin
And ending, here we shall return; reconnected we have learned
To know divinity inside and bring it forth with honored pride.
The key within our minds we hold, to mysteries we shall unfold;
Gateway to the worlds beyond,
In sacred space and peace we bond.

CHAKRA SEVEN
SYMBOLS AND CORRESPONDENCES

Sanskrit Name:	Sahasrara
Meaning:	Thousandfold
Location:	Top of head
Element:	Thought
Manifestation:	Information
Personal Function:	Understanding
Psychological State:	Bliss
Glands:	Pituitary
Other Body Parts:	Cerebral cortex, Central nervous system

Malfunction:	Depression, alienation, confusion, boredom, apathy, inability to learn
Color:	Violet to white
Seed Sound:	None
Vowel Sound:	Ngngng, as in sing (again, not really a vowel)
Petals:	Some say 960, some say 1,000. To the Hindus, numbers with ones and zeroes, as in 100, 1,000, or 10,000, indicated infinity. Therefore, the thousand petals is a metaphor for infinity whereas 960 is the mathematical equivalent of the first five chakras added together (4 + 6 + 10 + 12 + 16) multiplied by the two petals of chakra six, times ten.
Sephiroth:	Kether
Planet:	Uranus
Metal:	Gold
Foods:	none, fasting
Corresponding Verb:	to know
Yoga Path:	Jnana yoga, or meditation
Herbs For Incense:	Lotus, Gotu Kola
Guna:	Sattvas
Minerals:	Amethyst, diamond
Lotus Symbols:	Within Sahasrara is the full moon, without the mark of the hare, resplendent as in a clear sky. It sheds its rays in profusion, and is moist and cool like nectar. Inside it, constantly shining like lightning, is the triangle, and inside this, again, shines the Great Void which is served in secret by all the Suras."[1] Some say the petals turn upward, toward the Heavens.

Ancient texts say they turn downward, hugging the skull. The petals are believed to be a lustrous white.

Hindu Deities: Shiva, Ama-kala (upward moving shakti), Varuna

Other Pantheons: Zeus, Allah, Nut, Enki, Inanna, Odin, Mimir, Ennoia

THE THOUSAND-PETALED LOTUS

The universe is just the way we think it is—and that's why.
—John Woods[2]

At last we culminate the sevenfold journey, climbing to the thousand-petaled lotus blooming at the top of the head. Here we find the infinitely profound seat of cosmic consciousness known as the seventh or crown chakra. This chakra connects us to divine intelligence and the source of all manifestation. It is the means through which we reach understanding and find meaning. As the final goal of our liberating current, it is the place of ultimate liberation.

Like a king whose crown signifies order in the kingdom, the crown chakra represents the ruling principle of life—the place where the underlying order and meaning of all things is ultimately perceived. It is the pervading consciousness that thinks, reasons, and gives form and focus to our activities. It is the true essence of being as the awareness that dwells within. In the unconscious, it is the wisdom of the body. In the conscious mind, it is the intellect and our belief systems. In the superconscious, it is awareness of the divine.

In Sanskrit, the crown chakra is called Sahasrara, meaning thousandfold, referring to the infinite unfolding petals of the lotus. What brief glimpses I have been privileged to have of this chakra reveal a pattern of such magnitude, complexity, and beauty, that it is almost overwhelming. Its petals bloom in fractal-like patterns upon patterns, infinitely embedded in each other, drooping down like a sunflower to drop the nectar of understanding into the awareness of being. Each perfect petal is a monad of intelligence, which together form the gestalt of an overarching divine intelligence—sensitive, aware, responsive, and infinite. Its field is delicate, the slightest thought will ripple through the petals like wind in a field of grass. The shining jewels deep in the lotus shine forth only in a state of ultimate stillness. To witness this miracle is profound.

When we reach this level, the seed of our soul has sprouted from its roots in the earth, and grown upward through the elements of water, fire, air, sound, and light, and now to the source of all—consciousness itself, experienced through the element of thought. Each level brings us new degrees of freedom and awareness. Now the crown chakra blossoms forth with infinite awareness, its thousand petals like antennae, reaching to higher dimensions.

It is this chakra that yoga philosophy has deemed to be the seat of enlightenment. Its ultimate state of consciousness is beyond reason, beyond the senses, and beyond the limits of the world around us. Yoga practice advises withdrawing the senses (pratyahara) in order achieve the mental stillness necessary to perceive this ultimate state. Tantric philosophy, on the other hand, regards the senses as a gateway to awakening consciousness. Chakra theory tells us that it is both—a stimulation of intelligence to give us information, and a withdrawal to the interior where information is sifted into ultimate knowledge. Our thousand-petaled lotus must keep its roots in the Earth to maintain its blossom.

The element of this chakra is *thought*, a fundamentally distinct and unmeasurable entity that is the first and barest manifestation of the greater field of consciousness around us. Accordingly, the function of Sahasrara is *knowing*—just as other chakras are related to seeing, speaking, loving, doing, feeling, or having. It is through the crown chakra that we reach into the infinite body of information and run it through our other chakras to bring it to recognition and manifestation.

The seventh chakra relates to what we experience as the mind, especially the awareness that makes use of the mind. The mind is a stage for the play of consciousness, and can bring us comedy or tragedy, excitement or boredom. We are the privileged audience that gets to watch the play, although sometimes we identify so completely with the characters on stage (with our thoughts) that we forget it is only a play.

Through watching this play of thoughts, our mind assimilates experience into meaning and constructs our belief systems. These beliefs are the master programs from which we construct our reality. (In this way, the crown chakra is the master chakra, and relates to the master gland of the endocrine system, the pituitary.)

Physiologically, the crown chakra relates to the brain, especially the higher brain, or cerebral cortex. Our amazing human brain contains some thirteen billion interconnected nerve cells, capable of making more connections among themselves than the number of stars in the entire universe.[3] This is a remarkable statement. Our brains, as instruments of awareness, are virtually limitless. Yet there are 100 million sensory receptors *within the body*, and ten trillion synapses in the nervous system, making the mind 100,000 times more sensitive to its internal environment than to its external one.[4] So it is truly from a place *within* that we receive and assimilate most of our knowledge.

From within, we access a dimension that has no locality in time and space. If we postulate that each chakra represents a dimension of smaller and faster vibration, we hypothetically reach a plane in the crown chakra where we have a wave of infinite speed and no wavelength, allowing it to be everywhere at once. In this way, ultimate states of consciousness are described as omnipresent—by reducing the world to a pattern system occupying no physical dimension, we have infinite storage capacity for its symbols. In other words, *we carry the whole world inside our heads.*

This place within is the seat of consciousness and the origin of our manifesting current. All acts of creation begin with conception. We must first conceive of an idea before we can enact it. This begins in the mind and then descends through the chakras into manifestion. Conception gives us the pattern and manifestation fills it with substance, giving it form. Pattern implies order. To the Hindus, order is the underlying universal reality. Indeed, if we look at nature and the celestial universe, the apparent intelligence of its exquisite order is astonishing.

Pattern relates to the word for father, *pater*. The father gives the seed (the DNA), the information or pattern which stimulates the creation of form. Conception begins when a pattern is adequately received. It is then the maternal aspect that gives substance to the pattern (as well as half the DNA). Mother comes from *mater*, as does the English word: matter. To make something matter, it must materialize, manifest, be "mothered." In this way, Shiva provides the form or pattern, while Shakti, as the mother of the universe, provides the raw energy that materializes the form.

We may think that consciousness is invisible, but we only need to look around us—at the structure of our cities, the furnishings in our houses, or the contents of our bookshelves—to see the incredible versatility of consciousness in its manifested form. If we want to know what consciousness looks like, our world—both natural *and* manmade—is its expression. Consciousness is the field of patterns from which manifestation emerges.

What, then, is "higher" consciousness? Higher consciousness is the awareness of a higher or deeper order—one that is more inclusive. Higher consciousness is sometimes called cosmic consciousness, and refers to awareness of a cosmic or celestial order. Where the lower chakras are full of millions of bits of information about the physical world and its cycles of cause and effect, cosmic consciousness reaches far into the galaxies and beyond, opening to the awareness of unifying truths. It is the perception of meta-patterns, overarching organizational principles of our cosmic ordering system. From this place we can descend again to lesser orders with an innate understanding of their structure and function as subsets of these meta-patterns.

At Sahasrara, we are furthest removed from the material world—and with it the limitations of space and time. In this sense the seventh chakra has the greatest versatility and can encompass the greatest scope of any of the chakras, hence its state of liberation. Within our thoughts we can jump from ancient Stone Age to visions of the future. We can imagine being in our backyard or think of a distant galaxy, all in a mere instant. We can create, destroy, learn, and grow—all from a place existing within and requiring no movement or change without.

Some say Sahasrara is the seat of the soul, an eternal and dimensionless witness that stays with us throughout lifetimes. Others say it is the point through which the divine spark of Shiva enters the body and brings intelligence. It is the master processor of all awareness—the gateway to worlds beyond and worlds within, the dimensionless circumference that encompasses all that is. However we choose to describe it, we must remember that its scope is far greater than our words can convey. It can only be experienced.

CONSCIOUSNESS

The Universal Force is a universal Consciousness. This is
what the seeker discovers. When he has contacted this current
of consciousness in himself, he can switch on to any plane
whatsoever of the universal reality, to any point, and per-
ceive, understand the consciousness there, or even act upon it,
because everywhere it is the same current of consciousness
with different vibratory modalities.

—Satprem, on Sri Aurobindo[5]

Each of the chakras is a manifestation of consciousness at different layers of reality, with earth being the most dense, and the seventh chakra, as its opposite, the pure unmanifest consciousness, known in yoga philosophy as *purusha*. At chakra seven we must now ask the questions: What is this thing called consciousness? What is its purpose? How do we tap into it?

These are certainly big questions, and ones which have been asked by men and women since the beginning of time. And yet, to enter our last dimension—the dimension of mind, awareness, thought, intelligence, and information—we must begin the inquiry, *for the very faculty that is asking is consciousness itself—the object of our quest.*

It is when we ask ourselves, "Who is minding the store?" that we look inside and notice the awareness within. It does little good to gripe about the store's contents without asking this question. If we want a change, we must be willing to take it up with the manager. Some call this *the witness*, an aware being that is always present in the mystery of the Self. To witness our own awareness is to begin to fathom the mysterious possession of consciousness.

This phenomenon is nothing short of miraculous. A faculty that we all have—but cannot see, touch, measure, or hold—is the indelible reality that makes us alive. Its enormous capacity for regulating the body, playing music, speaking multiple languages, drawing pictures, reciting poetry, remembering phone numbers, appreciating a sunset, solving a puzzle, experiencing pleasure, loving, yearning, acting, seeing —the faculty of consciousness is endless in its remarkable abilities. To really turn our gaze of attention upon this miracle is to enter the endless unfolding petals of the lotus, and the true source of the Self.

That Self maintains a storehouse of memory, a set of belief systems, and a capacity to take in new data, while somehow integrating all this information into a coherent sense of *meaning*. This search for meaning is the driving force of consciousness and the search for the underlying unity of experience. When our own lives have meaning, they become part of a larger structure. When something lacks meaning, it doesn't match up with anything. Meaning is the pattern that connects. It brings us closer to unity. Meaning links the individual to the universal, the true meaning of yoga. I believe this search for meaning is the basic drive of the crown chakra in all experiences prior to *samadhi*, (where meaning becomes obvious).

From the mundane to the mystical, the search for meaning is behind most activities of the mind. If your boss is cross with you, you might ask, what does this mean? Is she having a bad day? Is it something you did wrong? Is she expecting too much from you? Are you in the wrong job? When people have accidents, illnesses, or auspicious coincidences, they search for meaning to help integrate the experience. As a therapist, I am told daily about events that occur in my clients' lives. Again and again, they ask the question, "What does this mean?"

Once we discern the meaning of a situation, we know better what to do, or how to operate, and we can again flow with the situation. This gives us our basic operating system. It connects us to an overarching sense of order, which can then integrate the rest of our experience into wholeness.

Consciousness is a force, related to the sattva guna. This force is one of unity, order, and organization. It is the design, the pattern, the intelligence. From crisscrossing wave forms in the brain to the structure of molecules, buildings and cities, consciousness is the ordering principle inherent in all things. Existence itself is but a vortex of conscious organization.

Tapping into this great field of consciousness causes it to descend, where it wraps itself around existing structures and becomes information. Information is the perceived lines of order that make up one's personal operating system. The very act of thinking is the process of following lines of order. As vehicles of consciousness, our natural inclination is to express that information—to use it and manifest it. The ultimate expression is physical form, yet it is the most limited. Because of its limitation, consciousness, after manifesting, wants to free itself from the binding of the physical and return again to its source—the nonphysical, where it can play in its infinite diversity. So the nature of consciousness is to both manifest and liberate, the eternal dance of Shiva and Shakti.

TYPES OF CONSCIOUSNESS

That within us which seeks to know and to progress is not the mind but something behind it which makes use of it.
—Sri Aurobindo[6]

Awareness implies the focus of attention. You may speak to me while I'm asleep, but I'm not aware of it—my attention is focused elsewhere. Scenes may drift by while I'm driving, but they escape my awareness and may be unfamiliar next time I see them. To open awareness we must notice where our attention goes. Then we can expand or focus it at will.

Information is around us in great multitude every moment of our lives. In order to use this information, we focus our attention on small amounts at a time. To be reading this book, you are focusing your attention on it, and away from other things, such as traffic, noisy children, or nearby conversation.

The consciousness of the crown chakra can be roughly divided into two types, depending upon where our attention goes: That which descends and becomes concrete information, useful for manifesting in the world, and that which expands and travels outward toward more abstract planes. The first is oriented toward the world of things, relationships, and the concrete self. It is a result of limiting attention. It is the consciousness that actively thinks, reasons, learns, and stores information. It is our *Cognitive Consciousness*. We can think of it as the lower focus of the crown chakra, organizing finite bits of detail into ever larger structures.

The second type of consciousness I call *Transcendent Consciousness*. It interfaces to a realm beyond the world of things and relationships. It is consciousness without an object, without awareness or reference to the individual self, and without the wide fluctuations that occur in the logical and comparative thought patterns of Cognitive Consciousness. Instead, this form of consciousness floats in a meta-awareness, encompassing all things simultaneously without focusing on any objects in particular. It floats because it lets go of the normal "objects of consciousness," and thus becomes weightless and free.

Cognitive Consciousness requires that awareness be focused on the finite and particular, sorted and assembled in logical order. Transcendent Consciousness requires opening awareness beyond cognition. To perceive higher order implies a greater distancing from the minute and particular. Paradoxically, this opening beyond cognition has the result of increasing the scope of our focused attention. By emptying the mind, that which remains is more pronounced, like watching someone alone on a field of snow as opposed to finding them on a crowded street.

INFORMATION

Space/time coordinates are not primary coordinates of physical reality, but are organizing principles invoked by consciousness to put its information in order.

—Robert Jahn[7]

Through our experiences, each one of us builds a personal matrix of information within our minds. From the first glimpse of our mother's face to our doctoral dissertations and beyond, we spend our lives trying to piece together some sense of order from what we see around us. Each bit of information we receive gets incorporated into that matrix, making it ever more complex. As it grows more complex it tends to periodically "reorganize" itself, finding higher levels of order which simplify its system. The bottom falls out, restructuring occurs, and with it a more efficient use of energy. This is the familiar "aha" reflex—the little enlightenments that come when some piece falls into place, allowing a new wholeness to be perceived. Enlightenment is a progressive understanding of ever greater wholeness. In our holographic paradigm, each new piece of information allows the basic picture to gain clarity.

Matrix structures are created from the meaning we derive from experience. They then become our personal belief systems and the ordering principles of our lives. We are part of this order and we organize all that we encounter according to this matrix, preferring to keep our inner and outer experiences coherent. If my belief system says that women are inferior, I will manifest that in all my actions, including finding people to corroborate it. If I believe this is my lucky day, I am more likely to manifest positive things in my life today.

Our belief systems are comprised of the various bits of meaning we have derived from our experience. If we repeatedly fail, and we tell ourselves that it means we are stupid, we eventually generate a belief in our own stupidity. These belief systems form the matrix into which all other information is funneled. If I tell you a bit of feedback, you run that piece of data against your background of knowledge and add it to your belief systems. You might say, "Oh, I can never do anything right or, I can never please you." That is a belief taken from what meaning you derive. Another person, with another belief system, may derive an entirely different meaning.

The relationship between meaning and belief is so strong that if some piece of data does not fit our inner matrix, we might say, "Oh, I don't believe you," and discard the information entirely. If I told someone I saw an extraterrestrial (I haven't), most people would not believe me, for they have no matrix for such an experience. If I told the same information to someone at a UFO conference, they might indeed believe me, or give the experience an entirely different meaning.

This is one of the traps of the mind. How do we take in new information and expand our consciousness, if we reject anything that does not fit the current inner paradigm? And if we disregard this inner matrix, how do we discern truth from fiction, or organize the vast amount of information that we receive at each moment?

The best answer to this lies in meditation, for it is a practice that allows the mind to sort through its data, discard outmoded belief systems and unnecessary information, and reset the personal matrix with an underlying unity. (Meditation is like defragmenting your hard drive —it leaves more room to operate and record new information without crashing your system.) It is meditation that allows our crown chakra to open the awareness ever wider without getting overwhelmed or lost in the infinite. It helps us retain our center, which is the primary organizing matrix of the Self.

Downloading Information

Parapsychological research, past life regression, and other studies have shown that there are certain qualities of the mind that exist independently of the brain. In some cases of past life regression, people have been able to remember facts that are objectively provable. They accurately describe a house they have never seen, they speak a foreign language, or they describe events that are later documented by journals, letters, or books. Obviously, since the human body/hardware has been completely made over, some information exists outside of the brain.

All this data implies that there is some kind of *information field* existing independently of its perceiver, much as radio waves exist independently of radios, or the Internet exists whether or not you have a computer. The body, with its amazing nervous system and reactive capacity, is the receiver of this information, just as your computer can receive and download information from the Internet.

This field, though it may be immaterial in the physical world, is nonetheless a very real and causative factor, just as an invisible magnetic field causes metal shavings to take a certain shape. This is why the higher planes are often called *causal planes.* When we "tune in" we can tap this information field and enter the realm of causality.

The biologist, Rupert Sheldrake, has coined a term that at least partially describes this phenomenon, called "morphogenetic fields," from *morphe,* "form", and *genesis,* "coming into being". The theory of morphogenetic fields postulates that the universe functions not so much by immutable laws as by "habits"—patterns created by the repetition of events over time. The repetition of these habits creates a field in a "higher" dimension which then increases the likelihood that events will fall into that pattern. Morphogenetic fields are characterisitic of objects and behaviors, and may explain much of what is called instinct.

The morphogenetic field for rabbits, for example, is created by the sheer number of rabbits that exist and have existed in the past. Anything that is coming into being that even closely resembles a rabbit will fall into the high probability of "rabbitness" created by that field. If you walked into a hardware store and said you wanted something with a handle that could drive nails, the likelihood that the manager would say "hammer" is very high—because so many already exist. Now that nail guns are more common, it's more likely, that, too, might be suggested. Twenty years ago it would have been unlikely, because there weren't very many nail guns.

Morphogenetic fields pertain to the relationships between con-sciousness and manifestation as they form a two-way link between the two worlds. The field is built up through what occurs in the tangible world, through repetition and habit. Then the field, once established, dictates future forms in the material world. The tendency to conform varies with the strength of the field. Says Sheldrake:

> It wouldn't be possible for a new field to set up in the presence of an overwhelming influence from a pre-existing habit. What can happen is that higher level fields can integrate lower level habits into new syntheses .... Evolution proceeds not by changing basic habits but by taking the basic habits it's given, and building more and more complex patterns out of them. [8]

An example of this is the overweight person who loses fifty pounds and has an insatiable desire to eat until just that amount of weight is regained. Have you ever noticed how heavy people tend to stay at about the same amount of heaviness most of the time, despite dieting or binges? The morphogenetic field of the body wants to maintain its familiar form. By reaching into a different level, "thinking thin" has been a more effective way to reduce, for it is changing the field that is causal to the form of the body.

When beliefs are held by large numbers of people, their field is stronger, lessening the chance for the survival of opposing beliefs. The field created by the belief in male supremacy is a primary example because it has been instilled so completely into our culture over the last several thousand years, offering greater advantages to men, who are then able to achieve more. As more women find their power through feminism, another field is being generated that allows the cultural belief system to change form. But this takes a long time and many, many women and men to involve themselves in building up the new field. As time goes by and the field gets stronger, it makes it easier for the next generation of women and men to hold a new belief system.

Thoughts are structures, just like bodies and buildings. Their details may change from moment to moment, but the overall structural matrix remains more or less the same over given amounts of time—especially when held by a large number of minds. If we wish to change our consciousness, we must tap into the fields from which it arises, and search for the higher degrees of order within them. From a transcendent level we can access new fields of higher order. Then we can change our matrix and its manifestations in the physical world. This is the process of self-conscious evolution, made possible only by journeys into consciousness.

TRANSCENDENCE AND IMMANENCE

When consciousness is released from the thousands of mental, vital, physical vibrations in which it lies buried, there is joy.
—Sri Aurobindo[9]

The crown chakra is a meeting point between finite and infinite, mortal and divine, temporal and timeless. It is the gateway through which we expand beyond our personal self, beyond the limits of space time and experience primordial unity and transcendent bliss. It is also the point at which divine consciousness enters the body and descends, bringing awareness to all the chakras, giving us the means to operate in the world around us.

We have described these two currents as creating two types of consciousness: cognitive and transcendent. In addition, the two currents produce two different but complimentary spiritual states: the *transcendent* and the *immanent.* Once again, it is the ascending current that brings us liberation and the descending current that brings us manifestation. To have a true theory of wholeness, one needs to cultivate both.

As we have worked our way through the seven levels of awareness related to each chakra, we have progressively transcended limitation, shortsightedness, immediacy, pain, and suffering. This is the direction most emphasized in Eastern thought, with the practice and philosophies of yoga comprising the essential gateway to universal consciousness. Pain and suffering, it is believed, occur through false identification with elements of the finite world, and obscure the ultimate reality of the infinite. It is attachment to limitation that forms obstacles to our spiritual growth, hence attachment is the primary demon of the crown chakra.

The most characteristic quality of Transcendent Consciousness is its emptiness. Therefore, we enter it by letting go of attachment. Transcendence carries us beyond the ordinary, to the broad expanse of unity. The observer is participant. There is no separation between self and the world, and no sense of time. Just as the emptiness of a cup allows it to be filled, the emptiness of our minds allows a clear channel through which to experience transcendence.

Transcendence brings liberation from the traps of illusion so that we can enter into a state of bliss and freedom. It is generally the ego that forms these attachments to maintain its sense of selfhood and safety—but that self is a smaller, more limited self, apart from the underlying unity of consciousness from which we are made.

The descending current of consciousness, having divine realization as its origin, brings *immanence.* Immanence is the awareness of the divine within, where transcendence is the awareness of the divine without. Immanence brings us intelligence, illumination, inspiration, radiance, power, connection, and finally manifestation. True self-knowledge is to understand that transcendence and immanence are complimentary and that inner and outer worlds are indelibly one.

While the liberating current brings us liberation or *mukti*, it is the descending current that brings enjoyment, or *bhukti*. As stated in Arthur Avalon's *Serpent Power,* the most fastidious translation of Tantric texts on the chakras:

> *One of the cardinal principles of the Sakti-Tantra is to secure by its Sadhana both Liberation and Enjoyment. This is possible by the identification of the self when in enjoyment with the soul of the world.*[10]

Just as the Muladhara chakra is both the source point of the rising Kundalini and the place where we press our roots deep into the ground, the Sahasrara is the origin of all manifestation and the gateway to the beyond. Transcendence and immanence are not mutually exclusive. They represent the basic oscillations of consciousness, the inhale and exhale of the crown chakra, the entry and exit point of human life.

MEDITATION: KEY TO THE LOTUS

> *Gracious One, pray your head is an empty shell, wherein your mind frolics infinitely.*
>
> —Old Sanskrit Proverb

There is no greater practice for developing the seventh chakra than meditation. It is the very act through which consciousness realizes itself. It is as essential to nourishing the spirit as eating and rest are to the body.

There are countless techniques for meditation. You can regulate your breath, intone mantras, visualize colors, shapes, or deities, move energy through your chakras, walk or move with awareness, hook yourself up to a brain machine, or just stare blankly in front of you. To be worthwhile, all of these forms must have one thing in common— they must enhance, soothe, and harmonize the vibrational aspects of the mind and body, cleansing the mind of its habitual clutter.

We take it for granted that we need to take showers, clean our houses, and wash our clothes. We'd be uncomfortable if we didn't, to say nothing of being the object of social criticism. Yet, the mind and its thoughts need cleansing, perhaps even more than our bodies. The mind works longer, encounters wider dimensions, and runs the operating system of our life as well! While few of us would consider eating dinner on yesterday's dirty dishes, we think nothing of tackling a new problem with yesterday's cluttered mind. No wonder we feel tired, confused, and ignorant!

Meditation is both an end and a means. We may achieve better clarity, mood elevation, or simply better physical coordination; but the mind, as an inseparable commander of all else, deserves the best treatment we can give it.

As the seventh chakra exists in the dimension of "withinness," meditation is the key to that inner world. Through meditation we can systematically tune out the outside world and cultivate sensitivity to the inner. Through that sensitivity we can then enter the point of singularity which connects all things. We are the vortex of all that we experience. At the center of that vortex lies understanding.

Through harmonization of our bodies, breath, and thoughts, we can line up our chakras and perceive the unifying essence of all creation. But this is not an alignment of physical reality as much as it is an inner alignment of archetypal energies, a spiritual alignment with the underlying unity we have come to discover in each chakra.

But what exactly does meditation do? What are the physiological effects, psychological states, and resulting benefits? And why is this strange practice of doing nothing so valuable?

The widespread practice of TM, or Transcendental Meditation, as taught by Maharishi Mahesh Yogi, has enabled some systematic study of mental and physical effects over a wide variety of subjects. Transcendental Meditation, as taught by the TM association, involves the simple practice of spending twenty minutes twice a day sitting quietly and internally uttering a mantra, given to the meditator by the teacher. There are no strange postures, breathing patterns or dietary recommendations, making this practice easy to learn and easy to study.

The most noteworthy finding of these studies seemed to show up in the EEG measuring of brain-wave patterns. In ordinary waking consciousness, brain waves are random and chaotic, and most commonly in the beta frequency. The two hemispheres of the brain may generate different wavelengths, and there may be further differences from the front to the back of the brain as well.

Meditation changes this dramatically. Immediately upon beginning, the meditation subjects showed increased alpha waves (brainwaves characteristic of a relaxed state of mind) which began at the back of the brain and moved forward. After a few minutes, the alpha waves increased in amplitude. The back and the front of the brain became synchronized in phase as did the left and right hemispheres. This resonance continued and in many cases theta waves appeared (a deeper state than alpha) especially in those more experienced with the practice. In the most advanced meditators, alpha was found to occur more frequently in a normal, waking state, and with greater amplitude. With these people theta was more prevalent during meditation, and even occurred during normal waking states.[11]

Meditation has physiological effects as well. Oxygen intake decreased by 16-18 percent, heart rate decreased by 25 percent and blood pressure was lowered, all of which are controlled by the autonomic nervous system, (the controller of involuntary processes).[12] This allows the body to enter a state of deep rest—far deeper than what it receives in sleep. This rest then allows for greater alertness in waking consciousness.

It is interesting to note that while meditators do enter a state of deep rest, the attention/awareness increases rather than decreases.

When a sound was produced periodically to a nonmeditator, the brain waves showed a gradual acclimation to the noise—less and less reaction until it was effectively "tuned out." The meditator, on the other hand, while meditating, reacted freshly to the sound each time it was made.[13] Therefore, while the body diminishes all its activities, the mind is essentially released from the body's limitations and freer to expand to new horizons.

It is suggested that meditation de-stimulates the cerebral cortex and the limbic system, and through brain-wave resonance heals the split between the old and the new brain.[14] This split has been suspected to be a cause of alienated emotional states and schizoid behavior, difficulties particular to humans and essentially nonexistent in animals. Better coordination between the two hemispheres can also lead to increased cognitive and perceptual ability.

And the psychological effects? Aside from a general feeling of relaxation, inner peace, and increased well-being, meditators were found to have improved academic performance, increased job satisfaction and production, a decrease in drug use (both prescription and recreational), and faster reaction times.[15] All this from simply sitting still and doing nothing!

In the face of this evidence it is hard to deny that meditation has great rewards. Who wouldn't want greater health, mood elevation, and increased performance? And all that for a practice that costs nothing, requires no equipment, and can be done anywhere! Yet why is it that so few people actually do take the time to meditate, and that even those who do find it difficult to practice as often as they would like to?

We have spoken of rhythms, resonance, and morphogenetic fields, and how all three of them tend to perpetuate themselves just as they are. In a world whose vibrational level is largely oriented around the first three chakras, placing greater value on materiality, it is difficult to find the time, validation, and even desire to go off and enter a different wavelength—especially one whose reward is so subjective. The idea that one "should" meditate, added to the thousands of other "shoulds" hammering on us each day, can almost make the practice repugnant.

Yet true meditation is a state of mind—not an effort. Once the state is achieved a few times, it begins to create its own self-perpetuating rhythms, its own morphogenetic field, and its own effect on the vibrations around us. Then it becomes an integral part of life, staying with us through waking consciousness, sleep, and all other activities. At this point meditation becomes a joy, not a discipline. But until then we can only describe the effects and hope they are enough to fire the will's curiosity. At least the price is right!

Meditation Techniques

So now we come to the how-tos. And here we find that meditation has as many techniques as there are meditators. I suggest that it is worthwhile to, at some point, give each of them a try, and from the experience tailor one to suit you exactly. Then stick with it for awhile, for it is over time that meditation practices show their greatest rewards.

It is important to find a quiet, comfortable environment where you won't be disturbed. Make sure you don't have clothing that is binding, that you won't be too hot or too cold, and that distracting noises are kept to a minimum. Meditation is generally better on a slightly empty stomach, though intense hunger pangs can also be distracting.

Most meditations are done while sitting comfortably with the spine straight, but not tense. This can be done in a chair, or sitting cross-legged on the floor—in either full or half lotus (see Figure 8.1, page 339.) or simple Indian style. The reason for this is that the body needs to be in a low-maintenance position so it can relax, yet not so comfortable that you fall asleep. Furthermore, a straight back allows alignment of all the chakras, and better transmission of energy up and down the Sushumna.

While in the half-lotus position, you can do any number of things: you can follow your breath in and out, tuning yourself to its rhythms; you can gaze at a mandala, a candle flame, or some other appropriate visual stimulus; or you can simply watch your thoughts as they go by, neither following them, stopping them, nor judging them. The separation of self and thoughts helps to achieve the Transcendent state.

As in the TM technique, you can internally utter a mantra and focus your mind on its vibration going through you. This harmonizes the vibrational states, as we have seen. You can watch your emotional states and achieve detachment from them, visualize various colors running through your chakras, or spend your time asking who it is that's meditating. A common Zen practice is to concentrate on a paradoxical statement, called a Koan, which de-intellectualizes the mind by its lack of logic. "What is the sound of one hand clapping?" is a typical Koan. Another is "What was the face you wore before you were born?" The idea is not to find an answer but to allow the question to knock down the barriers of your normal logical mode of thinking, and allow perception of something greater.

The commonality among these diverse forms is that they all involve focusing the mind on ONE thing. In normal, waking consciousness our mind flies to many things from moment to moment. The very one-pointedness of mind is the object in meditation. Each of these techniques—be it a sound, an object, or a Koan—is designed to be a focusing device for the mind to divert it from its normal, deeply rutted stream of chaotic consciousness.

It is difficult to compare one method to another and make any kind of value judgment. Different meditations affect people in different ways. The emphasis is not on the technique used, but on how well one is able to use it. No matter the technique, the act of repetition and concentration charges the act over time. It is a discipline, and like any other discipline becomes easier with practice.

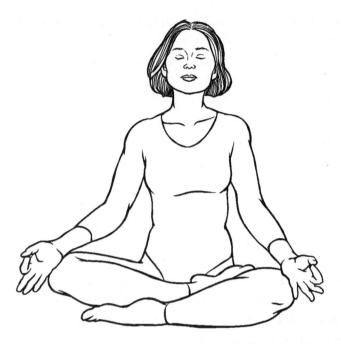

FIGURE 8.1
Half-Lotus Position.

ENLIGHTENMENT—
HOME AT LAST

Nirvana in my liberated consciousness turned out to be the beginning of my realization, a first step towards the complete thing, not the sole true attainment possible or even a culminating finale.

—Sri Aurobindo[16]

Enlightenment is not a thing, it is a process. A thing is something to acquire; a process is something to be. If enlightenment were a thing it would be a contradiction in terms to have "found" it, for it is inseparable from the self who is looking. Upon realization, we find that it was never lost!

Just as love is a difficult concept to describe, yet intrinsically part of a natural, healthy state, enlightenment can also be thought of as a natural state, and equally difficult to describe. In this way enlightenment would be achieved by a process of undoing rather than doing. We keep ourselves from enlightenment by our own mental blocks, just as a roof blocks the sun from shining down on us.

But to say that we have enlightenment already does not mean there is nothing to be gained from cultivating it. Just because it exists within us does not always mean it is intact. For there are always deeper states, higher places, and more to explore in the beyond. And when we can do this from where we are right now, we will indeed have achieved something!

While most people think of enlightenment as a state of knowing all the answers, we could also think of it as arriving finally at the right questions. In experiencing the beyond, we can only be left with a sense of awe and wonder. Answers can be things, but it is the questions that are the process.

In terms of the chakras, enlightenment occurs when the path through the chakras is complete. It is more than just an opening of the crown chakra, or of any other chakra on the Sushumna. It is an experience of unity among all things, and the integration of that experience with the Self. Only if the Self is connected can this occur. It is a process of becoming.

And so we come at last to the end and find that it is only another beginning. But for what other reason do ends exist?

SEVENTH CHAKRA EXERCISES

Following Your Thoughts

Lie or sit in a comfortable meditation position. Allow your mind to become relatively calm and quiet, using whatever technique is most effective for you.

Gradually let yourself pay attention to the thoughts that pass through your mind. Pick one and ask yourself where it came from, what thoughts preceded it. Then follow to the origin of that thought. It may be something that occurred years ago, or something that is pressing on you right now. Then again follow that thought to its source, and on to each thought's origin. Eventually we come to a kind of infinite source that has no objective origin.

Return and pick another thought that passes through. Repeat the same sequence, going further and further back. See how many of your thoughts emanate from a similar source—either an issue you are working with in your life right now, a past teacher, or your own place of connection with the infinite.

After following a few thoughts to their origin, begin watching your thoughts go by without tracing them. Simply let them pass, neither denying them nor retaining them. Let them return to their source until there are few or no thoughts passing through, and you too have returned to that source. Remain there as long as seems appropriate, and return slowly to normal consciousness.

Journey to the Akashic Records:

To be done as a guided meditation.

Lie comfortably on the floor, face up, head and neck relaxed, and slowly relax each part of your body. Let the floor beneath you give you support as you relax your legs . . . your back . . . your stomach . . . your arms and shoulders. Make fists with your hands and then release them, flexing each finger. Point your toes and release them, giving each foot a little wiggle. Slowly focus on the rhythm of your breathing . . . in . . . out . . . in . . . out. Let your body float lightly on the floor, each muscle letting go of its tension.

As you watch your breathing, become aware of your thoughts. Watch them as they slowly twist through your mind, effortlessly playing their images in your mind's eye. And as you watch your thoughts, become aware of some piece of information you would like to know—some question you have buried within you. It may be a question about a lover, a present dilemma, or information about a past life. Take a moment to focus on your question, to become clear on what it is you wish to know.

When your question is clear, let it go from your mind. It will return at the appropriate time.

As you lie effortlessly on the floor, imagine your body getting lighter. The solid mass of your flesh gradually lightens and you experience a swirling feeling, like rising into a mist. You fly upward, twisting and turning into this mist, shapeless and formless as it is. Eventually the mist begins to take more form and you perceive a spiral staircase leading upward. You follow the staircase higher and higher as it becomes more solid. Each step lets you feel a sense of your own destiny, each step brings you closer to that which you wish to know.

Soon your steps widen and you arrive at a large building, stretching as high and as far as you can see. It has one large door and you enter it, effortlessly. You see more stairways, long hallways, and many rooms with doors opening to them. You stand in the foyer and ask your question, hearing it echo throughout the whole building. The question comes back to you.

You begin to walk, listening to the echo of your question, following where the sound is the loudest and the clearest.

Follow your footsteps wherever they may take you, repeating your question as you walk. Eventually you will find yourself in a room. Notice the doorway, the furnishings. Is there anything written on the doorway? What colors are the furnishings, what time period are they from?

As you look around, you notice a large bookshelf with volumes and volumes of books. Examine the library and see if any book stands out, beckoning to you. Find one with your name on it. It may not be the name you use in this life, but it should fall into your hands effortlessly. Phrase your question once more and open the book, letting it fall open where it will. Read the passage you have opened to. Pause for a moment and reflect on its meaning, and then turn the next few pages, browsing. Open your awareness to the information around you—the rooms full of books, the ancient wisdom buried throughout the building, and pull it into your heart. Don't try to analyze it, just let it be.

Then when you are ready, return your book to its shelf, knowing that you can find it again whenever you want. Slowly turn and leave the room, walking back down the hallway full of doors. Enter the foyer and out the large columned door and step outside, reflecting, as you go, on the incredible view you can see from this height. Patterns upon swirling patterns ebb and flow at this place with every color and shape and rhythm you can imagine. Your body gets slowly heavier as you enter the atmosphere. Slowly you come down and down, sliding into the Earth plane where your body lies resting comfortably on the floor in this place now. Examine what you have brought with you, and when you are ready, return to the room.

Note: The actual significance of the information you have found is not always readily apparent. You may want to take time to reflect on it (perhaps even a few days) before sharing it.

ENDNOTES

1. Verse 41 of the Sat-Chakra-Nirupana, as translated by Arthur Avalon, *Serpent Power*, 428.

2. John Woods, personal conversation, 1982.

3. Bloomfield, et al. *Transcendental Meditation: Discovering Inner Awareness and Overcoming Stress*, 39.

4. Michael Talbot, *Mysticism and the New Physics*, 54.

5. Satprem, *Sri Aurobindo, or the Adventure of Consciousness*, 64.

6. Sri Aurobindo, in *Sri Aurobindo, or the Adventure of Consciousness*, 30.

7. Robert Jahn, from the "Foundation for Mind-Being Research" newsletter, *Reporter*. August, 1982, Cupertino, CA, 5.

8. Rupert Sheldrake, "Morphogenetic Fields: Nature's Habits," *ReVision*, Fall, 1982, Vol 5, No. 2., 34.

9. Ibid., p. 66.

10. Arthur Avalon, *Serpent Power*, 38.

11. Bloomfield, et al. *Transcendental Meditation: Discovering Inner Awareness and Overcoming Stress*. 75.

12. Ibid., appendix.

13. Ibid., 66.

14. Ibid., 78.

15. Ibid., appendix.

16. Sri Aurobindo as quoted by Satprem, *Sri Aurobindo, or the Adventure of Consciousness*, 153.

RECOMMENDED READING FOR CHAKRA SEVEN

Satprem, *Sri Aurobindo or The Adventure of Consciousness.* NY: Harper & Row, 1968.

Bloomfield, et al. *Transcendental Meditation: Discovering Inner Awareness and Overcoming Stress.* NY: Delacorte Press, 1975.

Feuerstein, Georg. *Wholeness or Transcendence: Ancient Lessons for the Emerging Global Civilization.* NY: Larson Publications, 1992.

Kabat-Zinn, John. *Wherever You Go, There You Are.* NY: Hyperion, 1994. (A book on keeping your mind present and focused.)

Le Shan, Lawrence. *How to Meditate.* NY: Bantam, 1974.(A good primer on many techniques and commonly asked questions about meditation.)

Suzuki, D. T. Shunryu. *Zen Mind, Beginner's Mind.* NY: Weatherhill, 1979.

Tart, Charles. *States of Consciousness.* NY: E. P. Dutton, 1975.

White, John, ed. *Frontiers of Consciousness.* NY: Julian Press, 1974. (A good and varied group of essays on various aspects of consciousness research.)

PART THREE

PUTTING IT
ALL TOGETHER

Chapter 9

THE RETURN JOURNEY

THE UNIVERSAL FORCE IS A universal consciousness. This is what the seeker discovers. When he has contacted this current of consciousness in himself, he can switch on to any plane whatsoever of the universal reality, to any point, and perceive, understand the consciousness there, or even act upon it, because everywhere it is the same current of consciousness with different vibratory modalities.

—Satprem on Sri Aurobindo[1]

We have climbed all the way up the chakra column. We have completed our ascending current but not our journey. We have climbed to the top of the spiritual mountain, and gained the view that is only possible from that perspective. But now our challenge is to get back down again, and to apply that new understanding to the world around us. Since we have brought the energies of the lower chakras to consciousness, it is now the task to bring that advanced consciousness back down to the lower chakras.

Pure consciousness, which enters the individual from the vast field of the supramental plane as *purusha,* condenses through the chakras as it falls downward to the plane of manifestation. Having climbed to the top to embrace Shiva, Shakti descends through the chakras by first entering the mind and senses, then the five elements of finite matter. When she reaches the final plane of Earth, there is nothing left for her to do, and she rests, becoming the coiled and dormant form of Kundalini-Shakti.[2]

In the journey upward, we used the chakras as stepping stones to our liberation, each step granting us more freedom from limited forms, repetitive habits, and worldly attachments. Each step expanded our consciousness and our horizons. In the downward current the chakras become "condensers" of the force of consciousness, organizing its energy for exchange on the various planes associated with each level. In the descent of consciousness, the chakras are analagous to pools that collect rainfall as it descends from heaven and runs down the mountains to the sea. Where there is a cavity, water collects in pools and can be used. Like pools, the chakras are chambers in the subtle body that allow the divine consciousness to collect and condense into progressively denser planes of manifesation. If a chakra is blocked, it is limited in the amount of energy it can gather.

This analogy also describes the different concepts of unity that can be understood at both ends of the spectrum. As the rain falls from heaven in a cloud of droplets, it is like a unified field of moisture. As it falls to earth, it breaks up into millions of tiny rivulets, which become larger but less numerous as thousands of little streams, and hundreds of even bigger tributaries, and tens of wide rivers, to a huge and single sea. The raindrops then rest in a unified body of water until they rise again to heaven as tiny droplets of evaporation. Each step downward creates something larger and coarser, yet moves toward simplicity and singularity.

So we begin our journey downward from pure consciousness—a field of nondimensionality that, in its highest state, is complete and unwavering. Transcendent Consciousness has risen past the ups and downs of differentiation until it is utterly smooth, without ripples or fluctuations. As soon as that consciousness begins to descend, however, we have a wave that ripples outward, a tiny point of awareness standing out against the void. This ripple is the first focus of consciousness—the first dawning of any existence.

As we focus our attention, waves of awareness emanate outward, forming tiny fluctuations in the fabric of space-time. These fluctuations are not isolated events but stimulate the creation of other waves, which propagate more waves. As they cross, these waves form interference patterns and the ethereal emanations of consciousness become more dense. The holographic principle discussed in chakra six is an example of such interference patterns. At each crossing of the waves is a node that draws awareness.

This is the level of chakra six. Raw information begins to have an image—something that consciousness can "recognize," or " re-know." Consciousness is now feeding back on itself. It perceives this image, reacts to it, perhaps alters it. The information is beginning to manifest but at this stage, it is little more than a well-formed thought.

As the mind focuses on these constructed images, it sends out more ripples, constructing more interference patterns for consciousness to recognize and react to. The fields become more dense. Our waves, now quite numerous, react to each other, generating fields of awareness, fields of ripples at varying frequencies or vibrations. Frequencies that are similar tend to harmonize and fall into resonance, deepening their amplitude.

Now we are at chakra five, where consciousness folds in on itself once again. Repeating images are given a name as they take on a particular vibrational quality. A name is a wave function that transports an idea from one mind to another. It can distinguish and delineate differences in our field of interference, drawing a border around them and making them distinct and specific.

As we name something, we define it within the world of relationships. At chakra four, we find that we perceive order among our named things. There are waves, and there are interferences. There are things and their relationships. In relationship, there must be balance for something to continue into manifestation.

We come now to chakra three and begin to enter the physical dimension of our bodies. Our ripples are becoming more dense, more ordered. We use our will to command raw energy to the shape and form of our intention. This creates a field that is charged with vital energy, a field that can direct and hold the shape of raw materials in accordance with a vision or intention. The vital energy of our life force holds our body together; the vital energy of love holds a relationship together; the vital energy of an idea evokes enthusiasm, which calls forth support from others.

We are now reaching a level of complexity and organization that approaches gravitational force. As energy and will pull random substance together, disparate energies become more dense. As they become more dense, they create their own gravitational field. The rest happens by itself, as raw energy gets pulled along the lines of cleavage set up long ago by the patterns of thought. Gravity pulls on our organized field, curving the fabric of space-time, pulling masses together, causing the movement that provides constant change. This movement seeks to balance difference, seeks to return the composite parts of our field to its initial unity.

And finally through this gravitational force, our ripples of constructive interference coalesce, creating mass. We have come to the world of material objects, with weight and volume. We have returned to the earth, one of innumerable masses floating in a sea of stars.

When we compare the downward current to the upward current, we find something very interesting. We find that the pattern is nearly the same. The two ends of the spectrum are remarkably similar.

From chakra one, we began with an initial unity, and moved from that unity into difference. From difference we moved to choice and to volition, and from volition to a three-dimensional world of space and time, full of precisely arranged relationships.

From chakra seven, we began with an initial unity as undifferentiated consciousness. As soon as that consciousness had the slightest ripple, the unity was shattered and difference was created. In the naming of thought patterns, volition was exercised, creativity was enacted, and that creativity set to organize its composite elements into precise patterns of relationships.

At the physical end of the spectrum, we have substances made of molecules and atoms. When we closely examine them, we learn that atoms are energy fields containing nodes of concentrated energy with large amounts of empty space between them. Upon examining subatomic particles, we notice that they appear more like waves, probabilities among conceptual variations of thought patterns.

At the ethereal end of our spectrum, we have consciousness. In its ultimate state it is undifferentiated, but in actuality it is a field outside of space-time with minute ripples of fluctuation—appearing more like waves, possibilities among conceptual variations of thought patterns.

Have we mistaken Kundalini for Ouroboros? Does the serpent have her tail in her teeth?

The Hindus talk about ultimate reality as being one of order. Things are not real, actions are not real, there is only divine order, the lines of which delineate all the Maya that we experience as the phenomenal world. This order is the organizing force acting upon all matter. The tantras describe the lines of force permeating all of space and time as the "hairs of Shiva." These hairs are the organizing principle in the Akasha, the world of nonmaterial spirit. As Shiva is the male principle of consciousness, the minute hairs of his head can only represent the first and barest emanations of thought which proceed from that consciousness. The initial difference is Shakti, the other, the female. With her the world is made. The dance is begun, but never concluded.

And so we find that the end is the beginning. We are not traveling a linear path, but an interpenetrating one. There is no destination, only the journey.

Now that we have considered the theoretical side of our descending current, we can apply it to our everyday lives.

We begin with raw information. The random buzzing of thoughts within our brain. Our thoughts play in the back of our heads—collecting other thoughts to help solidify them. Perhaps we meditate so our thoughts become more coherent. In meditation, some thoughts will catch our attention, and may even become an idea. As we focus on our idea, images form in the mind's eye. We may fantasize, daydream, or imagine various aspects of our idea. As we do, it takes on a mental image with form, shape, and color. Our random thoughts have begun to solidify, yet have a long way to go before they manifest.

Let's pretend that our idea is to build a house. As we think about it, we begin to visualize the size, shape, or color of the house. Perhaps we imagine walking in the front door or cooking in the kitchen. Our thoughts are starting to pool in chakra six, as we embellish our idea with imagination. As the images crystallize, we become able to tell someone else about our idea. We communicate about it (chakra five). We can now describe the size and shape of the house and we may begin to draw up plans, further concretizing our images. Next, we must bring our ideas into relationship (chakra four). We can't just build a house anywhere, we need to buy a piece of land, which is in a community that will have certain rules. We must be able to relate to architects and builders, planning commissioners and loan officers. *In order to manifest something, it must have some relationship to things that already exist.*

Our project will not happen by itself, merely from visualization and communication. We must apply our will, from chakra three. Our will directs raw energy, such as money, materials, and people, toward a certain goal. This takes energy, in the form of repeated and deliberate actions, guided by consciousness, and fueled by physical metabolic processes. As we invest this energy, our project begins to take form on the physical plane. We move things around, such as tools and building materials, and bring them together (chakra two) until finally we have manifested a finished building that rests on its foundation on the

Earth (chakra one). At this point we are complete, and like Shakti who rests in the first chakra, we get to rest and enjoy our manifestation.

Through this descent, a vast number of thoughts about the design of the house gradually evolves into a single building, made of many images, conversations, relationships, activities, movements, and materials. Manifestation involves distilling the many into one. Yet the house is only one of many other homes which were created by the same process.

To manifest is to allow our thoughts to become dense, to solidify. The more we think about something, the more we are likely to manifest it, but as we said in chakra one, manifestation requires that we accept limitation. This requires a certain amount of repetition. I can play a piano piece because I have practiced it many times. I can speak a language if I have repeated the vocabulary enough times to remember it. I have the deepest relationships with people I see most frequently.

The downward current is made from repeated patterns, which become dense. *If we cannot accept limitation or repetition, we won't manifest.* The upward current liberates us from the boredom of this repetition, and allows us to experience something new.

The journey upward expands our horizons, brings new insights and understanding. Shakti brings us *vital energy* as she reaches for Shiva, her lover. She is wild and fierce. The journey downward is marked by the presence of *grace,* the intelligent order that is the province of Shiva. The upward current brings us transcendence, the downward, immanence. It is these two highways that create our Rainbow Bridge—the connecting link between heaven and earth, mortal and divine. *It is only the two currents rushing past each other that creates the vortices that form the chakras.*

We now have the dance of liberation and manifestation, freedom and enjoyment, that form the basic polarities of human experience.

ENDNOTES

1. Satprem, *Sri Aurobindo, or the Adventure of Consciousness*, 64.
2. Arthur Avalon, *The Serpent Power*, 41.

Chapter 10

HOW
CHAKRAS
INTERACT

NOW THAT WE HAVE EXAMINED
EACH chakra in detail, our system is
complete. We can now examine ourselves as a whole, seeing how the various parts interact, both within ourselves, and with others. This chapter
will be an overview of how the chakras
work together. It will cover the common patterns among chakra interaction such as: relative strengths and
weaknesses between chakras, chakra
interaction in personal relationships,
and chakra patterns in culture. This
information helps pull together the

357

pieces of the system so that it can be understood as an integrated and interpenetrating whole.

As components of a comprehensive bio-psychic energy system, chakras do not function by themselves, but as wheels or gears in a larger machine—the machine being, of course, the human body/mind. The purpose of studying the wheels is so that we can know how they fit together—so that we know what parts go where, and we know how to troubleshoot when something goes wrong.

It cannot be stressed enough that with any use of the Chakra System, whether it be for therapy, personal growth, or medical diagnosis, the system must be considered as a whole. To diagnose yourself as having a third chakra malfunction without examining the part each chakra plays in the total structure of your personality would be a mistake. Any block that affects one part of the system will affect others. It would be like replacing the leading lady in a stage play when the director is at fault.

The fundamental theory of the Chakra System, at least in this writing, is that the chakras need to be in balance with each other. Ideally, there should be an even flow of energy through all of the chakras, neither favoring nor avoiding any particular one. Any imbalance in one end of the system is likely to create an imbalance in the other.

Personality characteristics, however, may tend to be somewhat dominant in one chakra or another. An artist might be highly visual, and a singer more oriented toward her fifth chakra. Within reason these discrepancies are natural expressions of individuality and should be left alone, or even enhanced, as long as the emphasis is not to the detriment of any other level of awareness.

The first thing to consider in examining any particular set of chakras is that each person has their own energy system with its own particular flavor and "quantity of flow." A half-inch copper pipe cannot handle as much water as a six-inch main line and should not be expected to. Therefore, we may as well dispense with the idea that there are any standards—that any chakras "should" be a particular way, or that people can accurately be compared to each other. This includes, in my opinion, thinking that we know which way chakras are supposed to spin.

We can only compare a person's chakras to the other chakras in their own system. We begin, then, by getting a feel for one's own particular flavor and flow—through interviewing them about their habits, desires, dreams, and the extent of their activities. Through this process certain patterns are bound to appear. One person may systematically suppress his emotions; another may continually exhaust herself, having a larger span of activities than her energy can handle. Still another avoids physicality and compulsively stays in the realm of spirit, while yet another clings to cynicism about anything that can't be seen in the material world.

As these patterns emerge, certain blockages may become apparent. A blockage can be due to a chakra that is "closed," i.e., unable or afraid to handle energy at that particular level; or it can be due to one that is too open, meaning that all attention and activity is consistently drawn to that level, at the expense of other levels.

Sandy, for example, has trouble with too little energy in her third chakra. She is easily intimidated, fearful of many things, and suffers from an inferiority complex. Because of this block, she is too shy to make many friends, she holds a low-paying job, and suffers from frequent illness. Thus, her third chakra block affects several other chakras as well, such as her fourth (love and friendship) and her first (survival) chakras. However, the treatment of her problem may lie in establishing a better relationship to her body, improving her health, giving her a firmer foundation from which to establish her self-esteem and personal power.

Frank, on the other hand, is also blocked in his third chakra, though in an opposite way. Frank is the type who acts as a bully, always having to be in control, always needing a new kind of stimulation, and enjoying his power over others. Because of his need for power, he has difficulty relating to people on an equal basis—he makes few friends, has trouble at work, and drinks himself to ill health. In both cases, the block affects the same chakra. But Frank's problem may lie in the emotional realm (second chakra) requiring healing on that particular level before other levels can be effectively dealt with, while Sandy needs grounding. There are no hard and fast rules—one must use intuition to assess the whole personality.

The best way to start chakra analysis is with ourselves—by examining our own energy system, our faults and virtues, and our wishes for change. The following set of questions may help to determine your own distribution. Answer them honestly, or ask a friend for their alternate viewpoint.

CHAKRA SELF TEST

Directions: Answer each question to the best of your abilities.

N = Never	P = Poor	1
S = Seldom	F = Fair	2
O = Often	G = Good	3
A = Always	E = Excellent	4

Score one point for the first column (N or P), two points for the second column (S or F), three points for the third column (O or G), and four points for the fourth column (A or E). Add up the points for each chakra and compare.

CHAKRA ONE: Earth, Survival, Grounding

	Answer	Score
How often do you go for a walk in the woods, park, or otherwise make contact with Nature?	N S O A	4
How often do you exercise consciously? (work out, do yoga, etc.)	N S O A	4

How would you rate your physical health?	P F G E	4
How is your relationship to money and work?	P F G E	2
Do you consider yourself well grounded?	N S O A	3
Do you love your body?	N S O A	4
Do you feel you have a right to be here?	N S O A	3
Total:		24

CHAKRA TWO: Water, Emotions, Sexuality

	Answer	Score
How would you rate your ability to feel and express emotions?	P F G E	3
How would you rate your sex life?	P F G E	1
How much time do you create for simple pleasure in your life?	N S O A	4
How would you rate your physical flexibility?	P F G E	3
How would you rate your emotional flexibility?	P F G E	3
Are you able to nurture and be nurtured by others in balance?	N S O A	3
Do you struggle with guilt about your feelings or sexuality?	A O S N	3
Total:		20

CHAKRA THREE: Fire, Power, Will

	Answer	Score
How would you rate your general energy level?	P F G E	4
How would you rate your metabolism/digestion?	P F G E	3
Do you accomplish what you set out to do?	N S O A	3

	Answer	Score
Do you feel confident?	N S O A	3
Do you feel comfortable being different (if need be) from those around you?	N S O A	4
Are you intimidated by others?	A O S N	3
Are you reliable?	N S O A	4
Total:	(29)	

CHAKRA FOUR: Air, Love, Relationships

	Answer	Score
Do you love yourself?	N S O A	4
Do you have successful long-term relationships?	N S O A	1
Are you able to accept others the way they are?	N S O A	2
Do you feel connected with the world around you?	N S O A	3
Do you carry a lot of grief in your heart?	A O S N	3
Do you feel compassion for those with faults and troubles?	N S O A	4
Are you able to forgive past hurts from others?	N S O A	2
Total:	(19)	

CHAKRA FIVE: Sound, Communications, Creativity

	Answer	Score
Are you a good listener?	N S O A	3
Are you able to express your ideas to others so that they are able to understand them?	N S O A	2
Do you speak the truth faithfully, speaking up when you need to?	N S O A	3

Are you creative in your life? (This is not limited
to doing an art form, it could be creative with
anything—setting the table, writing letters to
friends, etc.)   N S O A   3

Do you engage in an art form? (painting,
dancing, singing, etc.)   N S O A   3

Do you have a resonant voice?   N S O A   1

Do you feel "in synch" with life?   N S O A   2

           Total: (17)

CHAKRA SIX: Light, Intuition, Seeing

	Answer	Score
Do you notice subtle visual details in your surroundings?	N S O A	3
Do you have vivid dreams (and remember them)?	N S O A	4
Do you have psychic experiences? (intuitive accuracy, seeing auras, sensing future events, etc.)	N S O A	2
Are you able to imagine new possibilities as solutions to problems?	N S O A	3
Are you able to see the mythic themes (bigger picture) of your life?	N S O A	3
How would you rate your ability to visualize?	P F G E	4
Do you have a personal vision that guides you in life?	N S O A	3

           Total: (22)

CHAKRA SEVEN: Thought, Awareness, Wisdom, Intelligence

	Answer	Score
Do you meditate?	N S O A	1
Do you feel a strong connection with some kind of higher or greater power, God, Goddess, spirit, etc.?	N S O A	3
Are you able to work through and release attachments easily?	N S O A	2
Do you enjoy reading and taking in new information?	N S O A	3
Do you learn quickly and easily?	N S O A	3
Does your life have significant meaning beyond personal gratification?	N S O A	4
Are you open-minded in regard to other ways of thinking or being?	N S O A	4
	Total:	20

Scores of 22–28 indicate a very strong chakra; scores of 6–12 indicate a weak chakra. Scores between 13 and 21 are in the average range, but could use improvement. However, it is the *distribution* that is important. Compare your scores between different parts. Aside from the strongest and weakest chakras, is there a distribution pattern, such as higher scores in the lower chakras, or higher scores in the upper or middle chakras? Does this pattern coincide with your own views about yourself?

1. 24 = STRONG
2. 20 = Average
3. 24 = Strong
4. 19 = Average
5. 17 = Average
6. 22 = Strong
7. 20 = Average

Distribution Analysis

Energy flows in two ways in the chakra system—vertically, as it passes up and down connecting all the chakras, and horizontally, as it passes into and out from each chakra, interfacing with the world outside. The vertical channel can be thought of as the basic source, while the horizontal flow is the expression of that source.

The vertical channel is a polaric flow between the earth and the heavens—between matter and consciousness. In order for this flow to be full, each end of the spectrum must be open and connected to the raw energy source particular to it.

If the first chakra is closed, then the upward flow of liberating energy is blocked off. Cosmic energy may still come through the crown chakra, but it has no pull from the lower body to move toward manifestation. Ideas may proliferate, creativity and awareness may be high—but the person has a hard time finishing projects or directing his life. The consciousness may consist of loosely formed ideas or fantastic but impractical schemes that never come to fruition.

On the other hand, if the crown chakra is closed, while the first remains open, the problem is reversed. The earth energy has no pull toward expression, but sits like a wallflower waiting for a dance partner. The person may be highly practical, well-focused and secure financially, but lacking in creativity, hopes and dreams, or awareness of subtle planes. Plenty of plodding, but no dancing. Change is difficult, ruts and habits set in. The person has cut off his liberating current. The inability to manifest anything new results in an attachment to whatever security already exists.

These are, of course, extreme examples. Most situations are not so clear-cut. These combinations result in a dominant theme of either cosmic or earth energy. Some people are perfectly balanced, but this is the exception rather than the rule. Establishing the dominant theme is the first step in analyzing chakra blockages.

Both upward and downward currents can also be altered by imbalance in any of the chakras. If a person has a block in the second chakra, for example, with heavy emphasis on the cosmic energy, then most of the chakras are still well fed, with the greatest deprivation occurring in the first chakra. Opening the first chakra may then alleviate the problem by bringing energy up from the earth to meet and balance the cosmic energy trying to come down. Indeed, if the first chakra is closed, the cosmic energy will have a hard time filtering down as low as the second chakra.

If a person with predominantly physical energy has a second chakra blockage, then they are likely to be in sorrier shape. The five major chakras above will be blocked from their main source—the first chakra. In treating a person like this, one can work on opening the crown chakra (though it is likely to be difficult) or work on the second chakra directly to allow the earth energy to rise. This example illustrates why sex is often so important to physically oriented people. Aside from physical stimulation, it allows passage of energy to the rest of the body, otherwise malnourished.

Likewise, the middle chakras can be analyzed in terms of the directions of the vertical flows. Fifth chakra blocks in mental types result in an inability to manifest creativity and communicate ideas. In the physical type, they result in communication without content, or without knowledge or creativity to back them up.

In the third chakra blockages, a physical type may have power with no control over it. It may be intermittent, or insensitive. In a mental type, there may be a great deal of inner strength, but an inability to really accomplish anything in the "real" world— a lack of confidence in dealing with tangible things.

When the heart chakra is blocked, then energy from both ends is also blocked. The mind/body communication is shut down and needs to be re-established to open things up again. Likewise, if one or the other end points are blocked, the energy will balance itself in one of the other chakras, depending on which current is dominant.

Each chakra is a dynamic combination of earth and cosmic energy. The ratio between these two energies determines how the chakra expresses itself. This expression comprises the horizontal channel, branching out in a spherical fashion from each center. Each channel takes the source energy, both cosmic and material, and uses it to interact with the outside world. In this interaction, energy is also absorbed from the world and brought into combination with the source.

An earth-oriented fifth chakra might go in for sculpture, dance, or acting. A more mentally oriented fifth chakra would tend to go into writing or languages. An earth oriented third chakra would be interested in science and technology, while his more mental counterpart would be drawn toward executive functions.

In this way, each chakra perpetuates its patterns. A woman in technology will meet more people in technological fields than in political ones. Dancers are reinforced by other dancers to keep in shape, and writers are reinforced by other writers to read books.

I have seen only slight correspondence between gender and upper/lower chakra distribution. I believe most of this is cultural rather than biological in origin. Men, so typically blocked in the emotional center (which is the center chakra in the physical realm), are pushed into mental realms and out of the body. Women, typically assigned the job of physical maintenance, i.e., housework, cooking, and child raising (not to mention childbearing), get pushed into their lower chakras. Much of the imbalance between the genders fluctuates around the second chakra (emotions and sexuality)—resulting in a heavy emphasis in this area as the energy tries to balance itself out. Men, denied emotional release, put more emphasis on sexual contact as a way of reclaiming their bodies and re-establishing their physical connection. Women, often feeling oppressed by this, tend to shut down their sexuality and retaliate in emotional realms.

With more equality between the sexes, these patterns are changing. Nor are they so well established that exceptions are not almost as common as the rule. Many women spend a great deal of time in mental planes, while the men go out and work in the physical world. Many women tend to be more interested in spiritual pursuits, for instance, expressing themselves in intuitive fashion, while many men pursue more concrete goals, preferring to talk only about things that can be seen or heard in a tangible sense. As stated earlier, there are no hard and fast rules.

There is one more significant general pattern in chakra interaction—the spiral. As mentioned in the chapter on the heart chakra, the whole body/mind can be seen as a spiral emanating from or returning to the heart. If the initial outward movement of the spiral is toward communication, it will end in chakra one, manifestation. If the spiral initially goes toward the third chakra it will end in the seventh. In either cases, the channels connect chakras three and five, chakras two and six, and chakras one and seven.

The interrelationships of these combinations are not hard to see. Communication is facilitated by a sense of personal power and power is enhanced by effective communication. Psychic and intuitive faculties are enhanced by tuning into the emotions, and the emotions are strongly affected by subconscious information picked up psychically. Chakras one and seven are connected by their basic polarity; their dance creates the whole spectrum.

A thorough analysis of one's spiritual nature, physical problems, or general personality should encompass all these aspects. Again, the general rule for understanding and using a complex system is to look at the system as a whole, and analyze it with the faculties of all your chakras.

Chapter 11

CHAKRAS AND RELATIONSHIPS

CHAKRAS, AS THEY INTERACT WITH THE outside world, are constantly interacting with other chakras. Whether you're meeting someone on the street or having a long-term intimate relationship, each chakra reacts to the patterns of another's energy. In order to better understand our relationships and interactions with others, it is helpful to understand what is happening on a chakra level.

There are two basic principles governing interpersonal interaction. The first is that energy tends to balance itself; in other words, opposites attract. On a subconscious level, a person who is dominated by mental realms will unconsciously be attracted to others dominated by physical energy, even if they consciously seek out their own type. Often it is the differences rather than the similarities that make relationships last, because the differences are the meat of the growth. How often do you look at couples who are very different and wonder how they ever managed to get together in the first place, let alone stay together?

The second principle is that energy patterns tend to perpetuate themselves—two people who are mentally oriented will tend to stay in mental realms with each other, and those who are physically oriented will support each other in their physical pursuits.

So we have two kinds of interactions—those which are opposite and tend to balance and those which are the same and tend to perpetuate. A diagram of two people in a relationship might look like the one shown in Figure 11.1, page 371. The larger the circle, the more open the chakra, while the smaller circles represent closed chakras. Person B is largely oriented toward his upper chakras, somewhat open at the heart, though not aware of his intuitive faculties, probably due to the lack of grounding or lack of emotional information from chakra two. Person A is well grounded, open sexually and emotionally, highly intuitive, but somewhat closed on other levels with low confidence, and low self-esteem. In actuality, these two people are well balanced. The proximity of the three open chakras at the top would indicate a high degree of intellectual communication and learning: person A would be given information and communication stimulus to express her psychic faculties, perhaps awakening that quality in her partner. She would also be uplifted from her heavy grounding by her partner's emphasis on the upper chakras. He would be brought into the physical realms by her emphasis on earth energies and through sexual contact. The result is a balance in the heart chakra, opening each person on that level.

If this couple were to have problems, they would be in the realm of the third chakra, where neither is quite open, yet the crossing of energies indicates a high level of activity at this center. Due to the polaric differences between them, power struggles could become

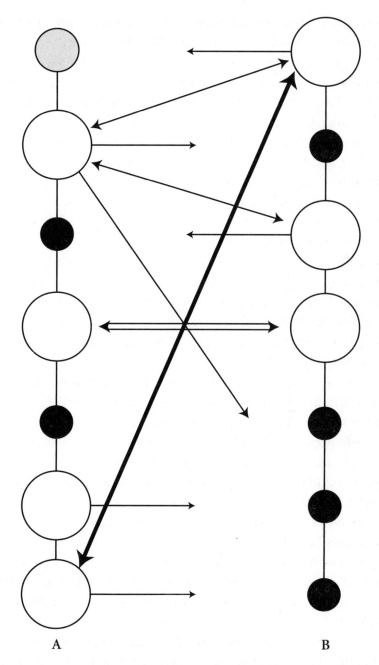

A   B

FIGURE 11.1
Chakras of two people whose opposite
chakra energies balance the relationship.

quite alienating if they become the focus instead of the balancing of energies in the heart chakra.

Another example appears in Figure 11.2, page 373. Here our two people are nearly alike. Both are open in the upper chakras as well as the heart, but are closed in the physical realm. These people would probably have a high degree of psychic communication, lots of shared knowledge, and a strong heart connection. Unfortunately, they would have a hard time manifesting this relationship, as neither one is grounded enough to bring it down into the real world. While she wants sexual contact to bring this about, his sense of power does not permit this, and neither has enough of the magnetic pull of the lower chakras to overcome the inertia of the set patterns. This couple would be likely to have a very strong and loving platonic relationship.

Chakras relate primarily on levels of their own vibration through resonance. Therefore, if one person has a fourth chakra that is very open and her partner has one that is closed, her very openness may serve to open his closed chakra. The reverse can also be true but is less often the case. An open chakra that finds no counterpart in the immediate vicinity will usually find outlets elsewhere. Heavy downward emphasis in one person's system, however, can pull energy out of another's upper chakras, resulting in what may feel like a closing down of those centers.

It is also possible that an open chakra may dominate another's closed chakra if it is on the same level. John, who is open in the fifth chakra, is paired with Paul, who is closed. John, therefore, does all the talking, and Paul retreats into greater silence. Or take the example of Bill and Mary. Bill's openness on the third chakra level keeps Mary, who is weak in that area, at a constant disadvantage, heightening her feeling of powerlessness. If he can be sensitive about this issue, she can learn from him and they will gradually balance out. If we are aware of the dynamics involved, we can better avoid the pitfalls.

The number of combinations that exist between people in relationships is infinite. If you want to examine a relationship, it can help to

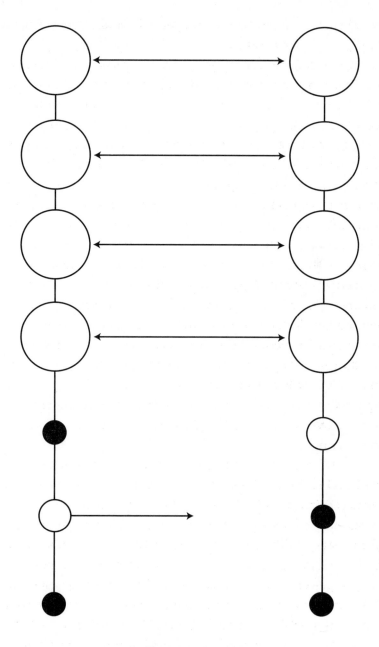

FIGURE 11.2
Chakras of a couple who have similar chakra energies.

make a diagram of where you feel each person is most open and most closed. Most information becomes apparent through keen observation. The chakras then become a metaphor for explaining those observations.

CULTURE—THE RELATIONSHIPS OF MANY

If two people in a relationship can have so many different patterns, what happens when we consider our culture as a whole? Aren't we all affected within our chakras by the culture at large?

The answer to this is a resounding *yes.* If one person can stimulate or depress another's energy on particular levels, several people can do it all the better. For this reason culture plays an important part in the state of our chakras, both positively and negatively.

Currently, Western culture appears to be heavily oriented toward the lower three chakras, with a predominant focus on money, sex, and power. It is tempting to interpret this as a need to deemphasize these chakras and become more "spiritual." In actuality, however, the sacredness of the first three chakras is already denied, and this promotes a fixation on their shadow aspects.

When there is undue fixation on a particular level, there is something basic that has not been fulfilled.

When the sacredness of our connection with the Earth is denied, it is replaced by materialism. Monetary empires become the means to security—having a bigger house, better car, or higher salary. This attachment perpetuates itself, since it defiles the planet, and takes us further away from our source. Like junk food, materialism does not satisfy the first chakra, but creates a greater hunger. Similarly, if we don't take care of our body, we eventually get sick and become preoccupied with our health. Over emphasis on the first chakra comes from a lack of energetic grounding and reverence for Nature. Western materialism can be seen as a cultural compensation for the loss of the Goddess as Mother Nature.

In chakra two, the sacredness of sexuality is denied publicly, while sexuality is used in most advertising, and annual sales of products to make us "sexier" rank in the billions. We are promised fulfillment through sexual attractiveness alone—not through the act of sex itself, or through ongoing relationship. The shadow side of denied sexuality is rape, child molestation, sexual harrassment, pornography, sexual addiction, and public fascination with political sex scandals. Our attachment at this level reflects a lack of fulfillment.

In the third chakra, issues of power and energy impact everyone's lives. Power is put in the hands of the few, and victimization and powerlessness become the cry of many. Power is seen as existing outside the self, and can be increased by having more money, being sexually attractive, or playing by the rules until someone higher up makes you a rule maker. As we said in Chapter 4, power tends to be modeled in terms of power-over, rather than power-with. In most situations, conformity is rewarded and individuation is discouraged. Our greatest public investment is the military, a system designed for one purpose only: to exert power and control when necessary through violence and intimidation.

There is less cultural conflict around the issue of love, as it is generally agreed by nearly everyone that love is one of the most important elements of life. However, the practice of love often falls short of the ideal. Money is poured into buying new bombers while the homeless sleep in doorstops on city streets. Racism, sexism, ageism, religious intolerance, and prejudice of every kind erode the practice of love and compassion that is the true realm of the heart. Love is reduced to fleeting romantic liasons between heterosexual adults, and even that is fraught with pain and frustration, with broken hearts, rampant divorce rates, and broken homes.

The fifth chakra is opening up widely on a cultural level. Mass communication of every kind connects each of us to the cultural matrix, and supplies us with instant information at every moment. Yet, the media, as we said earlier, pollutes our thinking with violence and sensationalism. We are polluted with noise in our daily life, from telephones and traffic to airplane and industrial noise. We fail to give this chakra the attention it needs and take care as to what we put on the airwaves and feed into the cultural nervous system.

The spiritual realms of chakra six and seven are just beginning to open up. Spiritual books have a greater market than ever before. People are learning to use their intuition and they are going to psychics for advice. More and more people are exploring religious diversity in their personal practice, incorporating Eastern and Western, ancient and modern techniques. Information is more accessible and plentiful than ever before.

Yet, there is still a long way to go before entry into the upper chakras is culturally sanctioned. There are far more people in commercial business than there are meditators. Psychics are suspected to be frauds. Spirituality often meets with cynicism, or outright judgment from those who see non-Christian practices as "going to the devil." The emphasis is so heavy on the lower chakras that the very rhythm of the culture makes it hard to meditate or find time for creative pursuits. Our language has few words to describe psychic phenomena, and the "spiritual type" is apt to find himself misunderstood. Our culture appears to suffer from spiritual poverty.

Different cultures have different chakra emphases. India, for example, emphasizes spiritual pursuits while de-emphasizing the development of personal power and materialism. India is known for its "upper chakra" orientation, and many people travel there to absorb spiritual teachings. Yet there is abject material poverty in India that is shocking to Americans.

Because cultural emphasis plays so large a role, those who wish to open up in new areas need to find people of similar temperament. Here they can find strength and support for their struggles as they learn and grow in new areas.

While we are each necessarily influenced by the culture around us, it also helps to realize that we can, by our own state of mind, affect our surroundings in return. Each time we raise or expand our own consciousness, we are making a cultural contribution. Each time we find others of like mind, we are strengthening that contribution. Every conversation contributes to the overall gestalt.

In understanding the relationships of our own chakras to the greater flow of culture around us, it helps to explore the evolutionary trends of consciousness throughout history. As we learn about what has come before, we can better project what probabilities the future may hold. Then our own part in that future is clarified.

Chapter 12

AN EVOLUTIONARY PERSPECTIVE

OF ALL THE IMPLICATIONS THE CHAKRA System suggests, perhaps the most exciting is its evolutionary perspective. As the chakras represent the organization of universal principles, it is no surprise that this profound formula for wholeness can be applied to cultural as well as individual progression. In perfect reflection of our psychological development, Western sociocultural history traces the progression of the chakras from bottom to top.[1] Using this formula as a lens from which to view our current millennial transformation, we find the Chakra System again provides an elegant map for the collective journey, shedding new light on the age old questions, *Where are we? How did we get here?* and *Where are we going?*

The first question, where are we?, can best be answered with a metaphor. It is generally agreed by anyone who keeps up with current events that we are in a state of massive global transformation. This transformation can be likened to a collective "coming of age" ritual—much like the tribal rituals that take an adolescent from childhood to adulthood. From the perspective of the Chakra System, the challenges that face us today can be understood as the passage through the chakra most associated with transformation itself, the fiery third chakra. We are burning the fuel of the past to illuminate the path of the future. Chakra three represents the current dominant values of power and will, energy and aggression, ego and autonomy, that must be incorporated, resolved, and transcended in our journey to the next level, chakra four, the realm of the heart, with its attributes of peace, balance, compassion, and love. We can look at this passage as a collective ritual of "coming of age in the heart."

Lest you think this sounds like a utopian fantasy hashed over from the sixties, let me put this in perspective with an evolutionary time line, dating back over the last 30,000 years of human history. This will then address the next question: How did we get here? which in turn brings us clues to that third and most important question: Where are we going? for out of that question arises the new global vision that is so desperately needed at this time.

How did we get here?

Chakra One: Earth and Survival

In chakra one the element "earth" and the instincts of "survival" are linked together to form the foundation of the entire Chakra System. On an individual level, we must insure our survival before we evolve to any other levels. Just as personal survival is dependent upon our connection to the Earth, so is our collective survival—specifically, the health of the biosphere—which we would do well to regard as the foundation for all future unfolding. As we personally reclaim the sacredness of the physical body, the Earth becomes the sacred body of planetary civilization, our collective first chakra.

We recall that the Sanskrit name of the first chakra is Muladhara, which means: "root." Our roots are found in the past, the *religio,* or re-linking, that brings us back to core principles, to simplicity, and unity. Our Paleolithic ancestors lived closer to the Earth, whose living web surrounded them as the ground of existence. They hunted game, gathered plants and lived in caves, sometimes traveling nomadically across the surface of the land, highly vulnerable to its moods and tides.

The Earth, as womb, was our origin, the mother that birthed us, our beginning, our foundation. The Earth, in her natural, numinous state, was the central religious influence of Paleolithic societies, worshipped by our ancestors as a living Goddess. Earth as life-giver and life-taker, and the Earth Mother as birther and regenerator, was synonymous with survival itself. Nature was the original template for the origin of life, the ground upon which it was formed, the very root of our existence.

With cultural values that debase both the body and the Earth, while simultaneously denying our past, *we have literally cut ourselves off from our roots.* In so doing, we are hindering our very survival and our ability to grow beyond this level. While the evolutionary direction of consciousness appears to be one that moves upward through the chakras, like living plants, we only grow taller by sending roots deep into the soil. Our growth must move in both directions simultaneously—upward toward the complexity of the future and downward, anchoring our roots in the simplicity of the past.

We cannot deny the roots of our past, nor our connection to the Earth, and have a future as a species. It is not surprising that movements abound reclaiming this ancient spiritual connection to the Earth, to Paleolithic mother goddesses, and to primal practices that link us directly and simply with this foundational level of mythic consciousness. This re-linking with Earth as a spiritual center can be a stabilizing influence in the massive changes that will indeed occur. It does not arrest our development, but secures it. As Marion Woodman has stated: "If we do not reclaim the sacredness within matter, this planet is doomed."[2]

When a child is an infant, he is bound to his mother for survival. His field can be conceived as a circle surrounding the mother as the center. He can only move just so far away from the center and still survive. This stage is characterized by the Jungian writer, Gareth Hill, as the *Static Feminine,* one of four states in the dialectic of static and dynamic masculine and feminine principles.[3] The symbol of the Static Feminine is a circle with a dot in the middle, much like the breast a child feeds upon. The circle is the limit that we can travel from the center and still survive. As we grow, that limit expands.

Just as the infant child is bound to the mother, our culture in its infancy was totally bound by the parameters of Mother Nature. She was the all-powerful center and ruler of our experience. As children of the Earth we were held by her rhythms of light and dark, warm and cold, wet and dry. She was the all-powerful good mother and bad mother who gave us bounty or destruction. Our spiritual roots are found in reclaiming the very sacredness within this phenomenal planet upon which we live.

Chakra Two: Water and Sexuality

Once an organism has secured its survival, it next turns to pleasure and sexuality. Chakra two, associated with the element water, represents the urge toward pleasure, the expansion of one's world through sensate exploration, the realm of emotions, and the play of opposites that occurs through sexuality.

The beginning of the second chakra cultural stage was marked by the climatic change that occurred at the end of the last great Ice Age, (10,000-8000 B.C.E.). This global springtime coincided with the beginnings of agriculture, the beginnings of seafaring, and the eventual development of irrigation technology—all aspects of the water element. Astrologically, it was the dawning of the age of *Cancer,* a cardinal water sign. The underlying theme of fertility, dominant in the Neolithic era, also fits with the watery aspect of procreation, and through its 7,000 years of stability, population estimates reveal a growth from 5 million to 100 million.[4] This marked increase brought its own challenges, further stimulating the growth of consciousness and culture.

The development of agriculture eased some of the demands of survival, enabling larger populations to be supported with relative stability. This created an enormous flowering of culture in terms of art, religion, trade, architecture, and early forms of writing. Because the archetype of the Great Mother was still the predominant principle during the Neolithic period, this stage is still characterized by the Static Feminine, though new elements were beginning to stir.

When fertility is worshipped, so is birth. With children come the growth of both males and females, and inevitably the worship of both genders. In the Great Mother mythology, there gradually emerged a mythical counterpart, the Son/Lover. As this archetype gained prominence, the inequalities in the mythical status between the sexes, as mother and child, would have become increasingly apparent. The role of the male, given a sacred honor as hunter in the Paleolithic, would have been much reduced in an agricultural society, whose emphasis is upon fertility. Much conjecture has been made about gender politics during this era and its ensuing downfall. Whether it was a balanced partnership society, as suggested by Riane Eisler,[5] or a golden age of matriarchy, as suggested by some wistful feminists, archeological research shows a general absence of fortifications or implements of war, instead revealing a peaceful, prosperous, and deeply religious growth of communities.[6]

However, inequalities cannot remain stable indefinitely, and whether by violent invasions from invading patriarchal tribes from the northern Steppes, as suggested by Marija Gimbutas,[7] or by gradual transformation of the culture from within, the mythical Son/Lover and the Great Mother as ruling principles of Nature, were brutally overthrown by a warrior Father God, leading us to the eventual replacement of the Goddess cultures by a ruling and aggressive patriarchy.

This violent and tumultuous change ushered in the beginning of our current era, the dawning of the third chakra.

Chakra Three: Fire and Will

Chakra Three is related to the element fire and marks the emergence of power that arises when consciousness awakens to individual autonomy and the development of personal will. Free will is a relatively new element that has only recently been introduced into the evolutionary mix. No other animals have fire, and none can transform themselves and their environment to the degree that humans can. Free will allows us to break away from passive habits, dictated by the past, and create a new direction. Free will is essential for breaking new ground, for the innovation that is the precursor to all change, and hence cultural evolution itself.

In child development, this stage is marked by the beginnings of impulse control, as the child learns to curtail his or her instinctual urges in favor of more socially acceptable behavior. This mastery also awakens the potential for individual autonomy, and the simultaneous need to determine one's own reality, which takes place, albeit clumsily, during the willful stage of the "terrible twos."

In a culture, this stage is marked by a civilization that is less deeply bound to the cycles of Nature, but has expanded, through progressively more complex technology, beyond the limitations that Nature imposes. It is unclear, during the Neolithic, how much individuals had a sense of their own autonomy, outside the mandates of the community. Anyone who has lived the life of a farmer knows how it binds one to the cycles and whims of Nature. My conjecture is that increased technological capability allowed the possibility of divergence from Nature which, in turn, awakened the potential for free will. Unfortunately, some individuals or tribes would have come to this realization before others, allowing them to use their new found will to control and dominate others who were weaker or who had not yet awakened their own will.

Over the next several millennia, rising masculine forces pushed against the dominant numinosity of the Mother Goddess and spawned an aggressive period of civilization that has continued into the present day. The force it must have taken to supplant the fundamental religious symbols that existed since the beginning of conscious time must have been considerable indeed. What could possibly equal the miraculous life-giving powers of the Goddess?

Death is the only power equal in strength to the ability to create Life. Thus the fear of death became a prime motivator of culture and behavior. The miracle of birth, which could only emerge from the feminine, became instead the *willed creation* of the masculine God. Thus the future emerged from the head, not the body, from fear rather than trust. The masculine archetype, in order to gain ascendance, was forced to prove an equivalent power through constant demonstrations of domination, war, and heroic activity.

The change from the peaceful Goddess cultures of the Neolithic to the aggressive sun-worshiping culture began with the invasions of the horse herders who descended from the northern steppes, around 4300 B.C.E.[8] Over a series of invasions and subsequent insurrections through the next three thousand years, this era was firmly established by the Iron Age, (circa 1500 B.C.E.), and the Goddess cultures had been sent to the Underworld of lost civilizations, to be replaced by an era typified by power, domination, and war. The Iron Age coincides with the astrological age of Aries, a cardinal fire sign, fire being the element of the third chakra. This change was made possible by the use of fire to forge metals, from which tools and weapons of war were made. Metal tools offered advantages in the struggle for survival, superiority over others, and a further stimulation of strategic thinking. The ability to do more with less enabled increased production that required greater coordination and governing by theocratic power structures, such as how to store and distribute grain, trade goods, or manage water resources. Weapons enabled the domination of one culture over another.

The third chakra heralded the birth of individualism, whose mythic theme was the Hero's Quest—the goal of which was to slay the dragons of the old ways (overthrow the unconsciousness of the past) and find one's individual power. This awakening of individualism occurred through heroic acts, the transcendent freedom brought by technology, and use of aggression as a basic mode of survival. Prometheus, who stole fire from the Gods, is a pivotal mythic figure of this age.

The most important thing to understand about this chakra—and its corresponding age—is that, for better or worse, *it is generally achieved through an **initial** rejection of the values associated with the previous two levels*—earth and water. Indeed, fire cannot burn if there is too much of either element. This denial of our underlying foundation is not a healthy way to grow. It reflects an immature, initial attempt to reroute the collective consciousness into a new direction from the passive, habitual tendencies of the lower chakras.

To the emerging patriarchal system, this meant a rejection and outright domination of the primary values of the previous Neolithic culture—which were the values of the first two chakras—the sacredness of the Earth, sexuality, emotion, women, community, and cooperation—essentially flipping all of these values into their opposites. Thus the peaceful Earth Goddesses were replaced by thunderous Sky Gods, the miracle of birth was supplanted by the fear of death, the sacredness of sexuality repressed, and cooperative partnership was replaced by hierarchical control. With this change, the basic order of life—as it had been known since the dawn of human consciousness, perhaps even hundreds of thousands of years—was broken.

In Hindu mythology this can be likened to the ascentionist approach, exemplified in Patanjali's Yoga Sutras, whose aim is to attain liberation by separating consciousness from its embeddedness in matter. As in most patriarchal religions, the direction emphasized was up, favoring heaven and devaluing the Earth. Indeed, this emphasis may have been necessary at the time to steer attention away from mundane concerns in order to realize there are other levels of reality. Opening up to another polarity in the cosmic dance expands our horizons and our choices. This polarity then allows the dynamic interplay of forces that is necessary to create power.

The third chakra age is characterized by the *Dynamic Masculine*, whose symbol is a circle with an arrow—the symbol we use for both the male and for the planet Mars, which represents aggressive energy. The arrow pushes away, in linear fashion, from the static circularity of the feminine in order to chart a new direction. Before the new direction can be established, however, the habits and customs of the old, which have been the ruling structures of consciousness, are often destroyed.

From the patriarchal domination of the Iron Age through the rising Scientific and Industrial revolutions, two world wars and countless other violent skirmishes, to the current creation of spacecraft and computer technology—the third chakra characteristics of aggression, technology, and political power still haunt us today. Issues of power and energy, excessive control and domination of others, are paramount in today's current events. Use of the world's resources for our incessant demands of energy production are central ecological concerns. Issues of reclaiming our personal wills which have been dominated by parents, schools, bosses, and government are central issues in the many twelve-step groups that assuage the victims of our current dominant paradigm. Empowerment is a buzzword of today's psychology, counteracting the "victim mania" that is such a central theme in today's recovery movement.

Aggression and violence dominate our newspapers, entertainment, and politics. The possibility of burning ourselves into blackened history through nuclear warfare, though receding since the retreat of the Cold War, still looms as a potential threat. Yet the fire of our time is also igniting new technologies, new channels of consciousness, heating up the chaotic motion of disjointed individuals in the planetary soup, moving them faster and faster as they converge upon each other toward a massive transformation to the next level.

The development of individualism, will, technology, and "empowerment" are essential steps in creating global consciousness. Individualism has brought us diversity, the possibility for greater novelty, and a sense of separateness that awakens individual will, necessary to become active co-creators of evolution rather than passive recipients. Where earth and water flow downward, passively following gravity, fire transforms the movement upward, enabling us to reach the upper chakras, collectively reaching toward an expanded global consciousness. It was perhaps the control of fire that initially stirred human consciousness into awakening, some half-million years ago. It is now the fires of our current technologies that are capable of awakening—or decimating—global consciousness. These are the uncertainties we face in this millennial transformation. But before we come fully into the present age, there is one more era that we must examine—humanity's first attempt to get to the heart—the Christian era.

Chakra Four : Love and Balance

Chakra four, in the original tantric diagrams, is depicted as the intersection of two triangles—the downward pointing triangle of spirit descending into matter, and the upward dissolution of matter into spirit. At the level of the heart chakra these polarities are perfectly balanced, and indeed balance is one of the central attributes to the heart chakra.

Though we are still struggling through the power and domination issues of the third chakra, I believe the rise of Christianity was initially an attempt to get to the fourth chakra. Its philosophical emphasis (even if it often failed in practice) was upon love, unity, forgiveness, and surrender of personal will to a "higher" power—a Father God who still carried some of the attributes of the angry patriarchal thunder gods, but who also carried a softer, more loving side. The birth of Christ, said to be the son of God, symbolized the blending of the divine and the mortal, characteristic of the half-way point that the fourth chakra represents.

The unfortunate thing about Christianity is that it was unable to truly reflect a religion of balance, emerging as it did at a time of intense patriarchy, where the presiding paradigm was still founded upon the denial of the lower chakras, and with it, denial of the sacred values placed on the feminine, on wildness, the earth, sexuality, and personal responsibility. Still, Christianity stabilized the predominant Dynamic Masculine, whose initial rejection of the old ways had produced a kind of social chaos of many divergent factions warring and competing with each other.

This stabilization turned the dynamic masculine into the *Static Masculine*, whose symbol is the cross, and whose emphasis is on stability through law and order. Thus the initial rejection of our basic nature is now regulated—it is no longer a reaction, but the permanent overvaluing of one part at the cost of another: light is good, dark is evil; male is powerful, female is weak; earth is transient and expendable, heaven is eternal and perfect. While this may produce the illusion of stability, it comes at the cost of intense repression, which is bound to surface wherever **there is** a weakness in the system. Thus the practice of love, balance, and forgiveness displayed miserable failures in the Crusades, the Inquisition, the witch burnings, and even today in the vicious demonization of cultural differences that occurs in some of the more extreme forms of Christianity. The repression of sexuality has created its shadow side of rape and incest. The repression of the sacredness of Earth has created shadow materialism, resulting in rampant ecological destruction.

Nonetheless, the Christian era, with its relative stability, allowed yet another proliferation of culture in terms of technology and growth of consciousness. During this time we produced the printing press, the telephone, radio, television and computer—all opening up communication possibilities that are a prerequisite for any kind of global unity to emerge. In fact, the industrial revolution, which took the dominant male out of the home and carted him off to work each day, allowed the first resurgence of feminism—where women were out from under the man's thumb long enough to compare notes and begin realizing who they were. This took a few generations, but eventually produced the consciousness-raising groups of housewives in the sixties and the opportunities for education and work that are necessary for any equality of the sexes to take place.

To truly come to balance in the heart requires an equal mixing of raw libido energy coming up from the lower chakras and conscious awareness coming down from the upper chakras. In other words, wholeness requires higher consciousness, vision, and communication, *balanced and integrated* with personal will, emotion, and primal instincts. I believe that a true awakening in the heart could not occur during the Christian era, because we had not yet achieved proficiency in the upper chakras. This in combination with the denial of the lower chakras created a system very out of balance.

In this light, let's now look at the achievements of upper chakra development that make it finally possible to weave, in balance and wholeness, a true culture of the heart.

Chakra Five: Sound and Communication

Chakra Five represents the symbolic representation of meaning, known as communication, an essential vehicle for the expansion of consciousness. Communication can be seen as the glue of evolution, continuously evolving in complexity from the reproductive language of DNA, to the earliest mating calls of animals, to the emergence of human speech, the advent of writing, publishing, broadcasting, and now the Internet. Each of these quantum leaps in communication can be seen as an evolutionary leap in consciousness. Each increases the capacity of information to travel more rapidly. Each is a step in building global consciousness.

By embracing communication in all its guises, we continue to reach toward greater consciousness as we learn, change, adapt, and create. Through communication, the network of global consciousness that Pierre Teilhard de Chardin referred to fifty years ago as the *noosphere*,[9] now commonly called the *global brain,* is taking shape. The noosphere can be seen as an organ of consciousness, analogous to a global cerebral cortex, that is now growing out of the body of the planet, Gaia.

The Internet is the clearest indication of this global brain, but the entire communication network is involved. It is indeed an evolutionary leap as potent to the evolution of global consciousness as the printing press was to the expansion of individual consciousness.

Chakra Six: Light and Intuition

A picture is worth a thousand words. With Chakra Six our method of portraying information jumps from the linear presentation of words on a page, or sound bites through time, to the holistic presentation of images in space. My words can only come to you sequentially, one at a time, but a picture enters through the eyes holistically, all at once. Through computer technology, mathematical equations can now be expressed as moving pictures, revealing dynamics of process that were previously hidden in piles of equations written on paper, giving birth to deeper understanding of chaos, complexity, and systems behavior. Pages on the World Wide Web can now include graphics and animation, as well as words. Books are sharing the market with videos and CD-ROMs, which provide a more rapid and whole brain way to absorb information. Television news comes to us in blasting images, letting us know more directly the realities of events across space and time—even as they are happening. The image is the message in television commercials, as creators adjust to their viewers' ability to use the "mute" button on their remote control and shut off sound altogether.

In the domain of spirituality, clairvoyance is making a comeback. New Age fairs are lined with booths of psychic readers who will intuit for you the unperceived patterns of your life and offer advice. The skill of creative visualization is employed by thousands as a means of bringing consciousness into manifestation, and in some quarters, intuition is even being admitted as a factor in scientific inquiry. A popular spiritual practice is to go on a "vision quest" for without a vision, how do we direct the course of our lives?

The ability to transmit images is indeed a quantum leap ahead of the communication of words, equal to previous jumps in communication technology. With images more can be communicated in less time, often with less ambiguity. Thinking in images, as a function of the right brain, is bringing a balance to the cognitive process of left brain logic which has dominated the collective consciousness over the last several centuries.

Chakra Seven: Thought and Consciousness

On a cultural level, chakra seven represents no less than the creation and functioning of the entire noosphere, the organization of information and consciousness itself on a planetary level. Is this global brain, with its infinitely vast network of unfolding information and awareness, not a metaphor for a collective thousand-petaled lotus, each petal a fractal point of connection to a larger matrix?

On the rational level, chakra seven is marked by the proliferation of knowledge and information, and on the mythic level, the increased interest in spirituality and consciousness expansion. The popularity of yoga and meditation, parapsychological research, mind-altering chemicals, and consciousness research is rapidly revealing consciousness to be the next frontier. Mind machines designed to alter the resonant frequencies of your brain waves initiating meditative states are increasing in sophistication and popularity. The creation of an information superhighway enables us to move consciousness around the globe at the speed of light. Computers, as the first instruments to extend the mind rather than just the body, can now take our consciousness beyond what is humanly possible, allowing vast increases of memory storage, computation ability, and creativity. As Al Gore has pointed out in *Earth in the Balance*[10] we have so much information, that we now have exformation—piles of data stored in computer disks that have never been reviewed by a human mind. As we enter the new millennium, we are overwhelmed with the vast abundance of information and potential for conscious understanding.

Yet it is essential that our developing consciousness be grounded in the body and in the Earth, that it have roots in our biological reality. Our consciousness carries our mythic structure, our values and directions, and shapes the interpretations of all that we see and the patterns of all that we do. The wisdom of this consciousness is of utmost importance at this time. What kind of operating system do we want? Do we need to evolve our own consciousness further before we can even answer that question?

Certainly, as consciousness evolves, the structure of our paradigms will change with it. The information we send out through the global network can be information that inspires global change or information that incites violence and aggression, such as the violent movies, and media sensationalism that pollute our communication networks. This information must be based on both fact *and* vision, feeling and understanding, embodying the balance, characteristic of chakra four. Our new mythology needs to be a paradigm of wholeness, one that embraces and integrates *each* of the levels we have encountered. Now we can ask our final question:

Where Are We Going?

To "come of age in the heart" is to fall in love with the world once again. It is to operate from love rather than guilt, devotion rather than duty, to interact with the world from the heart rather than the solar plexus. In order to awaken to the age of the heart, the entire thrust of our emerging era needs to be one of balancing polarities and integrating diversity.

We have never had a prevailing mythology where archetypes of both genders relate to each other from a position of equal maturity and strength. Now that we have experienced the maternal Earth Goddess, with her diminutive Son/Lover, and the complementary elevation of the Father God with his submissive Daughter/Wife, we are finally ready to hold each of these archetypal components in a kind of integrated balance. Now we can embrace *mature* elements of male and female, allowing these forms to dance with each other with equal power, at last removing the archetypal incest and allowing the younger offspring to embody the natural unfolding of the future that is their birthright. From this Sacred Marriage emerges the archetype of the Divine Child, which may very well be the future itself.

But these are not the only elements that are crying for balance in this emerging age. Mind and body, individual and collective, freedom and responsibility, light and shadow, progress and conservation, work and pleasure are all struggling for acknowledgment as equal qualities in a paradigm of wholeness. As long as we value one more than the other, we will be a culture out of balance.

The emerging age is characterized by the *Dynamic Feminine,* the final piece in the quaternity of static and dynamic feminine and masculine. The Dynamic Feminine is symbolized by a spiral, which moves from the center of the Static Masculine cross, pushing outward *without* limits, reintegrating the divided opposites of left from right and upper from lower, back toward the unifying circle. The Dynamic Feminine is characterized by creativity, chaos, and passion. By allowing spirit to move us into ecstasy, rather than using our heads to define spirit, it brings us ecstatic, rather than dogmatic religion. It connects rather than divides. As it spirals out into a circle, it connects inner with outer, individual with collective, up, down, left, right, mind and body, all into an inseparable dynamically moving whole.

It must be emphasized that in personal or collective systems, moving from one chakra to another does not require that we negate previous levels, but that we instead incorporate them. By reclaiming our bodies as individual temples, the Earth as a manifestation of living divinity, and the feminine as an equally important divine archetype, without negating the divine masculine, we are beginning to address the imbalances that have been imposed by the heavenly Father God over the last 3,000 to 5,000 years. By addressing social imbalances between races and genders, between work and leisure, between sacred and secular, between progress and conservation, individual and collective, we are approaching the balanced characteristics of the fourth chakra. Balance does not require a denial of anything, but an integration of everything, even light and shadow.

In Jungian theory, four is the completion of the quaternity, a stabilizing bringer of balance, a reintegration with the primal "one." In chakra four, the Hero's Quest of the third chakra era now moves to its next important stage—the Return Home. Here we reintegrate our technological prowess with the needs of the Earth, carrying with us the fruits of our heroic activity from chakra three, to now benefit the planetary culture we are struggling to evolve. We now enter the realm of reflexive consciousness, becoming aware of ourselves and our process.

The dawning of the age of Aquarius, a fixed air sign, marks the true arrival of the Age of the Heart Chakra, with an emphasis on humanitarianism, compassion, self-reflection, integration and healing. It is the peace that emerges within and without when essential balance has been achieved.

In 1969, with the advent of space technology reaching out beyond the limits of the planet, we were able to achieve a glimpse of our single, blue planet as if it were a political unity. As our astronauts and their cameras *returned home* with the global image they gleaned from their *heroic journey*, you could say that Gaia, through the eyes of humans, caught her first glimpse of herself. This moment, during the consciousness expanding period of the sixties, was a turning point in evolution. It was the beginning of the *Return Home,* the dawning of a global consciousness, the first collective awareness of ourselves as elements of a global entity.

Simultaneous to this dimmest dawning of planetary realization came the popularity of psychological inquiry, with a marked increase in people entering therapy, a process of deep self-reflection. It was in the same decade that James Lovelock first formed the Gaia Hypothesis, (the idea that the Earth is a colossal living being), that psychedelics opened people's awareness to the interconnected nature of all life, and that the new sciences of quantum physics, chaos theory, and dissipative structures began to leak into the mainstream and undermine the old scientific paradigms of reductionism and determinism. It was in the sixties that consciousness-oriented disciplines such as yoga became popular in the West, that people were tuning in, turning on, and dropping out, to reemerge later with the foundational principles for a new paradigm: the sacred principles of love, peace, and balance.

It was in the sixties that the Aquarian Age first began, but it is now, in the new millennium that we must anchor the Aquarian Age in the realities of our planetary parameters. It is time to become conscious agents in the dawning of planetary consciousness. It is time to realize ourselves as part of a living Earth, and offer our heroic achievements back home to the planet itself. For the outcome of a "coming of age" ritual is the formation of a new identity.

Our new evolutionary order must encompass and combine the planes and stages of all levels of consciousness. We can embrace Gaia as a mythological concept offering us a new identity as global participants. Benjamin Franklin once said that his greatest invention was of the term *American,* back in a time when the land was inhabited by French, English, German, Dutch, Indian, and others. The term American united this diversity in a single concept—united by the land they lived on. The word *Gaian,* can now provide a new identity—which includes all living beings—not only different races and genders, but different species, plants, and animals can all share this global identity.

The massive quantity of information generated by our observation of the natural world can steer us toward a more harmonious relationship with Gaia, using our growing technology in harmony and balance with the natural environment. To reclaim the body and its realm of feelings is important to physical health and personal empowerment, as is the reclamation of will that has been disowned by authoritarian cultural values. But the application of that will toward a new stage of love, compassion, and balance, rather than heroism and domination, is necessary to bring us to the dawning stage of the Heart Chakra, and the peace and healing we hope for in the future. Global communication, information networks, integration of spiritual values into everyday life, and the visioning of a sustainable future are upper chakra attributes that need to be brought "down" to the central point of the heart, in order to bring these changes about.

This is an exciting time of tumultuous changes and limitless possibilities. Because the future is uncertain, searching, visioning, and communicating are essential. For in the evolutionary drama, we are now simultaneously part of the audience, members of the cast, and authors of the drama itself. We are the co-creators of the evolutionary future.

ENDNOTES

1. For more information on chakras and individual childhood development, see my book: *Eastern Body, Western Mind.*

2. Marion Woodman, *Rolling Away the Stone,* (audio tape) (Boulder, Co: Sounds True Recordings, 1989).

3. These terms: static feminine, dynamic masculine, static masculine and dynamic feminine, used throughout this essay are derived from the work of Jungian analyst and Berkeley professor, Gareth Hill, in his book: *Masculine and Feminine: The Natural Flow of Elements in the Psyche* (Boston, MA: Shambhala, 1982).

4. Erich Jantsch, *Self-Organizing Universe,* (NY: Pergamom Press, 1980), 137.

5. Riane Eisler, *The Chalice and the Blade: Our History, Our Future,* (San Francisco, CA: Harper & Row, 1987).

6. Marija Gimbutas, *The Civilization of the Goddess,* (CA: Harper San Francisco, 1991).

7. Ibid.

8. Riane Eisler, *The Chalice and the Blade: Our History, Our Future,* (San Francisco, CA: Harper & Row, 1987), 44 ff.

9. Pierre Teilhard de Chardin, *The Phenomenon of Man,* (NY: Harper & Brothers, 1959), 200 ff.

10. Al Gore, *Earth in the Balance: Ecology and the Human Spirit,* (NY: Houghton Mifflin, 1992), 201.

Chapter 13

FOSTERING HEALTHY CHAKRAS IN CHILDREN

HOPE FOR A BETTER FUTURE
DEPENDS on raising children without the traumas and abuses that
plague so many people struggling
through recovery today. These
abuses often occurred at the hands
of well-meaning but ignorant parents, many of whom were simply
responding from their own
unhealed wounds, wounds they had
received from the previous generation, which may have been passed
on through family and culture for
many generations before that. As
adults today undergo the difficult

journey of healing these wounds, they understandably want to avoid at all costs, inflicting similar difficulties upon their own children.

Today's children need intelligent guidance that supports their growth and integration in body, mind, and spirit. Finding spiritual models that can be applied to children—models that address their development in a way that honors the different stages of a child's life can be difficult. Schools educate the mind, but suppress the body's natural urge to run and play. Daniel Goleman, in his best-selling book, *Emotional Intelligence*, illustrates the need to educate and mature the emotions before the intellect. Some children grew up completely eschewing religion, because they were made to sit on hard pews, or read books that were intellectually beyond their understanding, and thus have no interest in spiritual matters when they are older. Others, grow up to completely ignore the body, and incur health problems as a result. Still others, steer away from colleges and other intellectually demanding tasks because they grew up to believe they didn't have the necessary intelligence, often because they were given tasks as children that were beyond the abilities of their age.

The Chakra System, based on the seven wheel-like energy centers of the body, provides a profound mirror to the stages of childhood development. This system shows how the chakras develop sequentially, from bottom to top, as a child matures from birth to adulthood. In my personal growth seminars based on teaching this model as a way to heal adults from their past traumas and current difficulties, I am constantly asked by the parents in the audience, "I have a child who is at this stage right now. What do I do to support his development?"

This question goes beyond simply avoiding abuse—but moves into the creation of optimal human beings. This occurs through supporting children in all dimensions of their experience—physically, emotionally, mentally, and spiritually—and supporting them in ways that are appropriate for their current level of development.

What follows below is a brief introduction to the chakras and their childhood developmental stages, with simple advice for parents on how to support the unfolding of these important areas in a child's life.

CHAKRA ONE: WOMB TO 1 YEAR

Promote Embodiment

The most important thing you can do at this stage is to help your child come fully into her body. Frequent touch, holding, carrying, nurturing, and attendance to physical needs cannot be stressed enough. Your touch affirms your child's physicality. Your holding teaches her to hold herself. Playing with your child helps her develop motor coordination. Playing with her feet and hands, supplying toys she can grasp, playing when she's in the bath, all help stimulate motor development. Setting up an appropriate environment that is safe and comfortable, with age-appropriate toys helps the child relate to the outer world in a positive way.

Establish Trust by Allowing Attachment and Bonding

The child's only source of safety is through attachment to the primary caregiver. It is important for the mother (or father if he is primary parent) to be there as consistently as possible during the first year as a ground for the child. This means picking her up when she cries, frequently holding and cuddling her, talking to her, protecting her from loud noises, hunger, cold, or discomfort, and feeding her when she's hungry, rather than by a schedule. Some parents have difficulty allowing this attachment to form, because the child's natural neediness feels too demanding. Allowing this attachment to occur helps the child become more independent later.

Consistency of presence during infancy helps to reconcile the dilemma of trust vs. mistrust in a way that brings hope and confidence. Knowing that the parent is always there allows the child to relax into the development that needs to occur, rather than rise into tension and hypervigilance.

Appropriate Day Care

If the mother needs to work during the first year and can't be there with her child, she leaves her child at a disadvantage. Unfortunately, financial circumstances often make this the only option. The best parents can do is provide the healthiest child care possible, acting as advocates to make sure the child gets the care she needs. Making sure the child is touched frequently and appropriately, fed on demand, and cared for by competent adults in an age-appropriate environment are a few things the parents can look into when finding day care. Spending time at the day care with her child until she gets used to it is also helpful. Family day care and in-home babysitting are more likely to offer continuity and consistency. In addition, the mother needs to understand that the child may need extra nurturing, touch, and mother-child bonding in the evening at home. This is especially demanding on single and/or working mothers who are often exhausted at the end of the day. Yet, time taken for nurturing during the first year pays off in the long run with a calmer and healthier child who makes less demands later.

A feeling of safety comes from a safe environment. Peace in the home, protection from loud noises, sharp objects, falling, cold, and violence of adults or siblings is essential. Remember, environment is self to the infant. What they are embedded in is the first influence on who they are.

When a child is in an unfamiliar environment, such as a store, a park, a doctor's office, or a friend's house, the parent is an island of safety for the child. Understand that your child will be more insecure, and need to come to you again and again for reassurance.

Healthy Nourishment

Feeding schedules, though convenient for the parent, do not allow the child to establish her own rhythms, nor do they teach her that the world will respond to her needs. Breast feeding has been proven to be healthier emotionally and physically, as breast milk contains important antibodies, and the experience of breast feeding promotes mother child bonding, through physical closeness. But studies have shown that the emotional state of the mother while feeding is actually more important than whether it comes from a breast or a bottle. A bottle given lovingly is better than a breast given resentfully. Healthy nutrition on the part of the mother, refraining from harmful substances that flow into the milk, such as drugs and alcohol, and healthy nutrition when the child begins eating food are also essential to building a healthy body.

If you successfully handle this stage, you will give your child a healthy foundation from which to meet the many challenges that life will bring. She will have a sense of her own body and aliveness, and a sense of hope and optimism that the world can and will meet her needs.

CHAKRA TWO: 6 TO 18 MONTHS

Allow Separation and Attachment

Your child will now be in the hatching stage, beginning to separate from his parent as his body development allows him more and more movement. Because this is scary to him, he will go back and forth—moving away and coming back to see if everything's OK. In some ways he will seem even more attached, and this is natural. It is important to support both these movements—to encourage the separation by offering safe opportunities to explore, and by being warm and loving when reassurance is needed.

Provide Sensate Environment

Your child is exploring the world through his senses. This is his main mode of experience right now. It is important to provide colors and sounds, interesting toys, touch and pleasure through play, and a safe environment to explore. Your voice and attention are a major part of the sensate experience.

Support Exploration Through Movement

Your child wants to move about right now. This is not the time for a playpen, and if you must use one, use it only for short periods of time. Instead, find places where he can crawl and walk about safely, where he can run in the park, roll around in the yard, and learn to use his body in its new found joy of movement.

Reflect Emotions

Your child is learning his emotional language. If you want to teach emotional literacy, it's important to mirror his feelings. Be responsive to his cries and expressions of rage, fear, need or confusion. Don't negate or punish him for his emotions—he can't help what he feels. Reflect words to show him you understand: "How sad you look right now!" "Are you scared? Do you want Mommy to hold your hand?" Though he can't speak very well yet, he is beginning to understand words by listening. He will understand that his feelings have a name and that even without language he can communicate to someone what he needs or wants.

Be aware of your own emotional needs and states, as well as the emotional "field" in the household. Children pick up our rage and fear, anxiety and joy. Take care of your needs as much as possible so your unresolved emotions are not projected onto the innocent child. Create a positive environment.

CHAKRA THREE: 18 MONTHS TO 3 YEARS

Support Autonomy and Willfulness

As your child begins to separate, celebrate her independence. Try to support her in her willfulness, hard as it might be, by offering choices whenever possible. Instead of asking, "Do you want Cheerios?" "No!" "Do you want corn flakes?" "No!" "Do you want oatmeal?" "No!" and then getting exasperated, you can say "Do you want Cheerios, corn flakes, or oatmeal?" Or you can pick out two suitable outfits to wear, and give her a chance to choose. Give your child opportunities to feel willful in ways that are safe and appropriate.

Encourage Self-esteem

As the ego identity is forming at this stage, be sure to take delight in your child's accomplishments and make her feel appreciated. Support her independence without rejecting her. If you give your child tasks that she can successfully accomplish, she will develop confidence. Age-appropriate puzzles and toys, small jobs around the house, like putting toys in a box or picking up stuffed animals, can help to foster a basic sense of confidence. If she insists on doing a task that is beyond her abilities, such as tying her shoes, help her accomplish it. By all means, refrain from getting critical or overly frustrated by her awkward attempts to do simple things. Have patience. It will pay off in the long run.

Successful Toilet Training

Your child will indicate to you when she's ready for toilet training. She will show an interest in the toilet and adult bathroom activities. She may tell you when she's wet or resist diapers when you're putting them on. She will stay dry for longer periods of time. Sphincter muscles are not capable of holding on until the child is 18 months to 2 years. It may not be until age 3 that she can go all night without a diaper. If you wait until the time is right, she will feel a sense of pride over this new adult behavior, rather than engage in a fruitless battle of wills.

Rewards for successful behavior go farther than punishments for mistakes, which only create shame. Find treats that can be given as reinforcers, as well as hugging, clapping and verbal appreciation.

Appropriate Discipline

In supporting your child's autonomy and will, you obviously cannot relinquish all control. There needs to be appropriate limits, firmly given. Your child cannot understand sophisticated reasoning, but simple cause and effect statements, like: "Doggie bites! Don't touch!" can be understood. Severe punishment teaches aggressive behavior and fosters shame. Withdrawal of love puts the third and fourth chakras at odds, and stimulates the child's insecurity and need for approval.

Instead, try to divert your child's attention to something more appropriate. If you take the remote channel changer out of her mouth, don't yell at her when she cries. Give her something else to hold. Remove her from dangerous situations. Limits set firmly and consistently for short periods of time (such as time out in one's room alone for a few minutes) can be more effective than anger or withdrawal. Children are highly sensitive to parent's approval at this stage. When you must, disapprove of the behavior and not the child.

CHAKRA FOUR: 4 TO 7 YEARS

Pay Attention When Modeling Relationships

Children at this age are learning about social roles by identification and imitation. Parental identification allows children to feel that their parents are with them even when not physically present. This means your child will internalize your behavior as a part of himself. If you are angry and aggressive, you will teach him to be angry and aggressive in his relationship with himself and others. As he grows into an awareness of relationships around him, model balanced, loving relationships for him to observe and be a part of.

Model Empathy and Moral Behavior

Identification with you as parent will also give him a basis for moral behavior. Explain to him why you do certain things and refrain from others. "We're going to take cookies to Mrs. Smith, because she's all alone and it will make her feel better." "See how the baby likes it when you smile at her?" "We don't eat candy before dinner because it doesn't leave room for the food that makes bones and muscles."

Also, be aware that you are modeling gender behavior. Be careful not to support overly sexist or narrow interpretations of how men or women behave. Treat your boy and girl children with equal affection, responsibility, and respect. Allow your child to see a wide range of acceptable behavior. Let your daughter be aware of models of strong women. Let your son know that he won't lose his masculinity by showing his softer feelings.

Explain Relationships

Your child is trying to understand how everything he discovers goes with everything else. The more you can explain such relationships, the more secure he will feel. "We put the puzzle away so we don't lose the pieces." "We put gas in the car, so it will take us where we want to go, just like food gives us energy to run around." "Mommy has to work so she can get money to buy food."

Routine can be very important. If routine is interrupted explain why. "We can't go to the park today because Aunt Mary is coming to visit."

Support Peer Relationships

Your child can now relate to children his own age, with supervision. If he's not in school yet, find ways to get him together with other children. If he is in school, ask him about the other kids he interacts with. Find opportunities to foster friendships outside of school.

CHAKRA FIVE: 7 TO 12 YEARS

Support Communication

Your child has a solid command of language now. Help her use it. Have long discussions with her about the nature of the world. Encourage her to ask questions and take time to answer them. Ask her questions about herself, her feelings and her friends that she can talk about. Be an attentive listener.

Cognitive learning is enormous at this period. School is the major arena for learning and development of confidence. Show interest in your child's studies. Help her with her homework. Ask questions, supply added information, share what you know. Get involved in school projects. Model good study habits. Give rewards for good performance.

Stimulate Creativity

Success is the greatest motivator for developing competence. Supply your child with creative opportunities for industrious expression: art supplies, musical instruments, crafts, dance classes. Model the creative thinking process by searching for new ways to do things, even if it's something as mundane as setting the table. Teach her to use tools. Stimulate creativity with books and movies, concerts and plays.

When your child presents you with something she has created, be sure to appreciate it, even if it only looks like a silly blob. This teaches her that her creations have value, and supports her creative identity.

Show the drawing to others; put it up on the refrigerator; invite grandma to the school play.

Expose to Larger World

Take your child to new places. A trip to the museum, street fairs, the zoo, a traveling vacation, a campout in the mountains. Allow exposure to different ways of life and encourage her horizons to expand.

CHAKRA SIX: ADOLESCENCE

Support Identity Formation

Your adolescent is now searching for his own identity. This is not a time to become controlling over details that are not of direct harm, such as hair, clothing, or harmless activities, such as listening to music. Respect his expression of individuality. Encourage his own thinking by asking questions rather than giving answers. Instead of telling him what you did when you were his age, ask what he might tell his son if he were a father.

The roles he tries on will change many times before he settles into his adult identity. Don't worry about the ones you don't like. To strongly oppose it strengthens the likelihood that it will last longer.

Support Independence

Allow your child to have more of his own life. Encourage ways he can earn his own money, take responsibility for more aspects of his life, such as buying clothes, having his own transportation, creating activities. Let him make some of his own mistakes. If he feels you believe in him, he will more likely behave responsibly.

Set Clear Boundaries

Adolescents nevertheless must have a clear and consistent sense of limits. As they are now old enough for sophisticated reasoning, it is important to include them in the thinking behind those limits, even to the point of letting them suggest alternative ways to address these limits. My son, for example, got an F in English his first quarter of high school. He immediately lost television and computer privileges until the next grading period. Six weeks later, with four weeks left before the next report card was issued, he asked if he could resume some privileges by getting a note from his English teacher that said how much better he was doing. He took the initiative and brought home a note saying he was now doing "A" quality work. I rewarded him for the improvement by reinstating some privileges on a probationary basis.

CHAKRA SEVEN: EARLY ADULTHOOD AND BEYOND

Seventh chakra modeling actually occurs throughout childhood. By the time your son or daughter is truly at the seventh chakra stage, they are on their own and your influence will be minimal. But here's some general principles to practice beforehand:

Stimulate Questioning

Ask, don't tell. If your home is a safe place to question and discuss values, your child will learn to think for herself. If she is taught to think through her own problems, with support, learning that there may be many answers to a single situation, she will be more open minded. Involving her in intellectual discussions and asking for her opinion makes her feel that her thought processes are worthwhile.

Offer Spiritual Variety

Spirituality should not be forced on your child. It is better instituted by modeling conscious behavior, and sharing what you can as there is interest. In addition to exposing your child to whatever religion you practice, you can make their spirituality even more solid by giving them some exposure to other religions as well. Explain why your family has chosen the religion you practice. Allow your child to research other cultures and styles of worship. If your religion is best for her, she will come back to it on her own, more solid in her commitment because she's been offered choice. If she chooses another that she finds more fulfilling, it will be an informed choice, rather than a rebellious act.

Provide Opportunities for Education

Learning is the way we feed our seventh chakra and keep our operating system up-to-date. Support learning in whatever way you can, whether it's attending local community college, weekend workshops, a trek to the Himalayas, or a self-imposed course of study. Teach your child to find the lessons in experience. Ask what she's learning from different activities.

Let Go

When it's time for your young adult to leave home, support and celebrate their independence. It doesn't help to hang on to her nor does it help to push her out the door. As the parent withdraws control and attachment, the young person will naturally gravitate out into her own world.

CONCLUSION

As children grow up through the chakras, they don't immediately outgrow the needs of the previous chakra. Children need physical affection all through life, not just in the first and second chakras. They need continual approval for their self-esteem. They need to be talked to, engaged with, included in family councils and activities.

There is never justification for parents to inflict upon their children sexual activity, physical pain, or shaming criticism. If this occurs, find help for yourself immediately through local parent support groups or your own therapy. Break the cycle. Don't pass on abuse.

Children need love and attention, time and approval. They need to be encouraged, not discouraged. They need to be part of adult society, and they need their individuality to reform that society in ways that are in better harmony with the body, soul, and spirit. Children are the sacred beings of the future. They are the hope of humankind.

For more information on childhood developmental stages, see Judith's *Eastern Body, Western Mind.*

GLOSSARY
OF INDIAN
TERMS

Aditi: The Vedic goddess of space.

Agni: Hindu god of fire.

Ahimsā: The practice of non-harming.

Airāvata: The white, four-tusked elephant that emerged from the churning of the ocean. Animal in Muladhara chakra and Vissuddha chakra, Airavata draws water from the underworld to seed the clouds.

Ājñā: To know, to perceive, and to command. The name of the sixth chakra.

Ākāsha: Ether, space, vacuity; the place where traces of all existence and events remain.

Anāhata: Sound that is made without any two things striking; the name of the heart (fourth) chakra.

Ānandakanda lotus: A tiny eight-petaled lotus located on the Sushumna between the third and fourth chakras. It contains an altar and a "celestial wishing tree." Meditation on this lotus is said to bring liberation (moksa).

Āsana: Pose or posture comfortably held; refers to the various hatha yoga positions.

Ātman: Soul, self, eternal principle.

Avidyā: Ignorance, lack of understanding or knowledge.

Bhakti yoga: The yoga of devotion and service to another, usually a guru.

Bhukti: Enjoyment. That which takes place when higher consciousness descends to the lower chakras.

Bīja mantra: Seed sound; represented by a letter-symbol at the center of each chakra, this sound is believed to give one access to or control over the essence of that chakra.

Bindu: (1) Small dot on certain letters to represent the "mmm" sound; (2) mythical basic particle, a dimensionless monad from which matter is built; (3) a drop of semen.

Brahma: Creator god, partner to Sarasvati. Balancer of centripetal and centrifugal forces.

Brahma chakra: (1) Brahma's wheel, i.e., the universe; (2) the name of a particular magic circle. (p. 49, Stutley)

Chakra: (1)A center for the reception, assimilation, and expression of life-force energies; (2) any of the seven energy centers of the body; (3) a disc-like vortex of energies made from the intersection of different planes; (4) wheel, as on a chariot; (5) discus, favorite weapon of Visnu; (6) the revolving wheel of the gods; (7) the wheel of time; (8) the wheel of law and celestial order; (9) a tantric ritual circle of people, alternating male and female.

Chakrāsana: The Wheel Pose (backbend). An intermediate yoga pose that opens the front of all the chakras simultaneously.

Chakravāla: The nine mythical mountain ranges that surround the world, at the center of which is Mt. Meru.

Chakravartin: Ruler, king, superman. From early Vedic and pre-Vedic, pre-Aryan times, the all-powerful monarch who was allegedly preceded on his march by a luminous apparition in the form of a sun-wheel. The Chakravartin sees himself as the turner and the hub of the great wheel of karma, the ruler of the center of the universe. The chakra was one of seven symbols he was to receive when the moment arrived for him to fulfill his mission. (See Heinrich Zimmer, p. 130 ff.)

Chakreśvara: Lord of the discus, an epithet of Visnu.

Dākinī: One of the four elemental shaktis, associated with Earth in the Muladhara chakra.

Devī: Generic term for goddess.

Deva: Generic term for the god; also celestial power.

Dharma: (1) Divine cosmic order; (2) moral and religious duty, social custom, ethical principle; (3) the act of following religious duty.

Dhyāna: Meditation, contemplation.

Ganesha (or Ganapati): Elephant-headed god, remover of obstacles. Good-natured, he is associated with prosperity and peace.

Gaurī: "Yellow, brilliant one"—the name of a goddess, depicted in the Vissudha chakra (fifth), who is consort to Siva or Varuṇa. She is sometimes a fertility goddess, sometimes related to the primordial waters (apah), sometimes the sacred cattle. The Gauris are a class of goddesses which include Uma, Parvati, Rambha, Totala, and Tripura.

Guṇas: Qualities. The three threads that weave together the qualities found in all things: tamas, rajas, sattva.

Guru: A religious teacher, especially one who gives initiation.

Hākinī: The Sakti at the Ajna (sixth) chakra.

Haṁ: The seed sound of the Vissuddha (fifth) chakra.

Hanuman: Clever god in the form of a monkey.

Hatha yoga: The yoga through the path of training the body.

Idā: One of the three central nadis which represent the lunar, feminine energy of a person. It is also linked with the Ganges. Its color is yellow.

Indra: One of the chief sky gods in the Hindu pantheon. A god of healing and rain, he usually rides a bull.

Īsvara: God in the heart chakra, who represents unity. Literally, "Lord" he was the closest to a monistic god, though not due to importance.

Jaina: One of the heterodox post-Vedic Hindu systems, focusing mainly on asceticism and protection of all living things (ahimsā) for liberation from karma. The essence of its philosophy was the three ideals: faith, right knowledge, and right conduct.

Jīva: The individual soul or psyche, embodied as a life force, as opposed to atman, a more universal, spiritual sense of soul.

Jñāna yoga: The yoga of achieving liberation through knowledge.

Kākinī: The shakti at the anāhata (fourth) chakra.

Kali: Crone goddess, terrible mother, all powerful destroyer, consort of Siva. She is also the symbol of eternal time. She is usually black (the eternal night), open-mouthed with tongue hanging out, four armed, holding weapons and a bloody, severed head. She is the destroyer of ignorance and excess.

Kalpataru: The celestial wishing tree located in the Anandakanda lotus below the heart chakra.

Kāma: (1) Love, desire, lust—primal mover of existence. (2) the god of lust and love, Kama tried to entice Siva from his meditations and was reduced to a bodiless entity by the wrath of Siva, which is why he hovers over lovers when they are being sexual.

Karma, karman: Action; the continual cycle of cause and effect in which the individual is caught by the effects of past and present actions.

Karma-yoga: The path of yoga that approaches liberation through right action.

Kundalinī: (1) Serpent goddess who lies coiled three and one-half times around the Muladhara chakra. As she awakens she climbs the

Sushumna and pierces each chakra. (2) The activating energy force that connects and activates the chakras. (3) a kind of awakening, typified by rising currents of psychic energy.

Kuṇḍala: Coiled.

Lākinī: The Shakti at the Manipura (third) chakra.

Lakṣmī: Mother goddess of wealth and beauty, consort of Visnu, pervader and protector.

Laṁ: The seed sound of the Muladhara chakra.

Lingam: Phallic symbol, usually associated with Shiva. A sign of generative power, even though Shiva was believed to never ejaculate in his sexual activities. Symbol of male potential.

Maṇḍala: A round geometric design used as an aid in meditation.

Maṇipūra: Literally lustrous gem, this is the name of the (third) chakra located at the solar plexus.

Mantra: Literally "tool of thought"; denotes a sacred word, phrase, or sound, repeated internally or externally as a tool in meditation and ritual.

Māyā: Illusion, personified as a goddess. Magic, supernatural power, great skill.

Māhashakti: Literally, mother power. The great primordial energy field of constantly vibrating forces.

Mokṣa (also Mukti): Release, liberation. That which is obtained by releasing attachment, also by wishing on the Kalpataru.

Mudrā: A sign made by the particular positioning of the hands, sometimes used in meditation.

Mūlādhāra: Chakra one, base of the spine, element Earth. It means root support.

Nadīs: Channels of psychic energy in the subtle body. The root, nad, means motion or flow.

Ojas: Nectar of bliss. That which is distilled from bindu.

Padma: Lotus; sometimes used as an alternate name for the chakras.

Para śabda: Silent sound, thought form that precedes audible sound.

Pingalā: One of the three major nadis, representing the male or solar energy. Related to the Yamuna river, its color is red.

Prakṛti: Primal material nature, both active and passive. The basic stuff of which manifestation is made, the female counterpart to purusa.

Prāna: The breath of life, first unit, the five life winds (the pranas), the moving force of the universe.

Prānayama: The practice of controlling or exercising the breath for the purposes of purification and spiritual illumination.

Pūjā: Worship in the form of homage or ritual offering to a deity.

Puruṣa: The male principle, creative, active, mental. It is the consciousness that is counterpart to Prakrti. The two together create the world.

Rajas: The guna associated with raw energy, the mover, the changer, the fiery guna.

Rākinī: The form of Shakti in the Svadhisthana (second) chakra.

Raṁ: The seed sound in the Manipura (third) chakra.

Rudra: Alternate name of Shiva, one of the darker fire gods, associated with thunder and lightning, storms, cattle, and fertility.

Sahasrāra: Literally, thousandfold, the name for the seventh or crown chakra.

Śakti (also Shakti): Divine power or energy, female goddess, counterpart to Shiva. She is the active principle in all things, constantly changing. She is represented in many forms and by many names: in the lower chakras—Dakini, Rakini, Lakini, Kakini.

Samādhi: A state of enlightenment or bliss.

Samsāra: The flow and cycle of birth and death.

Sarasvatī: Literally, river goddess; the patroness of all the sixty-four arts, the mother of speech and writing, the epitome of purity, and the consort of Brahma.

Sattvas: The lightest of the gunas, associated with thought, spirit, and balance.

Siddhis: Magical powers believed attainable at certain stages of yoga practice and/or Kundalini awakening.

Śiva (also Shiva): One of the main Indian male gods, associated with the abstract and formless aspects of thought and spirit. The name means "auspicious." He is thought of as a burning white light, as a lightning bolt, as a lingam, as the Lord of Sleep, as the Destroyer (for he destroys form and attachments), as consort to Shakti and to Kali.

Sushumnā: The central vertical nadi that connects all the chakras. To have a full Kundalini awakening, the energy must travel up the sushumnā.

Svādhisthāna: The name for the second chakra, located in the lower abdomen and genital area. Early on the name meant "to drink in sweetness," from the root svadha, to relish, or sweeten. Later interpretations ascribe it to the root svad, meaning one's own, giving this chakra the name of "one's own place." Both are pertinent to describing the second chakra.

Tamas: The guna that represents matter, inertia at rest, resistance to opposing forces. It is the heaviest, most limited of the three gunas.

Tantra: (1) Literally weaving or loom. (2) refers to a large body of teachings woven from many threads of Indian philosophy that became popular around c.e. 600 to 700. (2) the practice of attaining liberation through the senses and through union with another.

Tantras: Doctrines referring to Tantric philosophy and practice.

Tapas: A heat force believed to be generated by ascetic practice, considered as a measure of personal power and advanced spirituality.

Tejas: Fiery energy, vital power, majesty authority. With tejas from the sun, Visnu's chakra was made. (p. 302, Stutley)

Trikona: Triangle that appears in several of the chakras and in other yantras. Pointing downward, it represents Shakti, pointing upward, Siva. In the heart chakra they are interlaced, representing sacred marriage.

Upanishads: A set of teaching doctrines that followed the Vedas, believed to be written between 700 and 300 b.c.e.

Vaikhari: audible sound.

Vam: The seed sound of the Svadhisthana (second) chakra.

Varuna: One of the earliest Vedic sky gods, father of many of the later gods, associated with law and divine order; he is associated with the stallion (from the early sacrifices) and the makara, as ruler of the primordial waters.

Vāyu: (1) Wind, and god of the wind, believed to have purifying powers. (2) Refers to one of five pranic currents in the body: udana, prana, smana, apana, and vyana.

Vedas: Literally, "knowledges," the earliest set of written doctrines, mostly sacred hymns and descriptions of rituals, originally coveted by the Aryan priestly class.

Vedānta: A post-Vedic philosophy accenting the sense of divinity within the self. "Thou art that."

Viṣṇu: Major Indian male deity, one of the major triad (Brahma, Visnu, Shiva), known as the Pervader and partner to Lakshmi.

Viśsuddha: Literally, purification; the name for the fifth chakra, located at the throat.

Yaṁ: The seed sound of the anāhata (fourth) chakra.

Y āma: God of death.

Yantra: Similar to mandala, a design used for meditation. (A yantra need not always be round.) Also a system of yoga based on meditation on visual symbols.

Yoga: Literally, yoke; a system of philosophy and techniques designed to link mind and body, and individual self to universal or god-self. There are many forms and practices of yoga; see Bhakti, Hatha, Jnana, Karma, Tantra, Mantra, Yantra, Pranayama.

Yoni: Female genitalia; sometimes depicted or worshiped in the form of a chalice; counterpart to lingam worship.

BIBLIOGRAPHY

Acharya, Pundit. *Breath, Sleep, the Heart and Life.* Clearlake, CA: Dawn Horse Press, 1975. A pleasant book about the benefits of taking life a little easier.

Arguelles, Jose and Miriam. *Mandala.* Boston, MA: Shambhala, 1972. A good introduction to mysticism in a non-esoteric way. A lovely book.

Asimov, Isaac. *The Human Brain: Its Capacities and Functions.* New York: Mentor Books, 1964.

Assagioli, Roberto, M.D. *The Act of Will.* New York: Penguin Books, 1974. Great for third chakra development of will.

Avalon, Arthur. *The Serpent Power.* New York: Dover Publications, 1974. A standard classic on the chakras, translates major tantric texts; scholarly with much Sanskrit—a wealth of information.

Babbitt, Edward D. *The Principles of Light and Color.* 1878. Reprint, New York: Citadel Press, 1980. Lots of interesting information written in semi-archaic style.

Baker, Dr. Douglas. *Anthropogeny,* Vol. VI of *The Seven Pillars of Ancient Wisdom* "Little Elephant" Essendon, England, 1975. Theosophical treatise on the seven rays and evolution.

———. *The Opening of the Third Eye.* York Beach, ME: Weiser, 1977. Theosophical approach to clairvoyance.

Ballentine, Rudolph, M.D. *Diet and Nutrition.* Honesdale, PA: Himalayan International Institute, 1978.

Bandler, Richard and John Grinder. *Tranceformations.* Moab, UT: Real People Press, 1981. Neuro-linguistic programming.

Barrie and Rockliffe. *The Sufi Message,* Vol 2., London, 1972.

Bentov, Itzhak. *Stalking the Wild Pendulum.* New York: Bantam Edition, 1979. A delightfully written book on the mechanics of consciousness.

Blair, Lawrence. *Rhythms of Vision.* New York: Schocken Books, 1976. A fascinating journey through physics and metaphysics.

Blawyn and Jones, *Chakra Workout for Body, Mind, and Spirit.* St. Paul: Llewellyn, 1996. A comprehensive series of exercises for rejuvenating subtle energies. Not particularly linked to the chakras, however.

Blofeld, John. *Mantras: Sacred Words of Power.* New York: E. P. Dutton, 1977. Mantras by a Buddhist scholar.

Bloomfield, et al. *Transcendental Meditation. Discovering Inner Awareness and Overcoming Stress.* New York: Delacorte Press, 1975. A good introduction to meditation and its benefits.

Buck, William, trans. *Mahabharata.* Berkeley: University of California Press, 1973, One of the classic myths of Hindu mythology.

Burton, Sir Richard F., trans. *The Kama Sutra of Vatsyayana.* New York: E.P. Dutton, 1962. The detailed text of Tantric sexual rituals.

Brughjoy, William, M.D. *Joy's Way.* Los Angeles, CA: J.P. Tarcher, 1979. A doctor's story of developing spiritual sensitivity and healing capacity and his discovery and description of the chakras.

Bruyere, Rosalyn. *Wheels of Light: Chakras, Auras, and the Healing Energy of the Body.* Vol I. Arcadia, CA: Bon Productions, 1994. Interesting smorgasbord of scientific and philosophical information on the chakras.

Capra, Fritjof. *The Tao of Physics.* New York: Bantam Books, 1975. A classic on physics and Eastern metaphysics.

Carlyn, Richard. *A Guide to the Gods.* New York: Quill, 1982. A nice reference book to the pantheons of different cultures.

Cecil. *Textbook of Medicine.* Philadelphia: W.B. Saunders Co., 1979.

Clark, Linda. *The Ancient Art of Color Therapy.* New York: Pocket Books, 1975. One of the standards on color therapy.

Collier's Encyclopedia. New York: MacMillan, 1981.

Crenshaw, Theresa L., M.D. *The Alchemy of Love and Lust.* New York: Pocket Books, 1996. An excellent and entertaining look at the hormone soup that runs our lives and our sexuality.

Crowley, Aleister. *The Book of the Law.* O. T. O. Grand Lodge, 1978.

———. *Eight Lectures on Yoga.* York Beach, ME: Weiser, 1974.

———. *Magick in Theory and Practice.* New York: Dover Publications, 1976.

———. *Magick Without Tears.* St. Paul, MN: Llewellyn, 1976. I refrain from too much comment on Crowley. Most people either like him or they don't. If you like him, there's much to learn.

Cunningham, Scott. *Crystal, Gem, and Metal Magic.* St. Paul, MN: Llewellyn, 1987.

———. *Incense, Oils, and Brews.* St. Paul, MN: Llewellyn, 1997.

———. *Cunningham's Encyclopedia of Magical Herbs.* St. Paul, MN: Llewellyn, 1985. Scott's books have been invaluable in coordinating herbs and stones to the elements and chakras.

Danielou, Alain. *The Gods of India.* Rochester, VT: Inner Traditions, 1985. An informative book on the Hindu pantheon, though rather short on goddesses.

Davis, Mikol and Earle Lane. *Rainbows of Life.* New York: Harper Colophon Books, 1978. A book on Kirlian photography and the aura of living things.

Dass, Ram. *The Only Dance There Is.* New York: Anchor Press, 1974. The first book I read with the word *chakra*. The book that got me started on all this.

DeBono, Edward. *Lateral Thinking.* Harper and Row, 1970. A great how-to book on unlocking creativity by changing the way you think.

Delangre, Jacques. *Do-in: The Ancient Art of Rejuvenation Through Self Massage.* Magalia, CA: Happiness Press, 1970. A simple way to care for your body.

Douglas, Nik and Penny Slinger. *Sexual Secrets.* New York: Destiny Books, 1979. A beautifully written and illustrated introduction to tantra practices for Westerners.

Dychtwald, Ken. *BodyMind.* New York: Jove Publications, 1977. A well-written book coordinating body and mind with good sections on the chakras.

Embree, Ainslie T. *The Hindu Tradition.* New York: Vintage Books, 1972. Informative and scholarly, well-written.

Evans, John. *Mind, Body and Electromagnetism.* Shaftesbury, Dorset: Element Books, 1986. Psychophysiology of human aura, energy concepts, consciousness, vibration, morphogenetic fields, etc.

Evola, Julius. *The Yoga of Power: Tantra, Shakti, and the Secret Way,* U.S. ed. Rochester, VT: Inner Traditions, 1992. Scholarly look at esoteric Tantric philosophy and practices.

Ferguson, Marilyn. *The Aquarian Conspiracy.* Los Angeles, CA: J. P. Tarcher, 1980. An excellent book for its time on changing trends in cultural thinking.

Feuerstein, Georg. *Tantra: The Path of Ecstasy.* Boston, MA: Shambhala, 1998. A well-written guide to Hindu Tantric philosophy.

———. *The Shambhala Encylopedia of Yoga.* Boston: Shambhala, 1997. A good source book for yoga terms and ideas.

Fortune, Dion. *The Cosmic Doctrine.* York Beach, ME: Weiser Publications, 1976. Thick with wisdom and metaphysical philosophy, much food for thought.

———. *The Mystical Qabalah.* 1935. Reprint, New York: Alta Gaia Books, 1979. A readable presentation of the Qabalah.

Frawley, David. *Tantra Yoga and the Wisdom Goddesses.* Salt Lake City: Passage Press, 1994. Traditional and modern Tantra focusing especially on the Hindu Goddesses.

Gach, Michael Reed. *Acu-Yoga.* Briarcliff Manor, NY: Japan Publications, 1981. A book of exercises designed to stimulate the chakras and acupuncture meridians for greater health.

Gardner, Joy. *Color and Crystals: A Journey through the Chakras.* Freedom, CA: The Crossing Press, 1988. For those into working with crystals, a handy guidebook.

Gawain, Shakti. *Creative Visualization.* San Rafael, CA: Whatever Publishing, 1978. A classic on the use of visualization for creating what you want.

Gerber, Richard, M.D. *Vibrational Medicine: New Choices for Healing Ourselves.* Santa Fe, NM: Bear and Co., 1988. A look at the subtle body and and how to use subtle vibrational energies to heal.

Greenwell, Bonnie, Ph.D. *Energies of Transformation: A Guide to the Kundalini Process.* Saratoga, CA: Shakti River Press, 1990. A commonsense guide to understanding kundalini awakenings. Highly recommended for those with spontaneous awakening and for therapists who may work with such.

Goldberg, B.Z. *The Sacred Fire.* New York: Citadel Press, 1974. A well-written documentary on the history of sex in ritual, religion, and human behavior (now out of print).

Guyton, Arthur C., M.D. *Textbook of Medical Physiology.* Philadelphia: W.B. Saunders Co., 1971.

Halpern, Steven. *Tuning the Human Instrument.* Belmont, CA: Spectrum Research Institute, 1978. An exploration of music and consciousness.

Hamel, Michael Peter. *Through Music to the Self.* Boston, MA: Shambhala 1976. More on music and consciousness, more scholarly than Halpern's *Tuning.*

Hampden-Turner, Charles. *Maps of the Mind.* New York: Collier Books, 1981. A delightful book with short essays and illustrations of the many models for the way the mind works.

Hills, Christopher. *Energy, Matter, and Form.* Boulder Creek, CA: University of the Trees Press, 1977. An exploration of some of the physical counterparts of psychic phenomenon.

————. *Nuclear Evolution.* Boulder Creek, CA: University of the Trees Press, 1977. A lengthy but worthwhile book on Hills' theory of chakras, evolution, and metaphysics.

Hubbard, Barbara Marx. *The Evolutionary Journey.* San Francisco, CA: Evolutionary Press, 1982. An early book from a delightfully inspired futurist.

Hunt, Roland. *The Seven Keys to Color Healing.* London: C. W. Daniel Company, Ltd., London, 1971. A good introduction to color healing.

Jahn, Robert: "Foundation for Mind-Being Research Newsletter," *Reporter,* August 1982. Cupertino, CA.

Jarow, Rick. *Creating the Work You Love: Courage, Commitment and Career.* Rochester, VT: Destiny Books, 1995. Career counseling from a chakra perspective, or how to be happy in each chakra in your work.

Jenny, Hans. *Cymatics.* New York: Schocken Books, 1975. Now out of print, however the following video features Dr. Jenny's work: *Cymatics: The Healing Nature of Sound.* Jeff Volk, series producer. MACROmedia, P.O. Box 279, Epping, NH 03042.1986.

Johnston, Charles. *The Yoga Sutras of Patanjali.* Albuquerque: Brotherhood of Life, 1983. A standard classic on yoga doctrine.

Judith, Anodea. *Eastern Body, Western Mind: Psychology and the Chakra System as a Path to the Self.* Berkeley, CA: Celestial Arts, 1996. Western psychology and chakra philosophy.

———— and Selene Vega. *The Sevenfold Journey: Reclaiming Mind, Body, and Spirit through the Chakras.* Freedom, CA: The Crossing Press, 1993. The workbook of exercises, rituals, and practices for opening the chakras taken from their Nine Month Chakra Intensive.

Jung, Carl Gustav. *The Psychology of Kundalini Yoga.* Sonu Shamdasani, ed. Princeton, NJ: Princeton University Press, 1996. Jung's lectures on Western psychology and the chakras.

Kahn, Sufi Inayat. *The Development of Spiritual Healing.* Geneva, Switzerland: Sufi Publishing Company, 1961. A nice little book on the essence behind healing.

Keyes, Ken. *Handbook to Higher Consciousness.* Mary, KY: Living Love Center, 1975. An extremely simplified, but relatively accurate view of the chakra levels of consciousness.

Keyes, Laurel Elizabeth. *Toning: The Creative Power of the Voice.* Marina del Rey, CA: Devorss and Company, 1978. The spiritual benefits of singing and chanting.

Khalsa, Dharma Singh, M.D. *Brain Longevity.* New York: Warner Books, 1997. A look at the chemicals that affect our brain and how to preserve it.

King, Frances. *Tantra for Westerners.* Rochester, VT: Destiny Books, 1986. A zippy little book on Tantra that combines Eastern practice with Western magical traditions.

Kramer, Joel and Diana Alstad. *The Guru Papers: Masks of Authoritarian Power.* Berkeley, CA: Frog, Ltd., 1993.

Krishna, Gopi. *Kundalini, The Evolutionary Energy in Man.* Boston: Shambhala, 1971. A classic on a yogi's struggle with the challenges and rewards of Kundalini awakening.

Leadbeater, C.W. *The Chakras.* 1927. Reprint, Wheaton, IL: Quest, 1974. The standard Western classic on chakras. For a long time this was the only Western book on the subject.

———. *Man, Visible and Invisible.* Wheaton, IL: Quest, 1971. A book about the human aura.

Leonard, George. *The Silent Pulse.* New York: E. P. Dutton, 1978. A wonderful book on resonance and fifth chakra theory.

Lewis, Alan E. and Dallas Clouatre. *Melatonin and the Biological Clock.* New Canaan, CT: Keats Publishing, Inc., 1996.

Love, Jeff. *The Quantum Gods.* York Beach, ME: Weiser, 1976. A very nice and original presentation of the Qabalah.

Lowen, Alexander, M.D. *The Betrayal of the Body.* New York: Collier Books, 1967. A good book on the relationship of mind and body, especially regarding natural pleasurable gratification.

———. *Bioenergetics.* New York: Penguin Books, 1975. A good introduction to bioenergetic therapy.

———— and Leslie. *The Way to Vibrant Health.* New York: Harper Colophon, 1977. A layman's manual to bioenergetic exercises. Recommended for those who want to work on the lower chakras, though it doesn't speak of chakras as such (now out of print).

MacDonnell, Arthur Anthony. *A Practical Sanskrit Dictionary.* New York: Oxford University Press, 1954.

Macy, Joanna Rogers. *Despair and Personal Power in the Nuclear Age.* Philadelphia: New Society Publishers, 1983. Well-written with numerous exercises and meditations for groups and for individuals relating to our current world situation.

McLuhan, Marshall. *Understanding Media.* New York: Mentor Book, 1964. A classic in its time.

Merrill-Wolfe, Franklin. *The Philosphy of Consciousness Without an Object.* New York: Julian Press, 1973. The title says it all. The pages are superfluous.

Mishlove, Jeffrey. *The Roots of Consciousness.* New York: Random House, 1975. An excellent book on the study of consciousness from ancient to modern times.

Monier-Williams, Sir Monier. *Sanskrit-English Dictionary.* New Delhi: Munshiram Manoharlal Publishers, 1976.

Montagu, Ashley. *Touching.* New York: Harper and Row, 1971. A wonderful book to validate the use and need for human touch.

Mookerjee, Ajit. *Kundalini, the Arousal of Inner Energy.* Rochester, VT: Destiny Books, 1982. A coffee table book on Kundalini, with theory, pictures, charts, and diagrams. A good introduction.

————. *The Tantric Way.* Boston, MA: New York Graphic Society, 1977. A nicely put together book on the art, science, and ritual of tantra philosophy.

Motoyama, Hiroshi. *Theories of the Chakras.* Wheaton, IL: Theosophical Publishing House, 1981. Chakras from the ascetic point of view. Includes translations of Tantric texts that talk about chakras.

Muktananda, Swami. *Play of Consciousness.* San Francisco, CA: Harper and Row, 1978. A guru's story of experiencing Kundalini awakening.

Muller, F. Max, trans. *The Upanishads.* New York: Dover Publications, 1962.

Mumford, Jonn. *A Chakra and Kundalini Workbook.* St. Paul, MN: Llewellyn, 1994. Psycho-physiological techniques for moving prana through the chakras.

Myss, Caroline. *Anatomy of the Spirit: The Seven Stages of Power and Healing.* New York: Harmony Books, 1996. Compares Quabalah, Christian sacraments, and chakras.

Oki, Masahiro. *Healing Yourself Through Okido Yoga.* Briarcliff Manor, NY: Japan Publications, 1977. A book of exercises for different aliments, it also focuses on different parts of the spine, so its good for working on your back or your chakras.

Organ, Troy Wilson. *Hinduism.* New York: Barron Educational Series, 1974. A lucid book on Hinduism.

Ott, John. *Health and Light.* New York: Pocket Books, 1973. Worth reading, this is a story of a man's discovery and self-healing through the effects of light on plants and animals.

Ozaniec, Naomi. *The Elements of the Chakras.* Shaftesbury, Dorset: Element Books, 1990. A brief introduction to the chakras.

Paulson, Genevieve Lewis. *Kundalini and the Chakras: A Practical Manual.* St. Paul, MN: Llewellyn, 1991. A manual of techniques for working with the chakras.

Peitsch, Paul. *Shufflebrain.* Boston, MA: Houghton Mifflin, 1981. A book supporting holographic theory by experiments in brain transplants in lower animals.

Pierrakos, John. *Core Energetics.* Mendocino, CA: Life Rhythm Publication, 1987. Bioenergetic theory, body armor, and chakras.

Prescott, James. "Body Pleasure and the Origins of Violence." *The Futurist* IX, no. 2 (April 1975): 64–75. The relation between sexual permissiveness and reduced violence.

Pribram, Karl. "Interview," *Omni Magazine,* October, 1982.

Radha, Swami Sivananda. *Kundalini Yoga For the West.* Palo Alto, CA: Timeless Books, 1996. Questions and things to think about regarding the chakras. Good charts and diagrams.

Radhakrishnan, Sarvepalli and Charles A. Moore. *A Sourcebook in Indian Philosophy.* Princeton, NJ: Princeton University Press, 1957. Translations and commentaries of major Indian texts.

Rajneesh, Bhagwan Shree. *Meditation: The Art of Ecstasy.* New York: Harper and Row, 1976. A fairly sensible book on the subject from a radical Indian guru.

Swami Rama, Rudolph Ballentine, M.D.; and Alan Hymes, M.D. *Science of Breath: a Practical Guide.* Honesdale, PA: Himalayan International Institute, 1979. Medical and Yogic information on the breath.

Rama, Swami; Rudolph Ballantine, M.D.; Swami Ajaya, M.D. *Yoga and Psychotherapy: The Evolution of Consciousness.* Honesdale, PA: Himalayan International Institute, 1976. A great introduction to the meeting of East and Western psychology.

Raymond, Lizelle. *Shakti—A Spiritual Experience.* New York: A. E. Knopf, 1974. A heartwarming book on the essential Goddess Shakti.

Reich, Wilhelm. *The Function of the Orgasm.* New York: World Pulications, 1942. One of Reich's most-read books, and a classic in studying Reichian theory.

Rele, Vasant G. *The Mysterious Kundalini.* Bombay: Taraporevala Sons and Company, 1970. A brief book of Kundalini, Yoga, and psychic anatomy.

Rendel, Peter. *Introduction to the Chakras.* London: Aquarian Press, 1979. This little 96-page book on the chakras is excellent.

Restak, Richard M., M.D. *The Brain, The Last Frontier.* New York: Warner Books, 1979. A doctor writes on the amazing capacities of the brain.

Samples, Bob. *The Metaphoric Mind.* Boston: Addison-Wesley, 1976. Lovely pictures, and lovely for the right brain.

Samuels, Mike. *Seeing with the Mind's Eye.* New York: Random House, 1976. A great book for exploring visualization techniques.

Sanella, Lee, M.D. *The Kundalini Experience.* Lower Lake, CA: Integral Publishing, 1987. A medical doctor takes a look at Kundalini experiences.

———. *Kundalini, Psychosis or Transcendence?* San Francisco, CA : H. S. Dakin Company, 1978. Examines non-classic Kundalini theory.

Satprem. *Sri Aurobindo, or the Adventure of Consciousness.* New York: Harper and Row, 1968. An excellent book encapsulating Aurobindo's teachings.

Scott, Mary. *Kundalini in the Physical World.* London: Routledge and Kegan Paul, 1983. A well-written and researched book on kundalini as an earth force.

Selby, John. *Kundalini Awakening: A Gentle Guide to Chakra Activation and Spiritual Growth.* New York: Bantam Books, 1992. A reasonable guide to the chakras. Takes a fair amount from *Wheels of Life.*

Sheldrake, Rupert. *A New Science of Life.* Los Angeles, CA: J. P. Tarcher, 1981. The theory of morphogenetic fields by the man who conceived the theory. Written for biologists, it doesn't describe the theory to laymen as well as more popular articles do. (See *ReVision Journal,* Vol. 5, No. 2, Fall 1982.)

Sherwood, Keith. *Chakra Therapy.* St. Paul, MN: Llewellyn, 1988. A gentle beginner's guide to combining psychology and metaphysics.

Silburn, Lillian. *Kundalini: Energy of the Depths.* Albany, NY: SUNY Press, 1988. Esoteric Kundalini practices and scriptural translation.

Slater, Wallace. *Raja Yoga.* Wheaton, IL: Quest Book, 1975. A series of lessons in yoga.

Starhawk. *Dreaming the Dark.* Boston: Beacon Press, 1982. An excellent book on reclaiming our power to make change in the world. This book has been an inspiration to me.

———. *The Spiral Dance.* San Francisco, CA: Harper and Row, 1979. A wonderful introduction to the elements of magic and Goddess religion.

Steiner, Claude. *Scripts People Live.* New York: Grove Press, 1975. A psychology text with some useful theories.

Stutley, Margaret and James. *Harper's Dictionary of Hinduism.* New York: Harper and Row, 1977. Nice, long entries on many things, with almost every major concept of Hinduism defined.

Talbot, Michael. *Mysticism and the New Physics.* New York: Bantam Books, 1980. One of the clearest and most interesting books I've read on this subject. More information than *Tao of Physics,* but just about as easy for the layperson.

Tansley, David V. *Chakras, Rays and Radionics.* London: C. W. Daniel Company, 1984.

Tart, Charles. *States of Consciousness.* New York: E. P. Dutton, 1975. A good scientific document on altered states of consciousness.

Teilhard de Chardin, Pierre. *Let Me Explain.* New York: Harper and Row, 1970. An inspiring book on human evolution.

Teish, Luisah. *Jambalaya.* San Francisco, CA: Harper and Row, 1985. Informative book on the Yoruba religion, from a dynamic priestess.

Tulku, Tarthang. *Kum Nye Relaxation.* Berkeley, CA: Dharma Publishing, 1978. Recommended for those who aren't into yoga but want to find a way to get similar relaxation benefits.

————. *Time, Space and Knowledge.* Berkeley, CA: Dharma Publishing, 1977. Stimulating thinking about the three words in the title.

Varenne, Jean. *Yoga and the Hindu Tradition.* Chicago: University of Chicago Press, 1976. An extremely lucid and well-written book on yoga philosophy and Indian metaphysics.

Vishnudevananda, Swami. *The Complete Illustrated Book of Yoga.* New York: Pocket Books, 1960. A good text with pictures of the various yoga postures.

Von Franz, Marie-Louise. *Time, Rhythm and Repose.* New York: Thames and Hudson, 1978. A lovely book.

Walsh, Roger, M.D. *Staying Alive.* Boston, MA: New Science Library, 1984. A really well-written and provocative book on our current world situation. One of the few books that gives some how-tos on the subject of cultural evolution.

Watson, Lyall. *Lifetide.* New York: Bantam Books, 1977. A fascinating journey into various aspects of life through the mind of a biologist.

Wauters, Ambika. *Chakras amd their Archetypes.* Freedom, CA: Crossing Press, 1997. A good introduction to archetypes, matching one negative and one positive to each chakra.

Welwood, John. *Challenge of the Heart.* Boston, MA: Shambhala, 1985. Essays on love from many authors—many are worth reading.

White, John, ed. *The Highest State of Consciousness.* New York: Anchor Books, 1972. More essays on transpersonal psychology and mystic religion.

————. *Kundalini, Evolution and Enlightenment.* New York: Anchor Books, 1979. An excellent selection of readings on Kundalini theory (not focused on practice).

White, Ruth. *Working with your Chakras: A Physical, Emotional, and Spiritual Approach.* York Beach, ME: Weiser, 1993. An English psychic's version of the chakras.

Wilbur, Ken. *The Atman Project: A Transpersonal View of Human Development.* Wheaton, IL: Quest Books, 1980. A look at human development through transpersonal models including the chakras.

Wilbur, Ken, ed. *The Holographic Paradigm and Other Paradoxes.* Boston: Shambhala, 1982. An excellent book on the holographic-mind theory.

Wilhelm-Baynes, trans. *I Ching.* Princeton: Princeton University Press, 1950.

Wolfe, W. Tomas. *And the Sun Is Up: Kundalini Rises in the West.* Red Hook, NY: Academy Hill Press, 1978. An interesting account of a man who raised Kundalini playing with a bio-feedback machine.

Wooldridge, Dean E. *The Machinery of the Brain.* New York: McGraw-Hill, 1963. A somewhat outdated but readable book on the brain.

Yeats, W.B. trans. *The Ten Principle Upanishads,* 1937. Reprint, New York: MacMillan, 1965.

Young, Arthur. *The Reflexive Universe.* New York: Delacorte Press, 1976. More models for consciousness and reality.

Zimmer, Heinrich. *The Philosophies of India.* Princeton, NJ: Princeton University Press, 1974. An excellent overview of the various currents that have contributed to Indian culture.

INDEX

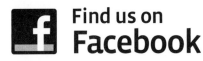
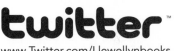

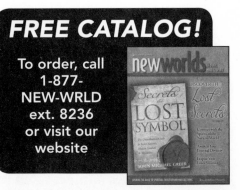

CHAKRAS FOR BEGINNERS

David Pond

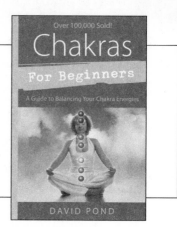

The chakras are spinning vortexes of energy located just in front of your spine and positioned from the tailbone to the crown of the head. They are a map of your inner world—your relationship to yourself and how you experience energy. They are also the batteries for the various levels of your life energy. The freedom with which energy can flow back and forth between you and the universe correlates directly to your total health and well-being.

Blocks or restrictions in this energy flow expresses itself as disease, discomfort, lack of energy, fear, or an emotional imbalance. By acquainting yourself with the chakra system, how they work and how they should operate optimally, you can perceive your own blocks and restrictions and develop guidelines for relieving entanglements.

The chakras stand out as the most useful model for you to identify how your energy is expressing itself. With *Chakras for Beginners* you will discover what is causing any imbalances, how to bring your energies back into alignment, and how to achieve higher levels of consciousness.

1-56718-537-1, 216 pp., 5³⁄₁₆ x 8   **$12.95**